quantitative medical data analysis using
mathematical tools and statistical techniques

quantitative medical data analysis using mathematical tools and statistical techniques

editors

don hong

Middle Tennessee State University & Vanderbilt University, USA

yu shyr

Vanderbilt University School of Medicine, USA

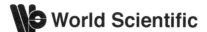 **World Scientific**

NEW JERSEY · LONDON · SINGAPORE · BEIJING · SHANGHAI · HONG KONG · TAIPEI · CHENNAI

Published by

World Scientific Publishing Co. Pte. Ltd.

5 Toh Tuck Link, Singapore 596224

USA office: 27 Warren Street, Suite 401-402, Hackensack, NJ 07601

UK office: 57 Shelton Street, Covent Garden, London WC2H 9HE

British Library Cataloguing-in-Publication Data
A catalogue record for this book is available from the British Library.

ISBN-13 978-981-270-461-0
ISBN-10 981-270-461-2

Printed in Singapore.

PREFACE

The increasing power and sophistication of computers over the past decade has placed many scientific disciplines in a position to incorporate formal mathematical tools, statistical techniques, and computer modeling and simulations into their methodologies. At the same time, there has been a growing interest among mathematicians, physicists, computer scientists, and engineers in the complex systems and databases of the life sciences. The resulting natural alliance of biologists with mathematicians, physicists, computer scientists, and engineers has led to the emergence of the rapidly growing and highly interdisciplinary field of Integrative Life Sciences. In today's environment, the volume of data available for medical research has increased dramatically. Quantitative Analysis can assist by applying advanced statistical analysis techniques and mathematical tools to help one get more information from the data sources. With quantitative biomedical data analysis, one can better understand the data and interpret the discovered biomarkers for diagnostic applications. In addition to traditional statistical techniques and mathematical models using differential equations, new developments with a very broad spectrum of applications, such as wavelets, spline functions, and learning theory, have found their mathematical home in Biomedical Data Analysis.

This book gives new and integrated introduction to quantitative medical data analysis from the viewpoint of the biomathematicians, biostatisticians, and bioinformaticians. Topics include mathematical models for cancer invasion and clinical sciences, data mining techniques and subset selection in data analysis, survival data analysis and survival models for cancer patients, statistical analysis and neural network techniques for genomic and proteomic data analysis, wavelet and spline applications for mass spectrometry data preprocessing, and statistical computing. The book offers a definitive resource to bridge mathematics, statistics, and biomedical sciences. It will be of interest to mathematicians, statisticians, and computer scientists working in biomedical data mining and analysis, disease modeling, and related applications. It will be also useful for biological and medical researchers who want an application-based introduction to current biomathematical models and statistical methods.

The contributors of this volume include experts in the fields. Besides the invited submissions for this review volume, selected papers presented at a workshop "Quantitative Medical Data Analysis", held at Johnson City, Tennessee from October 13-14, 2005 are included. All of the papers were peer reviewed. The workshop was sponsored by the National Security Agency. The Offices of the Vice Provost for Research and the Dean of Basic & Applied Sciences at Middle Tennessee State University (MTSU).

The editors gratefully acknowledge the support provided by the National Science Foundation (NSF), the National Security Agency (NSA), and the National Institutes of Health (NIH) during the past several years. The editors would also like to thank their colleagues: Maria A. Byrne, Curtis Church, Lisa Green, Robert Greevy, Changbin Guo, Peter Hinow, Aixiang Jiang, Cen Li, Anhua Lin, Yali Liu, Ginger Rowell, Ping Zhang, and Jan Zijlstra for their valuable suggestions and kind assistance in the editing of this book. The time and effort contributed by the anonymous reviewers to this edited volume for publication are greatly appreciated. We are also grateful to Jennifer Hong and Mindy Hong for their assistance on the proofreading of many articles. It is a pleasure to acknowledge the great support given to us by Ying Oi CHIEW and Lai Fun KWONG from World Scientific Publishing. Finally, we owe deep thanks to our families for their constant love, patience, understanding, and support. It is to them that we dedicate this book.

Don Hong and Yu Shyr
Nashville, Tennessee, USA

CONTENTS

Unit V. Computing and Visualization

UNIT I

STATISTICAL METHODOLOGY AND STOCHASTIC MODELING

CHAPTER 1

AN OVERVIEW ON VARIABLE SELECTION FOR LONGITUDINAL DATA

John J. Dziak[a] and Runze Li[b]

Department of Statistics and the Methodology Center,
The Pennsylvania State University,
University Park, PA 16802-2111, USA
E-mails: [a]jdziak@stat.psu.edu
[b]rli@stat.psu.edu

During the past two decades, there have been many new developments in longitudinal data analysis. Authors have made many efforts on developing diverse models, along with inference procedures, for longitudinal data. More recently, researchers in longitudinal modeling have begun addressing the vital issue of variable selection. Model selection criteria such as AIC, BIC, C_p, LASSO and SCAD can be extended to longitudinal data, although care is required to adapt the classical ideas and formulas to deal with within-subject correlation. This chapter presents a review on recent developments on variable selection criteria for longitudinal data.

1. Introduction

Since the 1980s, there has been considerable literature on the topic of longitudinal data analysis. Researchers have invested much effort in developing diverse models and proposing statistical inference procedures for longitudinal data (see, e.g., [12]). However, although variable selection is an essential part of statistical analysis, it has only recently received adequate attention in the context of longitudinal data analysis.

Often in longitudinal studies, many variables are measured. The number of potential predictors can be large, especially when nonlinear terms and interactions between covariates are introduced to reduce possible modeling biases. It is common in practice to include only a subset of important variables in the model, to enhance predictability and model parsimony. There are many existing subset selection criteria and procedures for linear regression models; for critical reviews see [5], [43], [19], and [33]. Some of the traditional variable selection criteria, including C_p, AIC, and BIC (see [31], [2], and [42], respectively), have been extended for longitudinal data. This chapter will give a systematic introduction of variable selection for longitudinal data.

In Section 2 we give an overview on variable selection for linear mixed effects models. Selecting significant fixed effect variables is relatively straightforward, but identification of significant random effects variables is very challenging; existing works dealing with this issue include Chen and Dunson[10] and Vaida and Blanchard[46]. Selection of significant random effects is closely related to covariance selection. Thus, we review some recent work on covariance selection in Section 3.

Generalized estimation equations (GEE) are very popular for analyzing binary, count and categorical longitudinal data. Penalized generalized estimating equations have recently been proposed for variable selection under the GEE framework (e.g., by Pan[36,37], Fu[18], and Dziak[13]). In Section 4 we present an overview of variable selection methods for GEE, and we explore their performance empirically in Section 5. In Section 6 we give an introduction to variable selection for partial linear models, which are useful for modeling longitudinal data semiparametrically.

2. Variable Selection for Linear Mixed Effects Models

Suppose that we have a sample of n subjects. For the i-th subject, we collect the response variable y_{ij}, the $d \times 1$ covariate vector $\mathbf{x}_{ij}$, and the $q \times 1$ covariate vector $\mathbf{z}_{ij}$, at various times t_{ij}, $j = 1, \cdots, n_i$, where n_i is the number of observations on the i-th subject and $N = \sum_i n_i$ is the total number of observations. Covariates may be constant within each subject, or may change over time.

For succinct presentations, we will use matrix notation. Let $\mathbf{y}_i = (y_{i1}, \cdots, y_{in_i})^T$, $\mathbf{X}_i = (\mathbf{x}_{i1}^T, \cdots, \mathbf{x}_{in_i}^T)^T$ and $\mathbf{Z}_i = (\mathbf{z}_{i1}^T, \cdots, \mathbf{z}_{in_i}^T)^T$. In general, the **linear mixed effects model** is defined as

$$\mathbf{y}_i = \mathbf{X}_i \boldsymbol{\beta} + \mathbf{Z}_i \boldsymbol{\gamma}_i + \boldsymbol{\varepsilon}_i, \qquad (2.1)$$

where $\boldsymbol{\beta}$ is the fixed effect parameter vector, $\boldsymbol{\gamma}_i$ is subject-specific random effects with $\boldsymbol{\gamma}_i \sim N(0, \mathbf{A})$, and $\boldsymbol{\varepsilon}_i$ is a random error vector following $N(0, \sigma^2 \mathbf{I})$. In the context of (2.1), model selection is a broader issue than variable selection; for example, one may choose the best among several candidate mean structures[50]. However, for simplicity we focus only on variable selection in this section, and in Section 3 we will review some methods for covariance selection problems.

There are two kinds of variable selection problems for linear mixed effects models: identifying significant fixed-effects variables when the random effects are not subject to selection, and identifying both significant fixed effects and random effects. We may select significant fixed effects covariates by using a relatively straightforward penalized likelihood approach, but selection of significant random effects is more challenging. Let us begin with selection of fixed effects covariates.

2.1. *Fixed effects variable selection*

When the random effects are not subject to selection, we rewrite the mixed effects model as

$$\mathbf{y}_i = \mathbf{X}_i \boldsymbol{\beta} + \boldsymbol{\xi}_i, \tag{2.2}$$

where $\boldsymbol{\xi}_i \sim N(0, \Phi_i(\boldsymbol{\theta}))$ with $\Phi_i(\boldsymbol{\theta}) = \mathbf{Z}_i \mathbf{A} \mathbf{Z}_i^T + \sigma^2 I$. Here $\boldsymbol{\theta}$ consists of all unknown parameters in $\mathbf{A}$ and σ^2. Thus, (2.2) is a linear model with correlated errors. This enables us to modify variable selection procedures for ordinary linear regression models to select significant variables for (2.2). Liu, et al.[30] proposed a leave-one-out cross validation method to estimate the predicted residual sum of squares (PRESS) and select significant variables for model (2.2) via minimizing the PRESS. Let us assume for the moment that $\boldsymbol{\theta}$ is known. Let $\mathbf{e}_i = \mathbf{y}_i - \mathbf{X}_i \widehat{\boldsymbol{\beta}}$ be the ordinary residuals, with $\widehat{\boldsymbol{\beta}}$ being the maximum likelihood estimate (MLE, equivalently the weighted least squares estimate) of $\boldsymbol{\beta}$. Define $\mathbf{e}_{(-i)} = \mathbf{y}_i - \mathbf{X}_i \widehat{\boldsymbol{\beta}}_{(-i)}$ to be the deleted residual with $\widehat{\boldsymbol{\beta}}_{(-i)}$ defined as the parameter estimate when the i-th subject is deleted from the analysis. Define

$$\text{PRESS} = \sum_{i=1}^{n} \|\mathbf{e}_{(-i)}\|^2, \tag{2.3}$$

where $\| \cdot \|$ is the Euclidean norm. As for the ordinary linear regression model, a fast algorithm can be developed here to calculate the PRESS statistic. Let $\mathbf{X} = (\mathbf{X}_1, \cdots, \mathbf{X}_n^T)^T$, $\Phi = \text{diag}\{\Phi_1(\boldsymbol{\theta}), \cdots, \Phi_n(\boldsymbol{\theta})\}$, $\mathbf{H} = \mathbf{X}(\mathbf{X}^T \Phi^{-1} \mathbf{X})^{-1} \mathbf{X}^T \Phi^{-1} = \{\mathbf{H}_{ij}\}$, with $i, j = 1, \cdots, n$, be one version of the hat matrix for model (2.3), where $\mathbf{H}_{ij}$ is $n_i \times n_j$. Define $\mathbf{Q} = \mathbf{I} - \mathbf{H}$ and let $\mathbf{Q}_{ii}$ be the i-th diagonal block of $\mathbf{Q}$. As shown in [30],

$$\mathbf{e}_{(-i)} = \mathbf{Q}_{ii}^{-1} \mathbf{e}_i.$$

Thus,

$$\text{PRESS} = \sum_{i=1}^{n} \|\mathbf{Q}_{ii}^{-1} \mathbf{e}_i\|^2. \tag{2.4}$$

Then the PRESS statistic can be calculated without fitting the model n times. Although the parameter $\boldsymbol{\theta}$ is unknown in practice, we replace $\boldsymbol{\theta}$ in PRESS by its MLE or residual maximum likelihood estimate (REMLE). Then one selects the best subset by minimizing the PRESS statistic over all 2^d possible subsets. Liu, et al.[30] also studied the theoretical properties of PRESS. For linear regression models, leave-one-out cross-validation is asymptotically equivalent to the C_p criterion and the AIC criterion (see [43]), and intuitively such a relationship should still hold for model (2.2). Thus, the PRESS variable selection criterion will be asymptotically *inconsistent*, i.e., the probability of selecting the smallest correct model does not converge to 1 as either n or N go to ∞.

We then introduce penalized likelihood approaches, such as AIC and BIC for model (2.2). Pauler[38] derived the BIC and its modifications for linear mixed effects models, and Vaida and Blanchard[46] proposed conditional AIC for mixed effects models. Let $\ell_i(\boldsymbol{\beta}, \boldsymbol{\theta})$ be the logarithm of the conditional likelihood function of $\mathbf{y}_i$ given $\mathbf{x}_i$ and $\mathbf{z}_i$. Then define a `penalized conditional log-likelihood function` as

$$\frac{1}{n} \sum_{i=1}^{n} \ell_i(\boldsymbol{\beta}, \boldsymbol{\theta}) - \sum_{j=1}^{d} p_{\lambda_j}(|\beta_j|), \tag{2.5}$$

where $p_{\lambda_j}(\cdot)$ is a penalty function with a regularization parameter λ_j. Maximizing (2.5) yields a penalized likelihood estimate. λ_j controls model complexity, and can be set to a fixed value (as in AIC or BIC) or chosen adaptively by a data-driven method such as the generalized cross-validation (GCV)[11]. In fact, the tuning parameters λ_j need not be the same for all j; this allows us to incorporate prior information for the unknown coefficients by using different λ values for each predictor. For instance, we may wish to be sure of keeping certain theoretically important predictors in the model, so we might choose not to penalize their coefficients.

Residual (restricted) maximum likelihood (REML) is often used to construct an unbiased estimate for $\boldsymbol{\theta}$ in mixed effects models. Thus, we might consider penalized residual likelihood instead of penalized conditional likelihood, see [20] for a discussion of penalized REML. As yet another alternative, we may consider penalized profile likelihood by replacing the conditional likelihood $\sum_i \ell_i(\boldsymbol{\beta}, \boldsymbol{\theta})$ by the profile likelihood $\sum_{i=1}^{n} \ell_i(\boldsymbol{\beta}, \boldsymbol{\theta}(\boldsymbol{\beta}))$, where $\boldsymbol{\theta}(\boldsymbol{\beta})$ is the MLE of $\boldsymbol{\theta}$ given $\boldsymbol{\beta}$. Throughout this paper, we focus on the penalized likelihood (2.5).

Let the penalty function be the entropy or L_0 penalty, namely,

$$p_{\lambda_j}(|\beta_j|) = \frac{1}{2}\lambda^2 I(|\beta_j| \neq 0),$$

where $I(\cdot)$ is an indicator function and all $\lambda_j = \lambda$. The penalized likelihood with the entropy penalty can be rewritten as

$$\frac{1}{n}\sum_{i=1}^{n}\ell_i(\boldsymbol{\beta},\boldsymbol{\theta}) + \frac{1}{2}\lambda^2|M|, \qquad (2.6)$$

where $|M| = \sum_j I(|\beta_j| \neq 0)$, the size of the candidate model. The AIC[2] and AIC_C (the finite sample correction of AIC, see [23]), have been extended to linear mixed effects model in [46], and the BIC[42] was extended for the linear mixed effects model in [38], in which two modifications of the BIC were further proposed by considering an arbitrary, possibly informative prior and the generalized Cauchy prior of Jeffreys[24]. Both AIC and BIC can be written as the penalized likelihood (2.6) with certain values of λ. Specifically, the AIC corresponds to $\lambda = \sqrt{2/n}$ in (2.6). Classical BIC corresponds to $\lambda = \sqrt{\log(n_e)/n}$, where n_e is the effective number of observations and may be taken to be either n or N, based on the model structure of interest[38]. Theorem 1 of Jiang and Rao[25] gives conditions on λ, under which the resulting criterion is asymptotically consistent. Using Jiang and Rao's results, it may be verified that if n_i is uniformly bounded, the BIC (by either formula) is asymptotically consistent, while the AIC is not.

Many other penalties have been considered in the penalized least squares case, i.e., for linear regression models with *iid* error, and they can be extended to the longitudinal case. The form of $p_{\lambda}(\cdot)$ determines the general behavior of the estimator. Define the L_p penalty to be $p_{\lambda_j}(|\beta_j|) = \lambda_j p^{-1}|\beta_j|^p$, $p > 0$. It is well known that the L_2 penalty with least squares results in a ridge regression estimator[21]. The L_p penalty with $0 < p < 2$ yields bridge regression[17], with properties intermediate between best-subset and ridge regression. With the L_1 penalty specifically, the penalized likelihood estimator is the LASSO of Tibshirani[45]. Antoniadis and Fan derived characterizations of penalized least squares with orthonormal design matrix, and Li, Dziak and Ma[28] extended these to non-orthogonal design matrices and explored the insights they provide into choice of penalty functions. Fan and Li[15] suggested using the `smoothly clipped absolute deviation` (SCAD) penalty, defined by

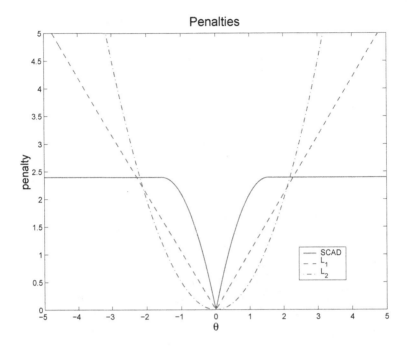

Fig. 1.   Penalty Functions

$$p_\lambda(|\beta|) = \begin{cases} \lambda|\beta|, & \text{if } 0 \le |\beta| < \lambda; \\ \frac{(a^2-1)\lambda^2 - (|\beta|-a\lambda)^2}{2(a-1)}, & \text{if } \lambda \le |\beta| < a\lambda; \\ \frac{(a+1)\lambda^2}{2}, & \text{if } |\beta| \ge a\lambda. \end{cases}$$

The SCAD uses two tuning parameters, λ and a. Fan and Li[15] suggested fixing $a = 3.7$ based on a Bayesian argument. They also found that in terms of empirical performance in simulations, the SCAD estimate using $a = 3.7$ was as good as the SCAD estimate with the value of a chosen by GCV. The SCAD penalty, the L_1 and L_2 penalty functions are depicted in Figure 1. The SCAD estimator is similar to the LASSO estimator since it gives a sparse and continuous solution, but the SCAD estimator has lower bias than LASSO. Directly applying Theorems 1 and 2 of Fan and Li[15], it can be shown that under certain regularity conditions and with proper choice of penalty functions and tuning parameter, the SCAD-penalized estimate is $\sqrt{n}$−consistent and possesses the oracle property asymptotically. In particular, when $\lambda \to 0$ and $\sqrt{n}\lambda \to \infty$, maximizing the penalized likelihood function with the SCAD penalty yields an estimate $\widehat{\boldsymbol{\beta}} = (\widehat{\beta}_1, \cdots, \widehat{\beta}_d)^T$ and $\widehat{\boldsymbol{\theta}}$ such that with probability tending to one, $\widehat{\beta}_j = 0$ if the true value of β_j is 0, while for those β_j with nonzero true value of β_j, the coefficient estimates enjoy the same asymptotic efficiency as that of the oracle estimator (i.e., an estimator that knows in advance which β_j are 0).

The penalties in the penalized likelihood can be viewed as a prior for β (see [45]). The penalized likelihood estimate is the posterior mode, which is much easier to compute than the posterior mean. Weiss, Wang and Ibrahim[48] proposed Bayesian variable selection procedure using Bayes factors. They specified a multivariate normal prior for β given σ^2 and $\mathbf{A}$, an inverse gamma prior for σ^2, and a Wishart prior for $\mathbf{A}$.

2.2. *Random effects covariate selection*

Vaida and Blanchard[46] proposed conditional AIC (cAIC) for choosing significant random effects covariates. They focus on prediction at the cluster level, conditioning on the clusters, so that the random effects $\boldsymbol{\gamma}_i$ act as parameters. Therefore the relevant likelihood is the conditional likelihood given the $\boldsymbol{\gamma}_i$'s. Their proposed cAIC is distinguished from the AIC defined in the last section, in that the model likelihood is conditional on $\boldsymbol{\gamma}_i = \widehat{\boldsymbol{\gamma}}_i$ and the number of parameters is related to the effective degrees of freedom ρ, defined by $\rho = \text{tr}(H_1)$, where H_1 is the hat matrix mapping the observed data vector $\mathbf{y}$ into the fitted vector $\widehat{\mathbf{y}} = H_1\mathbf{y}$. In practice, H_1 depends on $\mathbf{A}/\sigma^2$ and needs to be estimated. Note that both σ^2 and $\mathbf{A}$ are nuisance parameters. We estimate them using the MLE or REMLE under the full model. As in [46], let us treat both σ^2 and $\mathbf{A}$ as known. Consider a given submodel of the linear mixed effects model (2.1):

$$\mathbf{y}_i = \mathbf{X}_{is}\boldsymbol{\beta}_s + \mathbf{Z}_{is}\boldsymbol{\gamma}_{is} + \boldsymbol{\varepsilon}_i. \tag{2.7}$$

We first estimate $\boldsymbol{\beta}_s$ by using its MLE or REMLE $\widehat{\boldsymbol{\beta}}_s$ and predict $\boldsymbol{\gamma}_{is}$ using $\widehat{\boldsymbol{\gamma}}_{is} = E(\boldsymbol{\gamma}_i | \widehat{\boldsymbol{\beta}}, \mathbf{y})$, the empirical Bayes estimator. Thus, twice the conditional log-likelihood is

$$2\ell_c(\mathbf{y}|\widehat{\boldsymbol{\beta}}_s, \widehat{\boldsymbol{\gamma}}'_{is}s) = -\sum_{i=1}^{n}[n_i\{\log(2\pi) + \log\sigma^2\} + \|\mathbf{y}_i - \mathbf{x}_{is}^T\widehat{\boldsymbol{\beta}}_s - \mathbf{z}_{is}^T\widehat{\boldsymbol{\gamma}}_{is}\|^2/\sigma^2].$$

$$\tag{2.8}$$

Then the cAIC proposed by Vaida and Blanchard[46] is defined to be

$$\text{cAIC} = -2\ell_c(\mathbf{y}|\widehat{\boldsymbol{\beta}}_s, \widehat{\boldsymbol{\gamma}}'_{is}s) + 2\rho.$$

In practice, we may replace σ^2 by its MLE under the full model, denoted by $\widehat{\sigma}_F^2$. To select the best subset of random effect covariates, we then minimize

$$\sum_{i=1}^{n} \|\mathbf{y}_i - \mathbf{x}_{is}^T \widehat{\boldsymbol{\beta}}_s - \mathbf{z}_{is}^T \widehat{\boldsymbol{\gamma}}_{is}\|^2 + 2\widehat{\rho}\widehat{\sigma}_F^2$$

over all possible subsets, where $\widehat{\rho}$ is an estimate of ρ; this approach is similar to the C_p criterion for the linear regression model[31].

Alternatively, we may replace σ^2 by its conditional MLE, the maximizer of the conditional likelihood (2.8), i.e.,

$$\widehat{\sigma}_{cs}^2 = \frac{1}{N} \sum_{i=1}^{n} \|\mathbf{y}_i - \mathbf{x}_{is}^T \widehat{\boldsymbol{\beta}}_s - \mathbf{z}_{is}^T \widehat{\boldsymbol{\gamma}}_{is}\|^2,$$

where $N = \sum_{i=1}^{n} n_i$. Then we find a subset of $\mathbf{x}$ and $\mathbf{z}$ which minimizes

$$N \log \widehat{\sigma}_{cs}^2 + 2\widehat{\rho}$$

and this can be viewed as an extension of AIC for linear regression models. Vaida and Blanchard[46] also proposed a finite sample correction for cAIC; here we omit the details.

Chen and Dunson[10] propose a hierarchical Bayesian model to identify random effects having zero variance. A key step in their approach is to apply a `modified Cholesky decomposition` for the covariance matrix $\mathbf{A}$ of the random effects:

$$\mathbf{A} = \mathbf{D}\boldsymbol{\Gamma}\boldsymbol{\Gamma}^T \mathbf{D}, \tag{2.9}$$

where $\mathbf{D} = \text{diag}\{d_1, \cdots, d_q\}$ is a diagonal matrix, and $\boldsymbol{\Gamma}$ is a lower triangular matrix with one on its diagonal. Represent $\boldsymbol{\gamma}_i = \mathbf{D}\boldsymbol{\Gamma}\mathbf{v}_i$, where $\mathbf{v}_i = (v_{i1}, \cdots, v_{iq})^T$ is a vector of independent standard normal latent variables. Thus, model (2.1) can be rewritten as

$$\mathbf{y}_i = \mathbf{X}_i \boldsymbol{\beta} + \mathbf{Z}_i \mathbf{D}\boldsymbol{\Gamma}\mathbf{v}_i + \boldsymbol{\varepsilon}_i.$$

Thus, we can select significant random effects variables by identifying nonzero diagonal elements of $\mathbf{D}$. This can be done by choosing mixture priors with positive point mass at zero for d_j under the Bayesian variable selection framework. Following standard convention, Chen and Dunson[10] choose conjugate priors for $\boldsymbol{\beta}$ and σ^2. The modified Cholesky decomposition allows us to choose the prior for nonzero off-diagonal elements of $\boldsymbol{\Gamma}$, given $d_1, \cdots, d_q$, to be a normal distribution. With these priors, we are ready to run MCMC to get the posterior distribution of the parameters, including posterior probabilities for models. Since the priors for the d_j's have point mass at zero, non-significant random effects can be estimated at zero variance (i.e., removed from the model).

3. Covariance Selection

As demonstrated in the last section, selection of significant random effects is closely related to covariance selection. A modified Cholesky decomposition, slightly different from (2.9), is the main device for handling covariance selection problems. There are a number of works on applications of Cholesky decomposition to longitudinal data analysis and estimation of large covariance matrices[39,40,35,49,22,28]. In this section, we introduce the covariance selection problem in general terms. The methods described here can be directly applied to longitudinal data analysis and parsimonious estimation of large covariance matrices.

Suppose that $\mathbf{e}_1, \cdots, \mathbf{e}_n$ are a m-dimensional random sample from a population with mean zero and covariance matrix $\boldsymbol{\Sigma}$. Using the modified Cholesky decomposition, we have

$$\mathbf{L}\boldsymbol{\Sigma}\mathbf{L}^T = \boldsymbol{\Lambda},$$

where $\mathbf{L}$ is a lower triangular matrix having ones on its diagonal, and $\boldsymbol{\Lambda} = \text{diag}\{\sigma_1^2, \cdots, \sigma_d^2\}^T$ is a diagonal matrix. Note that $\boldsymbol{\Sigma}$ is symmetric and positive definite. The modified Cholesky decomposition allows us to use m parameters in $\boldsymbol{\Lambda}$ and $m(m-1)/2$ parameters in $\mathbf{L}$ to model $\boldsymbol{\Sigma}$. Parsimonious estimation of $\boldsymbol{\Sigma}$ can be done by imposing sparsity on the elements of $\mathbf{L}$. Smith and Kohn[44] assumed that the random samples follow a m-dimensional normal distribution, and applied a Bayesian variable selection approach for $\boldsymbol{\Sigma}$ by specifying prior distribution for $\mathbf{D}$ and $\mathbf{L}$ and by allowing l_{ij} $(i > j)$, the strictly lower diagonal elements of $\mathbf{L}$ having a positive mass at 0. Following a typical Bayesian variable selection for linear regression models, they obtained the posterior distribution using MCMC. Since the prior for l_{ij} has positive mass at 0, the Bayesian approach may yield a sparse model for $\mathbf{L}$.

Let $-\phi_{tj}$, $1 \leq j < t \leq m$, be the (t,j)th of $\mathbf{L}$, Denote $\mathbf{u}_i = \mathbf{L}\mathbf{e}_i = (u_{i1}, \cdots, u_{im})^T$. Thus, for $2 \leq t \leq m$

$$e_{it} = \sum_{j=1}^{t-1} \phi_{tj} e_{ij} + u_{it} \tag{3.1}$$

where $(e_{i1}, \cdots, e_{im}) = \mathbf{e}_i$. That is, the e_{it}, $t = 2, \cdots, m$, is an autoregressive (AR) series, which gives an interpretation for elements of $\mathbf{L}$ and $\mathbf{D}$. Huang et al.[22] imposed a normality assumption on the population, and implemented covariance selection by minimizing the following negative penalized likelihood function with L_q penalty:

$$\sum_{t=1}^{m} \left(n \log \sigma_t^2 + \sum_{i=1}^{n} \frac{\{e_{it} - \sum_{j=1}^{t-1} \phi_{tj} e_{ij}\}^2}{\sigma_t^2} \right) + \lambda \sum_{t=2}^{m} \sum_{j=1}^{t-1} |\phi_{ij}|^q.$$

Note that since $\mathbf{D}$ is diagonal, $u_{i1}, \cdots, u_{id}$ are uncorrelated. The AR representation for elements of $\mathbf{L}$ and $\mathbf{D}$ allows us to use penalized least squares for covariance selection (see [28]). Thus, without the normality assumption, we are still able to parsimoniously estimate the covariance matrix. We first estimate σ_t^2 using the mean squared errors from model (3.1). For $t = 2, \cdots, m$, covariance matrix structure can be selected by minimizing the following penalized least squares functions:

$$\frac{1}{2n} \sum_{i=1}^{n} (e_{it} - \sum_{j=1}^{t-1} \phi_{tj} e_{ij})^2 + \sum_{j=1}^{t-1} p_{\lambda_{t,j}} (|\phi_{tj}|), \qquad (3.2)$$

where $p_{\lambda_{t,j}}(\cdot)$'s are penalty functions with tuning parameter $\lambda_{t,j}$. This reduces the non-sparse elements in the lower triangle matrix $\mathbf{L}$. With estimated $\mathbf{L}$ and $\mathbf{D}$, $\boldsymbol{\Sigma}$ can be easily estimated by $\widehat{\mathbf{L}}^{-1} \widehat{\mathbf{D}} (\widehat{\mathbf{L}}^{-1})^T$.

4. Variable Selection for GEE Model Fitting

The generalized estimating equations (GEE) approach of Liang and Zeger[27] provides a unified way to fit regression models with clustered/longitudinal data for discrete or continuous y. It can be viewed as an extension of quasi-likelihood approach for generalized linear models (GLIM; see [1], [32]) to allow longitudinally correlated clusters. Let $\mu_{ij} = E(y_{ij}|\mathbf{x}_{ij}) = g(\mathbf{x}_{ij}^T \boldsymbol{\beta})$ for known link function $g(\cdot)$, and $\mathrm{Var}(y_{ij}|\mathbf{x}_{ij}) = \phi \mathrm{V}(\mu_{ij})$ for a scale parameter ϕ and variance function $\mathrm{V}(\cdot)$. Let $\boldsymbol{\mu}_i = (\mu_{i1}, \cdots, \mu_{in_i})^T$, $\mathbf{x}_{ij} = [x_{ij1}, ..., x_{ijd}]^T$, and $\mathbf{D}_i$ be a matrix with (j,k)-element $\partial \mu_{ij}/\partial \beta_k$. Liang and Zeger[27] proposed estimating $\boldsymbol{\beta}$ by solving the following generalized estimating equations

$$\dot{G}(\boldsymbol{\beta}) \stackrel{\mathrm{def}}{=} \sum_{i=1}^{n} \mathbf{D}_i^T \mathbf{A}_i^{-1/2} \mathbf{R}_i^{-1} \mathbf{A}_i^{-1/2} (\mathbf{y}_i - \boldsymbol{\mu}_i) = 0, \qquad (4.1)$$

where $\mathbf{A}_i$ is a $n_i \times n_i$ diagonal matrix with elements $\phi \mathrm{V}(\mu_{ij})$, and $\mathbf{R}_i$ is the working correlation matrix.

4.1. *Extensions of traditional variable selection procedures*

Since a GEE model does not specify a likelihood structure, traditional measures of model fit and of degrees of freedom are not well defined in the GEE approach. Thus, extending traditional variable selection criteria, such as C_p, AIC and BIC, to the GEE approach is challenging. Different measures of model fit and degrees of freedom lead to different variations upon traditional variable selection procedures.

Let us begin with the cross-validation method, which is conceptually simple, but computationally expensive. To extend cross-validation to GEE, we first need to define a measure of model fit. A simple measure is the residual sum of squares, defined by

$$RSS_S = \sum_{i=1}^{n} \sum_{j=1}^{n_i} \{y_{ij} - g(\mathbf{x}_{ij}^T \widehat{\boldsymbol{\beta}})\}^2,$$

where $\widehat{\boldsymbol{\beta}}$ is the resulting estimate of the GEEs (4.1). Based on the RSS_S, the cross-validation method can be extended for GEE methods by leaving one-subject out rather than leaving one-observation out so that no cluster is broken up. To reduce computational cost, one may apply k-fold cross-validation rather than leave-one-out cross validation (in fact, this may improve performance, see [4], [43]). The marginal RSS criterion does not take into account the heteroscedasticity of observations. Cantoni, Field, Flemming and Ronchetti[8] considered generalized least squares loss. Let $r_{ij} = \{y_{ij} - g(\mathbf{x}_{ij}^T \widehat{\boldsymbol{\beta}})\}/\{\widehat{\phi}V(\widehat{\mu}_{ij})\}$ and define the generalized residual sum of squares

$$RSS_W = \sum_{i=1}^{n} \sum_{j=1}^{n_i} w_{ij} r_{ij}^2.$$

where w_{ij}'s are weights, which can be specified based on data analyst's experience and simply set to be 1. Replacing RSS_S by RSS_W, we also can extend the cross-validation method for longitudinal data.

Another cross-validation approach was suggested by Pan[37], who proposed choosing a model to minimize some linear combination of the expected predictive bias

$$\text{EPB} = E_x E_y \mid \dot{G}(Y|\mathbf{X}, \widehat{\boldsymbol{\beta}}(\mathbf{X}) \mid \tag{4.2}$$

on new data. This is a generalization of the C_p in that Pan[37] tries to predict a risk function for future data, but is much more general than quadratic loss. Pan's scheme for finding the model which minimizes EPB involves cross-validation and bootstrapping. Perhaps because (4.2) is rather abstract and estimating it requires computational effort, this criterion has unfortunately received little attention.

For linear regression models with independent observations, leave-one-out cross validation is asymptotically equivalent to two simple and easily implemented criteria, Mallows' C_p and AIC. To extend C_p and AIC for GEE methods, we need to define degrees of freedom for model fit. A simple but reasonable (see [52]) definition of degrees of freedom is the number of regression coefficients used in the model, denoted by df_S; we define others later. It is also necessary to choose a goodness of fit measure. It is known that Mallows' classical C_p for linear regression models estimates a quadratic predictive risk. Cantoni, Flemming and Ronchetti[9] extended the C_p criterion to GEE fit using a weighted quadratic predictive risk, resulting in a generalized C_p, denoted as GC_p. The weights allow data analysts to incorporate their professional experience easily and incorporate robustness (see [7]), but implementing the GC_p with a general weighting scheme requires bootstrapping or Monte Carlo simulation to estimate the effective degrees of freedom of the model fit. This is very computationally expensive and may become infeasible in practice. Fortunately, the GC_p with all weights equal has a simple, closed form. Let

$$\mathbf{M} = n^{-1} \sum_{i=1}^{n} \mathbf{D}_i^T \mathbf{V}_i^{-1} \mathbf{D}_i, \quad \text{and} \quad \mathbf{N} = n^{-1} \sum_{i=1}^{n} \mathbf{D}_i^T \mathbf{A}_i^{-1} \mathbf{D}_i,$$

where $\mathbf{V}_i = \mathbf{A}_i^{1/2} \mathbf{R}_i \mathbf{A}_i^{1/2}$. Cantoni, Flemming and Ronchetti[9] set the degrees of freedom for GEE model fit to be

$$df_C = \text{tr}(\mathbf{M}^{-1}\mathbf{N}).$$

The GC_p is then

$$GC_p = \sum_{i=1}^{n} \sum_{j=1}^{n_i} r_{ij}^2 - \sum_{i=1}^{n} J_i + 2\, df_C. \tag{4.3}$$

The definition of degrees of freedom is motivated by the definition of robust sandwich formula for the GEE estimate, and if working independence is used then $df_C = df_S$, see [9] for a more detailed derivation of the degrees of freedom.

The classic AIC is asymptotically equivalent to C_p for linear models, but applies more generally. It estimates the relative Kullback-Leibler distance of the likelihood function specified by a model, from the true likelihood function which generated the data. AIC cannot be used directly in GEE since the likelihood is not specified (although a quasi-likelihood may be implicitly specified). Pan[36] considered the problem of extending Akaike's derivation of AIC to GEE models. Pan's procedure works best with a working independent correlation matrix, so we use this formulation. With working independence, the GEE model fit can be seen as a maximum pseudo quasi-likelihood fit. To take into account the within-subject correlation, Pan[36] sets the degrees of freedom for a GEE estimate $\widehat{\beta}$ with working independent correction matrix to be

$$df_P = \text{tr}(\widehat{\Omega}\widehat{V}),$$

where $\widehat{\Omega}$ is the observed Fisher information matrix for the logarithm of pseudo quasi-likelihood denoted by $QL(\beta)$, i.e., $\widehat{\Omega} = -\partial^2 QL(\widehat{\beta})/\partial\beta\partial\beta^T$, and $\widehat{V}$ is the estimated covariance matrix of $\widehat{\beta}$ using robust sandwich formula. Pan[36] thus suggests selecting significant variables by minimizing the following the `quasi-AIC` (QIC)

$$QIC = -2QL(\widehat{\beta}) + 2df_P. \tag{4.4}$$

See [36] for heuristic derivation of these formulas. This QIC is similar to Takeuchi's information criterion, a more general form of Akaike's information criterion in the classical case; it is also closely related to earlier adjustments to AIC for overdispersion (see [6, pp. 65-69]). If the responses are independent and the model is adequate, then QIC is equivalent to AIC. However, QIC's reliance on working independence may make it less effective if within-subject correlation is high.

Ad hoc generalization of the BIC is possible along the same lines, although the ambiguity of the sample size becomes a difficulty (see [38] and [20]). Naïve possibilities include $-2QL(\widehat{\beta}) + \log(n)df$ and $-2QL(\widehat{\beta}) + \log(N)df$, but more research is needed.

We conclude this section with a remark. Although several authors have made efforts in developing variable selection for GEE model fit, it is not clear which measure of model fit is the best or which definition of degrees of freedom will perform best. Further research to provide both theoretical insights and empirical justification for extending traditional variable selection procedures to longitudinal data are clearly needed. Some other practical remarks on GEE model selection are found in [3].

4.2. *Penalized GEE*

In this section, we extend the non-concave penalized likelihood approach[45,15] to GEE model fitting. We combine selection and estimation by solving the following **penalized generalized estimating** equations:

$$\dot{Q}(\boldsymbol{\beta}) \overset{\text{def}}{=} \dot{G}(\boldsymbol{\beta}) + N\dot{\mathcal{P}}(\boldsymbol{\beta}) = \sum_{i=1}^{n} \mathbf{D}_i^T \mathbf{A}_i^{-1/2} \mathbf{R}_i^{-1} \mathbf{A}_i^{-1/2}(\mathbf{y}_i - \boldsymbol{\mu}_i) + N\dot{\mathcal{P}}(\boldsymbol{\beta}) = 0,$$

$$(4.5)$$

where $\dot{\mathcal{P}}(\boldsymbol{\beta}) = [p'_{\lambda_1}(|\beta_1|)\text{sgn}(\beta_1), \cdots, p'_{\lambda_d}(|\beta_d|)\text{sgn}(\beta_1)]^T$.

Fu[18] studied the asymptotic properties of these penalized generalized estimating equations with L_q penalties, including L_1 as a special case. He further addressed practical implementation issues and recommmended an adaptation of the GCV (see [11]) to select the regularization parameter λ_j.

As demonstrated in Fan and Li[15], the SCAD penalty defined in Section 2.1 retains the main virtues of L_1 while reducing estimation bias. Here we suggest using the SCAD penalty instead of the L_1 penalty in (4.5). The oracle property for penalized GEE with the SCAD penalty can be established using the same strategy as that in [15], see [13] for more details. Since the SCAD penalty is singular at the origin, and is nonconvex over $(0, \infty)$, it is not straightforward to solve the penalized GEE with the SCAD penalty.

For practical implementation, we use a modified Newton-Raphson algorithm to solve the penalized GEEs, with iterative local quadratic approximation (LQA, [15]) to approximate the SCAD penalty. Given an initial value $\boldsymbol{\beta}^{(0)}$ that is close to the solution of (4.5), for coefficient estimates not too close to zero ($|\hat{\beta}_j| \geq \eta$ where in practice η could be .001, or smaller if the standard error of $\hat{\boldsymbol{\beta}}$ is very small), the penalty $p_{\lambda_j}(|\beta_j|)$ can be locally approximated by the quadratic function as

$$[p_{\lambda_j}(|\beta_j|)]' = p'_{\lambda_j}(|\beta_j|)\text{sgn}(\beta_j) \approx \{p'_{\lambda_j}(|\beta_j^{(0)}|)/|\beta_j^{(0)}|\}\beta_j.$$

With the local quadratic approximation, the Newton-Raphson algorithm can be implemented directly to solve the penalized GEE (4.5). When the algorithm converges, the solution satisfies the penalized GEE equations $\dot{Q}(\boldsymbol{\beta}) = 0$. Of course, for $|\hat{\beta}_j| < \eta$ we set $|\hat{\beta}_j|$ to zero. Following conventional techniques in GEE approaches, we may use a sandwich formula to estimate the standard error of the coefficient estimates in the final model. A similar LQA algorithm can be used to find L_q-penalized estimates also; this is very similar to the adjusted iterative algorithm mentioned by Fu[18].

To implement penalized GEE in practice, it is desirable to have an automatic data-driven method for selecting the tuning parameters $\boldsymbol{\lambda} = (\lambda_1, \cdots, \lambda_d)$. Fan and Li[15] chose the tuning parameters by minimizing a GCV criterion. Wang, Li and Tsai[47] later proposed a BIC-like tuning parameter selector. They demonstrate that the BIC selector performs better than the GCV selector, in that selecting the tuning parameters by BIC guarantees that the resulting estimator possesses the asymptotic oracle property, while using GCV does not. Thus, we will use the BIC selector for the SCAD in our numerical comparison.

By some straightforward calculation, the effective number of parameters in the last step of the Newton-Raphson algorithm is

$$e(\boldsymbol{\lambda}) = \text{tr}[\{\ddot{G}(\boldsymbol{\beta}) + N\boldsymbol{\Sigma}_{\boldsymbol{\lambda}}(\widehat{\boldsymbol{\beta}})\}^{-1}\ddot{G}(\boldsymbol{\beta})],$$

where $\ddot{G}(\boldsymbol{\beta}) = \partial G(\boldsymbol{\beta})/\partial\boldsymbol{\beta}$, corresponding to the nonzero components of $\widehat{\boldsymbol{\beta}}$ and $\boldsymbol{\Sigma}_{\boldsymbol{\lambda}}(\widehat{\boldsymbol{\beta}})$ is a diagonal matrix with diagonal elements $p'_{\lambda_j}(|\widehat{\beta}_j|)/|\widehat{\beta}_j|$ for nonzero $\widehat{\beta}_j$'s.

Parallel to two extensions of the BIC proposed in [38], the BIC statistic can be defined as follows:

$$BIC_1(\boldsymbol{\lambda}) = \frac{1}{N}\log(\frac{1}{N}\sum_{i=1}^{n}\sum_{j=1}^{n_i} r_{ij}^2) + \log(n)e(\boldsymbol{\lambda}), \qquad (4.6)$$

or

$$BIC_2(\boldsymbol{\lambda}) = \frac{1}{N}\log(\frac{1}{N}\sum_{i=1}^{n}\sum_{j=1}^{n_i} r_{ij}^2) + \log(N)e(\boldsymbol{\lambda}), \qquad (4.7)$$

where r_{ij} is the Pearson residual corresponding to $\widehat{\boldsymbol{\beta}}$, given $\boldsymbol{\lambda}$. One may replace the Pearson residuals with deviance residuals if they are available. The BIC_2 is more compatible with the original definition of the BIC (and is equivalent under working independence), but in practice it tends to be a little too strong, and it tends to give somewhat poorer empirical performance than BIC_1. Both presumably have similar asymptotic behavior if the n_i are bounded (see [43]).

We can select $\boldsymbol{\lambda}$ by minimizing, say, BIC_1. To find an optimal $\boldsymbol{\lambda}$, the BIC selector needs to be minimized over a d-dimensional space, an unduly onerous task. However, it is intuitively expected that the magnitude of λ_j should be proportional to the standard error of estimate of β_j. Therefore, we may set $\boldsymbol{\lambda} = \lambda\,\text{se}(\widehat{\boldsymbol{\beta}}_{GEE})$ in practice, where $\text{se}(\widehat{\boldsymbol{\beta}}_{GEE})$ stands for the standard error of the unpenalized GEE estimate. Thus, we minimize the BIC score over the one-dimensional space, saving a great deal of computational cost. This scheme is used in our simulations.

5. Numerical Comparison

This section presents some comparisons of variable selection procedures for longitudinal data. Comparisons of variable selection procedures for linear mixed models can be found in [20], and some comparisons of covariance selection are found in [28].

Example 1. In this example, we generated 200 data sets using Octave code (a free version of Matlab), each consisting of $n = 50$ subjects with each subject having $J = 5$ observations (i.e, all n_i equals $J = 5$), from the following linear model:

$$y_{ij} = \mathbf{x}_{ij}^T \boldsymbol{\beta} + 3\varepsilon_{ij},$$

where $\boldsymbol{\beta} = (3, 1, 0, 0, 2, 0, 0, 0)^T$ (i.e., there were 5 inactive and 3 active predictors), and $\mathbf{x}_{ij} \sim N_8(\mathbf{0}, \boldsymbol{\Sigma})$, where the diagonal elements of $\boldsymbol{\Sigma}$ all equal 1, and all off-diagonal elements equal 0.6. Furthermore, $(\varepsilon_{i1}, \cdots, \varepsilon_{iJ})^T$ are multivariate normal with AR(1) true correlation structure with $\rho = 0.7$.

In our simulation, we compare the following GEE model selection criteria:

(1) naïve AIC ignoring correlation, defined as $N \log(RSS_S/N) + 2df_S$;
(2) naïve C_p, defined to be $RSS_S + 2df_S \hat{\sigma}^2$, where $\hat{\sigma}^2$ is the MSE under the full model;
(3) Cantoni's C_p defined in (4.3);
(4) Pan's AIC, defined in (4.4);
(5) Fu's penalized GEE with L_1 penalty. The λ_j were proportional to the unpenalized standard errors; their magnitude was chosen using the modified GCV-like statistic defined in [18].
(6) Penalized GEE with the SCAD penalty. The tuning parameters are selected by using BIC_1 and BIC_2 tuning parameter selectors described in Section 4.2. Corresponding to the BIC_1 and BIC_2, this procedure is referred to as SCAD$_1$ and SCAD$_2$ in Table 1, respectively.

To find the subset which minimizes AIC and C_p criteria in (1)—(4), we exhaustively search all 2^8 possibilities. Thus, the corresponding results represent best subset variable selection with the underlying criterion.

We compare each variable selection procedure in terms of model complexity and model error, defined by $\mathrm{ME}(\hat{\beta}) = (\hat{\beta} - \beta)^T E(\mathbf{x}\mathbf{x}^T)(\hat{\beta} - \beta)$ (see [15]). Table 1 depicted the mean of model error for each procedure and summarized model complexity in terms of *correct deletions*, the average number per simulation of truly zero coefficients correctly estimated as zero, *erroneous deletions*, the average number of truly nonzero coefficients erroneously set to zero, and *proportion correct models*, the proportion of trials in which exactly the true subset of nonzero predictors was chosen.

To study the impacts of choice of working correlation structure, we compare every procedures under three working correlation structures: working independence, AR(1) and compound symmetry; these are abbreviated as Ind, AR, CS in Table 1.

Table 1. Comparison of GEE Model Selection (Continuous Response)

Criterion	10 × Mean ME			Prop. True Models		
Working Corr. Matrix:	Ind	AR	CS	Ind	AR	CS
Full	2.87	1.25	1.69	0.00	0.00	0.00
Naïve AIC	1.87	0.77	1.13	0.63	0.65	0.63
Naïve C_p	1.87	0.77	1.13	0.63	0.66	0.63
AIC (Pan)	1.87	0.85	1.11	0.58	0.35	0.41
C_p (Cantoni)	1.87	0.80	1.08	0.63	0.44	0.42
LASSO (Fu)	2.18	1.14	2.03	0.08	0.40	0.25
SCAD$_1$	1.68	0.64	1.04	0.50	0.41	0.33
SCAD$_2$	1.73	0.64	1.12	0.70	0.62	0.50
	Correct Deletions			Erroneous Deletions		
Working Corr. Matrix:	Ind	AR	CS	Ind	AR	CS
Full	0.00	0.00	0.00	0.00	0.00	0.00
Naïve AIC	4.59	4.60	4.59	0.06	0.03	0.06
Naïve C_p	4.59	4.61	4.59	0.06	0.03	0.06
AIC (Pan)	4.53	4.08	4.21	0.04	0.01	0.02
C_p (Cantoni)	4.59	4.26	4.24	0.06	0.01	0.02
LASSO (Fu)	2.66	4.14	3.70	0.00	0.00	0.01
SCAD$_1$	4.26	4.17	4.04	0.03	0.00	0.01
SCAD$_2$	4.63	4.51	4.39	0.03	0.00	0.01

From Table 1, taking correlation into account led to much better estimation performance than using working independence. Not surprisingly using the correct correlation structure, AR(1), was better than using an incorrect (compound symmetric) correlation structure. In general, parsimonious methods outperformed less parsimonious ones, partly because the true model in this example is rather simple. SCAD tended to give smaller models than LASSO, and generally better estimation performance. Overall, SCAD outperforms the other procedures in terms of model errors and model complexity.

Example 2. In this example, we compare the variable selection procedures for data with correlated binary responses. The simulations were conducted using R code since we used the correlated random binary data generator by Leisch and Weingessel[26]. We conducted 200 simulations, and in each simulation, $n = 100$ subjects with $J = 10$ observations (i.e., all n_i equals

10). We generated correlated binary response with marginal distribution:

$$y_{ij}|\mathbf{x}_{ij} \sim \text{Bernoulli}\{p(\mathbf{x}_{ij})\},$$

where $p(x) = \exp(-0.5 + \mathbf{x}_i^T \boldsymbol{\beta})/\{1 + \exp(-0.5 + \mathbf{x}_i^T \boldsymbol{\beta})\}$, $\boldsymbol{\beta}$ is the same as that in Example 1, $\mathbf{x}_{ij} \sim N_8(\mathbf{0}, \boldsymbol{\Sigma})$, where the diagonal elements of $\boldsymbol{\Sigma}$ all equal 1, and all off-diagonal elements equal 0.5. The binary responses were exchangeably correlated (i.e., with compound symmetry).

Since the classic C_p criterion is not well defined for binary data, we do not include it in our comparison. Simulation results are summarized in Table 2, in which MSE is the mean squared error in coefficient estimation.

Table 2.   Comparison of GEE Model Selection (Binary Response)

Criterion	10 × Mean MSE			Prop. True Models		
Working Corr. Matrix:	Ind	AR	CS	Ind	AR	CS
Full	1.11	0.87	0.82	0.00	0.00	0.00
Naïve AIC	0.88	0.62	0.66	0.38	0.53	0.46
AIC (Pan)	0.88	0.64	0.69	0.38	0.41	0.31
LASSO (Fu)	0.77	0.65	0.63	0.01	0.00	0.00
SCAD$_1$	0.78	0.62	0.66	0.69	0.72	0.70
SCAD$_2$	0.86	0.76	0.79	0.61	0.57	0.56
	Correct Deletions			Erroneous Deletions		
Working Corr. Matrix:	Ind	AR	CS	Ind	AR	CS
Full	0.00	0.00	0.00	0.00	0.00	0.00
Naïve AIC	4.09	4.41	4.34	0.07	0.10	0.10
AIC (Pan)	4.07	4.22	4.05	0.07	0.08	0.09
LASSO (Fu)	1.92	1.70	1.63	0.00	0.01	0.01
SCAD$_1$	4.83	4.93	4.88	0.23	0.22	0.23
SCAD$_2$	4.94	4.97	4.98	0.38	0.41	0.43

The SCAD with BIC_2 had a false deletion rate higher than we would wish; the SCAD with BIC_1 had almost as good a correct deletion rate but a noticeably lower false deletion rate. In general, then, the lighter version seems to be better. Pan's AIC does fairly well. The LASSO provides good estimation performance but not very sparse models.

6. Variable Selection for Other Models

Although mixed effects models and GEE are very popular formulations for analyzing longitudinal data, many other models have also been used. In this section, we will briefly introduce variable selection procedures for a partial linear model, a semiparametric approach highly relevant to longitudinal data (see [51], [34], [29], and [16]).

Suppose that we have a sample of n subjects. For the i-th subject, the response variable $y_i(t)$ and the covariate vector $\mathbf{x}_i(t)$, are collected at times $t = t_{i1}, \cdots, t_{in_i}$, where n_i is the total number of observations on the i-th subject. The **partial linear model** for longitudinal data has the following form:

$$y_i(t_{ij}) = \alpha(t_{ij}) + \boldsymbol{\beta}^T \mathbf{x}_i(t_{ij}) + \varepsilon_i(t_{ij}) \tag{6.1}$$

for $i = 1, \cdots, n$, and $j = 1, \cdots, n_i$. As before, variable selection is important in the partial linear model, because the number of available x variables in (6.1) can be large.

Fan and Li[16] proposed a class of variable selection procedures via the **nonconvex penalized quadratic loss**

$$\frac{1}{2n} \sum_{i=1}^{n} (\mathbf{y}_i - \boldsymbol{\alpha}_i - X_i \boldsymbol{\beta})^T W_i (\mathbf{y}_i - \boldsymbol{\alpha}_i - X_i \boldsymbol{\beta}) + \sum_{j=1}^{d} p_{\lambda_j}(|\beta_j|). \tag{6.2}$$

where $\boldsymbol{\alpha}_i = [\alpha(t_{i1}), \cdots, \alpha(t_{in_i})]^T$. We can then implement entropy, L_q, or SCAD penalties for the $p_{\lambda_j}(|\beta_j|)$. Since $\alpha(t)$ is an unknown nonparametric smooth function, (6.2) cannot directly be minimized in $\boldsymbol{\beta}$. Therefore, Fan and Li[16] proposed eliminating the nuisance function $\alpha(\cdot)$ using a profiling technique; see [16] for details. Then the resulting estimate of (6.2) is a penalized profile least squares estimate. The sampling properties of the penalized profile least squares estimate were studied by Fan and Li[16], who demonstrated that with a proper choice of regularization parameters and penalty functions, the proposed variable selection procedures perform as well asymptotically as an oracle estimator.

More research is needed to study how to choose significant variables for other existing models for longitudinal data. For example, there is little or no existing work in the literature on variable selection for generalized linear mixed effects models and generalized partial linear models for longitudinal data.

Acknowledgements

This research was supported by a NSF grant DMS-03048869 and a National Institute on Drug Abuse (NIDA) grant P50 DA10075.

References

1. A. Agresti, *Categorical Data Analysis*, (2nd ed.), Wiley, Hoboken, NJ, 2002.
2. H. Akaike, A new look at the statistical model identification. *IEEE Trans. on Automatic Control*, **19** ((1974)), 716-723.
3. G.A. Ballinger, Using generalized estimating equations for longitudinal data analysis, *Organizational Res. Meth.*, **7** (2004), 127-150.
4. L. Breiman, Heuristics of instability and stabilization in model selection. *Ann. Statist.*, **24** (1996), 2350-2383.
5. S.T. Buckland, K.P. Burnham, and N.H. Augustin, Model selection: An integral part of inference, *Biometrics*, **53** (1997), 603-618.
6. K.P. Burnham and D.R. Anderson, *Model Selection and Multimodel Inference: a Practical Information-Theoretic Approach*, (2nd ed.), Springer-Verlag, NY, 2002.
7. E. Cantoni, A robust approach to longitudinal data analysis, *Canad. J. Statist.*, **32** (2004), 169-180.
8. E. Cantoni, C. Field, J.M. Flemming, and E. Ronchetti, *Longitudinal Variable Selection by Cross-Validation in the Case of Many Covariates*, Technical Report, University of Geneva, Econometrics Dept. URL: http://www.unige.ch/ses/metri/cahiers/2005_01.pdf, 2005.
9. E. Cantoni, J.M. Flemming, and E. Ronchetti, Variable selection for marginal longitudinal generalized linear models, *Biometrics*, **61** (2005), 507-514.
10. Z. Chen and D.B. Dunson, Random effects selection in linear mixed models, *Biometrics*, **59** (2003), 762-769.
11. P. Craven, and G. Wahba, Smoothing noisy data with spline functions, *Numerische Mathematik*, **31** (1979), 377-403.
12. P.J. Diggle, P. Heagerty, K.Y. Liang, and S.L. Zeger, *Analysis of Longitudinal Data*, (2nd ed.), Oxford University Press, Oxford, 2002.
13. J.J. Dziak, *Variable Selection for Longitudinal Data by Penalized Quadratic Inference Functions*, Ph.D. dissertation, Department of Statistics, The Pennsylvania State University, 2006.
14. J.W. Eaton, *GNU Octave Manual*, Network Theory Ltd., URL http://www.octave.org, 2002.
15. J. Fan and R. Li, Variable Selection via Nonconcave Penalized Likelihood and its Oracle Properties, *J. Amer. Statist. Assoc.*, **96** (2001), 1348-1360.
16. J. Fan and R. Li, New estimation and model selection procedures for semiparametric modeling in longitudinal data analysis, *J. Amer. Statist. Assoc.*, **99** (2004), 710-723.
17. I.E. Frank and J.H. Friedman, A statistical view of some chemometrics regression tools. *Technometrics*, **35** (1993), 109-148.
18. W. Fu, Penalized estimating equations, *Biometrics*, **59** (2003), 126-132.
19. E. I. George, The variable selection problem. *J. Amer. Statist. Assoc.*, **95** (2000), 1304-1308.
20. M.J. Gurka, Selecting the best linear mixed model under REML, *American Statistician*, **60** (2006), 19-26.

21. A.E. Hoerl and R. Kennard, Ridge regression: Biased estimation for nonorthogonal problems, *Technometrics*, **12** (1970), 55-67.

22. J. Z. Huang, N. Liu, M. Pourahmadi, and L. Liu, Covariance selection and estimation via penalised normal likelihood. *Biometrika*, **93** (2006), 85-98.

23. C.M. Hurvich and C. Tsai, Regression and time series model selection in small samples. *Biometrika*, **76** (1989), 297-307.

24. H. Jeffreys, *Theory of Probability*, (3rd Ed.), Oxford University Press, Oxford, 1961.

25. J. Jiang and J.S. Rao, Consistent procedures for mixed linear model selection, *Sankhyá*, **65** (2003), 23-42.

26. F. Leisch and A. Weingessel, bindata: Generation of Artificial Binary Data. R package version 0.9-12, 2005.

27. K.-Y. Liang and S.L. Zeger, Longitudinal data analysis using generalized linear models, *Biometrika*, **73** (1986), 13-22.

28. R. Li, J.J. Dziak, and Y. Ma, Nonconvex penalized least squares: Characterizations, algorithm and application, manuscript, 2006.

29. D. Y. Lin and Z. Ying, Semiparametric and Nonparametric Regression Analysis of Longitudinal Data (with discussion), *J. Amer. Statist. Assoc.*, **96** (2001), 103-126.

30. H.H. Liu, R.E. Weiss, R.I. Jennrich, and N.S. Wenger, PRESS model selection in repeated measures data, *Comput. Statist. & Data Anal.*, **30** (1999), 169-184.

31. C.L. Mallows, Some comments on C_p, *Technometrics*, **15** (1973), 661-675.

32. P. McCullagh and J.A. Nelder, *Generalized Linear Models*, (2nd ed.), Chapman & Hall, New York, 1989.

33. A.J. Miller, *Subset Selection in Regression*, (2nd ed.), Chapman & Hall, NY, 2002.

34. R. A. Moyeed and P.J. Diggle, Rates of Convergence in Semiparametric Modeling of Longitudinal Data, *Australian Journal of Statistics*, **36** (1994), 75-93.

35. J. Pan and G. MacKenzie, Model selection for joint mean-covariance structures in longitudinal studies, *Biometrika*, **90** (2003), 239-244.

36. W. Pan, Akaike's information criterion in generalized estimating equations. *Biometrics*, **57** (2001), 120-125.

37. W. Pan, Model selection in estimating equations, *Biometrics*, **57** (2001), 529-534.

38. D.K. Pauler, The Schwarz criterion and related methods for normal linear models, *Biometrika*, **85** (1998), 13-27.

39. M. Pourahmadi, Joint mean-covariance models with applications to longitudinal data: unconstrained parameterization. *Biometrika*, **86** (1999), 677-690.

40. M. Pourahmadi, Maximum likelihood estimation of generalized linear models for multivariate normal covariance matrix, *Biometrika*, **87** (2000), 425-435.

41. R Development Core Team, R: A language and environment for statistical computing, R Foundation for Statistical Computing, Vienna, Austria. URL http://www.R-project.org, 2005.

42. G. Schwarz, Estimating the dimension of a model, *Ann. Statist.*, **6** (1978), 461–464.

43. J. Shao, An asymptotic theory for linear model selection, *Statistica Sinica*, **7** (1997), 221-264.
44. M. Smith and R. Kohn, Parsimonious covariance matrix estimation for longitudinal data, *J. Royal Statist. Soc., B*, **97** (2002), 1141-1153.
45. R.J. Tibshirani, Regression shrinkage and selection via the LASSO, *Journal of Royal Statistical Society, B*, **58** (1996), 267-288.
46. F. Vaida and S. Blanchard, Conditional Akaike information for mixed-effects models, *Biometrika*, **92** (2005), 351-370.
47. H. Wang, R. Li, and C.-L. Tsai, A consistent tuning parameter selector for SCAD. *Biometrika*, (2006), To appear.
48. R.E. Weiss, Y. Wang, and J.G. Ibrahim, Predictive model selection for repeated measures random effects models using Bayes factors, *Biometrics*, **53** (1997), 592-602.
49. W.B. Wu and M. Pourahmadi, Nonparametric estimation of large covariance matrices of longitudinal data, *Biometrika*, **90** (2003), 831-844.
50. A. Yafune, T. Funatogawa, and M. Fshiguro, Extended information criterion (EIC) approach for linear mixed effects models under restricted maximum likelihood (REML) estimation. *Statist. Med.*, **24** (2005), 3417-3429.
51. S.L. Zeger and P.J. Diggle, Semiparametric Models for Longitudinal Data With Application to CD4 Cell Numbers in HIV Seroconverters, *Biometrics*, **50** (1994), 689-699.
52. H. Zou, T. Hastie, and R. Tibshirani, On the "Degrees of Freedom" of the Lasso, Technical Report paper, Department of Statistics, Stanford University, Stanford, CA: www-stat.stanford.edu/~hastie/Papers/dflasso.pdf, 2004.

CHAPTER 2

SOME RECENT RESULTS IN MODEL SELECTION

Xiaoming Huo[a,b] and Xuelei (Sherry) Ni[b,c]

[a]*Department of Statistics, University of California at Riverside,*
Riverside, CA, USA
[b]*School of Industrial and Systems Engineering,*
Georgia Institute of Technology,
765 Ferst Dr. Atlanta, GA 30332-0205, USA
E-mails: [a]*huo@gatech.edu*
[c]*xni@isye.gatech.edu*

In statistics, model selection has a long standing history, while new results in this area still keep coming. At this point, it is nearly impossible and not helpful to give a comprehensive survey on all the available theorems. We take a special angle: from where more results are likely to be generated. Our perspective is based on some recent interesting findings in applied mathematics; namely, in some cases a subset of NP hard problems can be solved effectively by some convex optimization approaches, which only require polynomial time. We discuss the potential of this approach. For users who would like to know more about the existing ideas in model selection, we provide a summary in the end.

1. Introduction

Model selection is a classical topic in statistics. Here, for simplicity, we restrict to an ordinary linear regression model. For classical results, an excellent survey is given by George[22], while Kadane and Lazar[29] give a superior survey from a Bayesian viewpoint. Since their appearance, many new interesting results have come out. Presenting all of them here is nearly impossible and also distractive. As anticipated, researchers have taken different angles in tackling the model selection problem.

The perspective taken in this paper is new. It can be summarized into the following three steps.

- First of all, it is proven (see [28]) that many *classical* criteria in model selection require solving NP-hard problems. Hence, in general, there is no efficient algorithmic solution.

In fact, the state-of-the-art algorithm in solving this problem is still the leaps-and-bounds [18], which was proposed in 70's and basically utilizes the branch-and-bound technique that is widely used in combinatorial optimization. There are some recent improvements; for example LBOT[38]. However, when the number of predictors is more than 40 to 50, most of these methods will take intolerable amount of time.

- In applied mathematics, it is found that even though some problems are NP-hard in general, there are special cases, under which they are solvable in polynomial time. A case that has been cited for many times is Donoho and Huo[11]. This motivates us to search for special conditions, which (a) can be verified in polynomial time and (b) indicate that a model selection problem has polynomial time solution.

- The above leads to the action: finding a group of conditions, which help to identify solvable model selection problem. See some initial results in [28].

The above differs from many existing works in the following way: we consider the computational aspect, in particular the *solvability* of model selection problems, assuming that the model selection criteria are based on a prefixed class of optimization problems; while other works may emphasize more on the statistical properties of the results of model selection approaches, as we will summarize in Section 5.

Another difference (from many existing statistically algorithmic papers) is that instead of considering a particular numeric method, we abstract them into two types of problems: **(P0)** and **(P1)**, which will be defined in the next section. Instead of finding an efficient algorithm for either of them, we consider when do these two problems have the identical solutions. Such an equivalence is argued to establish an efficient algorithm to solve the model selection problem. More details will be articulated.

As a fundamental tool, progress in model selection is likely to improve the methodologies in biostatistics. This paper does not focus on biostatistical applications in particular.

This chapter is organized as follows. We give an overview of our perspective in Section 2. Details on related literature and formulation are presented in Section 3. In Section 4, we use two extreme examples to illustrate the model selection problem. Section 5 summarizes various interesting findings/ideas that have been published recently — for obvious reasons, we give an emphasis on publications that come after the two survey papers mentioned at the beginning of this article.

2. Our Perspective

We consider two types of optimization problems:

- one optimization problem that is based on a counting measure,

$$(\textbf{P0}) \qquad \min_x \quad \|y - \Phi x\|_2^2 + \lambda_0 \cdot \|x\|_0,$$

where $\Phi \in \mathbb{R}^{n \times m}, x \in \mathbb{R}^m, y \in \mathbb{R}^n$, notation $\|\cdot\|_2^2$ denotes the sum of squares of the entries of a vector, constant $\lambda_0 \geq 0$ is an algorithmic parameter, and quantity $\|x\|_0$ is the number of nonzero entries in vector x;

- one optimization problem that depends on a sum of absolute values,

$$(\textbf{P1}) \qquad \min_x \quad \|y - \Phi x\|_2^2 + \lambda_1 \cdot \|x\|_1,$$

where $\|x\|_1 = \sum_{i=1}^m |x_i|$ for vector $x = (x_1, x_2, \ldots, x_m)^T$, and constant $\lambda_1 \geq 0$ is another algorithmic parameter whose role will be discussed later.

Note $\|x\|_0$ (respectively, $\|x\|_1$) is a quasi-norm (respectively, norm) in $\mathbb{R}^m$. In the literature of *sparse signal presentation*, they are called ℓ_0-norm and ℓ_1-norm, respectively. The numbers "0" and "1" in the notations (**P0**) and (**P1**) follow such a convention in Donlho and Huo[11], Donoho, et al.[10], and Chen and Huo[4,5].

Model selection in regression is equivalent to *subset selection*. In subset selection under linear regression, many well known criteria – including C_p statistic, Akaike information criterion (AIC), Bayesian information criterion (BIC), minimum description length (MDL), risk inflation criterion (RIC), and so on — are special cases of (**P0**), by assigning different values to λ_0. Details regarding the foregoing statement will be provided later. It is shown that problem (**P0**) in general is NP-hard (Theorem 1; also see Huo and Ni[28]).

On the other hand, (**P1**) is the mathematical problem that is called upon in Lasso[47]. Recent advances (whose details and references are provided in Section 3.2) demonstrate that some stepwise algorithms (e.g., least angle regressions (LARS) presented in Efron, et al.[14]) reveal the solution paths of problem **(P1)**, while parameter λ_1 takes a range of values. More importantly, most of these algorithms only take polynomial number of operations — i.e., they are polynomial-time algorithms. In fact, the complexity of finding a solution path for **(P1)** is the same as implementing an ordinary least square fit[14].

The main objective of this chapter is to find when **(P0)** and **(P1)** give the same result in the subset selection. Following Huo and Ni[28], a subset that corresponds to the indices of the nonzero entries of the minimizer of **(P0)** (respectively, **(P1)**) is called a *type-I* (respectively, *type-II*) *optimal subset with respective to* λ_0 (respectively, λ_1). A subset that is both type-I and type-II optimal is called a *concurrent optimal subset*. It is known that there exists a necessary and sufficient condition for the type-II optimal subset, and this condition can be verified in polynomial time. However, in general, there is no polynomial-time necessary and sufficient condition for the type-I optimal subset. Therefore, we search for easy-to-verify (i.e., polynomial-time) sufficient conditions for type-I optimal subsets. Two types of results are derived in Huo and Ni[28]. The first is based on the assumption that the covariates whose correlations with the response vector are higher than the others form the optimal subset. The second result is motivated by a new advance in sparse signal representation, and is rather general. Since this is not the theme of this chapter, we omit further details.

3. Formulation and Related Literature

We review more literature in *subset selection*. Recall in a regression setting, $\Phi \in \mathbb{R}^{n \times m} (n > m)$ denotes a model matrix. Vectors $x \in \mathbb{R}^m$ and $y \in \mathbb{R}^n$ are coefficient and response vectors. The columns of matrix Φ are *covariates*. A regression model is $y = \Phi x + \varepsilon$, where ε is a random vector. Let $\mathbf{I} = \{1, 2, \ldots, m\}$ denote all the indices of the coefficients. A subset of coefficients (or, covariates) is denoted by $\Omega \subseteq \mathbf{I}$. Let $|\Omega|$ denote the cardinality of set Ω. Let x_Ω denote the coefficient vector that only takes nonzero values when the coefficient indices are in the subset Ω. A subset selection problem has two competing objectives in choosing a subset Ω: firstly, the residuals, which are in the vector $y - \Phi x_\Omega$, are close to zeros; secondly, the size of the set Ω is small.

3.1. *Subset Selection Criteria and (P0)*

Rich literature can be found on the criteria regarding subset selection. Miller[36] and George and Foster[22] provided an excellent overview. An interesting fact is that a majority of these criteria can be unified under **(P0)**, where $\|y - \Phi x\|_2^2$ is the residual sum of squares (denoted by RSS(x)) under the coefficient vector x, and constant λ_0 depends on the criteria. The following summarizes some well-known results:

- Paper [1] defines its criterion by maximizing the expected log-likelihood $E_{X,\hat{\theta}}(\log f(X|\hat{\theta}))$, where $\hat{\theta}$ is the estimation of parameter θ, $f(X|\theta)$ is the density function. This is equivalent with maximizing the expected Kullback-Leibler's mean information for the discrimination between $f(X|\hat{\theta})$ and $f(X|\theta)$, i.e.: $E_{X,\hat{\theta}}(\log \frac{f(X|\hat{\theta})}{f(X|\theta)})$, for a known true θ. Under a Gaussian assumption in the linear regression, the above leads to the Akaike information criterion (AIC) that minimizes

$$\text{AIC} = \frac{\text{RSS}(x)}{\sigma^2} + 2 \cdot \|x\|_0,$$

  where σ^2 is the noise variance, and other notations have been defined at the beginning of this section. It is a special case of **(P0)** by assigning $\lambda_0 = 2\sigma^2$.

- Mallows' C_p (see [35, 24]), which is derived from the unbiased risk estimation, minimizes

$$C_p = \frac{1}{\hat{\sigma}^2} RSS(x) + 2 \cdot \|x\|_0 - n,$$

  where $\hat{\sigma}$ is an estimate of parameter σ. When $\hat{\sigma}^2 = \sigma^2$ is assumed, Mallows' C_p is equivalent to AIC. Again, C_p is a special case of **(P0)**.

- Motivated by the asymptotic behavior of Bayes estimators, Bayesian information criterion (BIC)[43] chooses to select the model that maximizes

$$\log f(X|\hat{\theta}) - \frac{1}{2} \cdot \log n \cdot \|x\|_0.$$

  Here, under the squared error loss and the Gaussian model assumption with known variance σ^2, BIC is to minimize

$$\text{BIC} = \frac{RSS(x)}{\sigma^2} + \log n \cdot \|x\|_0.$$

  The above is again a special case of **(P0)** by assigning $\lambda_0 = \sigma^2 \log n$.

- The equivalence between BIC and the minimum description length (MDL) is well known, see Hastie, et al.[27] . Hence, MDL is a special case of **(P0)** as well.

- Risk inflation criterion (RIC) is suggested in George and Foster[19] from a minimax estimation vantage point. RIC recommends the model that minimizes

$$\text{RIC} = \frac{RSS(x)}{\sigma^2} + 2\log p \cdot \|x\|_0,$$

  where p is the number of available predictors. This is derived from selecting the model with minimum risk inflation. Readers can see that RIC is another special case of **(P0)**, by taking $\lambda_0 = 2\sigma^2 \log p$.

Although **(P0)** is a fine compendium of many subset selection criteria, solving **(P0)** generally requires exhaustive search of all the possible subsets. When $\|x\|_0$ (i.e., the number of the selected covariates) increases, the methods based on exhaustive search become rapidly impractical. In fact, solving **(P0)** in general is an NP-hard problem. The following theorem can be considered as an extension of a result that was originally presented by Natarajan[37].

Theorem 1: Solving the problem **(P0)** with a fixed λ_0 is an NP-hard problem.

Using the idea of Lagrange multiplier, we can see that solving **(P0)** with λ_0 is equivalent to solving the **sparse approximate solution** (SAS) problem in Natarajan[37] with ε, which is proven in Natarajan[37] to be NP-hard. Hence, in general, solving **(P0)** is NP-hard.

3.2. *Greedy Algorithms and (P1)*

Due to the hardness of solving **(P0)**, a *relaxation* idea has been proposed. The relaxation replaces the ℓ_0 norm with the ℓ_1 norm in the objective, which leads to **(P1)**. The idea of relaxation started in *sparse signal representation*[6]. Theoretical properties are derived later in [11, 10]. A partial list of new representative results includes Tropp[49,48], Gribonval and Nielsen[25], and Chen and Huo[4,5]. Being compared with the problem in this chapter, the problem of sparse signal representation has a different objective. In sparse signal representations, researchers consider a redundant *dictionary*[33,23] and the conditions under which the sparsest representation can be solved via a linear programming. Their formulations of **(P0)** and **(P1)** are slightly different from ours. However, a group of results in this chapter are certainly motivated by some recent results in **sparse representation**. More connections are discussed in Huo and Ni[28].

At the same time, **(P1)** has been proposed in statistics as a way of subset selection. The method is named Lasso[47]. An interesting recent development — the least angle regressions (LARS)[14] — demonstrates that certain greedy algorithms can reveal the solutions to **(P1)** with varying values of λ_1, based on the idea of *homotopy*[39]. More recent analysis demonstrates further that greedy algorithms can literally render the entire solution path in a large class of problems, referring to Hastie, et al.[26] and the references therein. A recent conference presentation[32] gives the most succinct solution in generating solution paths, utilizing a homotopy continuation method[40] and an analysis of *subdifferential*. A standard reference for the background of this material is Rockafellar[42].

4. Case Study

To illustrate further the necessity and feasibility of deriving equivalence conditions between **(P0)** and **(P1)**, we describe two extreme examples. In the first example, solutions of **(P1)** and **(P0)** completely disagree. In the second example, **(P1)** and **(P0)** share the same subset.

4.1. *An Extreme Example for the Least Angle Regressions*

Least Angle Regression[14] is a forward variable selection method. An extensive manual regarding forward selection can be found in Atkinson, et al.[2]. As been indicated previously, LARS can give the solution path of **(P1)**. However, this homotopy does not guarantee that LARS always reveal the optimal solutions of **(P0)**; i.e., **(P0)** and **(P1)** could disagree. In this subsection, we present one particular case, in which LARS choose wrongly in the first iteration and end up correcting it inefficiently. As a result, LARS do not include the correct covariates until the last step. Initially, such an example motivated us to consider the conditions of equivalence.

Details of LARS algorithm can be found in Efron, et al.[14] . In a nutshell, LARS start with zero coefficients, select the most correlated covariates with the signal (i.e., the response) s, then move along the direction that is equiangular among the selected covariates until some other covariates have as much correlation with the current residual, add these new covariates under consideration and move along the new equiangular direction. When the covariates and the response are standardized to have mean 0 and unit norm, correlation between vectors is proportional to the inner product. In the following, for clarity, we first give an example with nonstandardized vectors, and choose the covariates according to the inner products. The corresponding example with standardized covariates and signal is presented later in Section 4.1.1. Section 4.1.2 shows how to use the result to come up with a dramatic example for presentation.

The first example is generated as follows. Let $\phi_i \in \mathbb{R}^n, i = 1, 2, ..., m$, denote the ith column of the model matrix Φ. Hence, $\Phi = [\phi_1, \phi_2, ..., \phi_m]$. Let $\delta_i \in \mathbb{R}^n, i = 1, 2, ..., m$, denote the dirac vector taking 1 at the ith position and 0 elsewhere. For $i = m - A + 1, m - A + 2, ..., m$, let $\phi_i = \delta_i$, where A is a positive integer. Consider a special signal $s = \frac{1}{\sqrt{A}} \sum_{i=m-A+1}^{m} \phi_i$. Obviously, in this case, the optimal subset is $\{m - A + 1, ..., m\}$. For the first $m - A$ columns of Φ, make $\phi_j = a_j \cdot s + b_j \cdot \delta_j$, where $1 \le j \le m - A$ and $a_j^2 + b_j^2 = 1$. Note ϕ_i's and s are all unit-norm vectors. From now on, for simplicity, we always assume $1 \le j \le m - A$ and $m - A + 1 \le i \le m$. It is easy to verify that

$$\langle s, \phi_j \rangle = a_j \qquad \text{and} \qquad \langle s, \phi_i \rangle = 1/\sqrt{A}.$$

In this example, we choose $1 > a_1 > a_2 > \cdots > a_{m-A} > 1/\sqrt{A} > 0$.

Now we consider the procedure of LARS. In the first step, since ϕ_1 has the largest inner product with s, evidently column ϕ_1 will be chosen. The residual will be $r_1 = s - c_1\phi_1$, where c_1 is the coefficient to be determined. The following result about the consequent step in LARS is proved in the Appendix of [28].

Lemma 2: *In the consequent step of LARS, covariate ϕ_2 is chosen, with* $c_1 = \frac{a_1 - a_2}{1 - a_1 a_2}$.

Hence, the residual of the first step becomes

$$
\begin{aligned}
r_1 &= s - c_1\phi_1 \\
&= s - \frac{a_1 - a_2}{1 - a_1 a_2}(a_1 s + b_1 \delta_1) \\
&= \frac{b_1^2}{1 - a_1 a_2} s - \frac{(a_1 - a_2)b_1}{1 - a_1 a_2}\delta_1 \\
&= \frac{b_1^2}{1 - a_1 a_2}[s - \frac{a_1 - a_2}{b_1}\delta_1].
\end{aligned}
$$

Note that in LARS, only the direction of a residual vector determines the selection of the next covariate(s). The amplitude of a residual vector does not change the variable selection. Hence, we introduce a surrogate residual with a simpler form:

$$\widetilde{r}_1 = s - \frac{a_1 - a_2}{b_1}\delta_1.$$

Residuals $\tilde{r}_1$ and r_1 have the same direction. This is an important step to simplify our analysis.

As a sanity check, the following calculations are performed:

(1) For i, $\langle \phi_i, \tilde{r}_1 \rangle = 1/\sqrt{A}$.

(2) For j,

$$\langle \phi_j, \tilde{r}_1 \rangle = \langle a_j s + b_j \delta_j, s - \frac{a_1 - a_2}{b_1} \delta_1 \rangle$$

$$= a_j - \frac{b_j(a_1 - a_2)}{b_1} \langle \delta_j, \delta_1 \rangle.$$

As special cases: $\langle \phi_1, \tilde{r}_1 \rangle = a_2$, $\langle \phi_2, \tilde{r}_1 \rangle = a_2$, and for $j \geq 3$, $\langle \phi_j, \tilde{r}_1 \rangle = a_j$.

The above analysis demonstrates some basic techniques that will be used in the consequent LARS steps. Now we can use induction to show the following.

Theorem 3: In the example described in the beginning of this section, LARS choose covariates $\phi_1, \phi_2, ..., \phi_{m-A}$ one by one sequentially in the first $m - A$ steps.

It takes some energy to verify the above theorem. We skip it. Readers can find the proof in Huo and Ni[28]. This example shows that LARS can choose all the covariates outside an intuitively optimal subset before it reaches any covariate inside the optimal subset.

4.1.1. *Standardized Covariates*

Readers may notice that LARS should proceed along the direction that depends on the correlations between ϕ_i's and the residual. Meanwhile, in our previous case study, the proceeding direction is determined due to the inner product. The inner product is not proportional to the correlation since the response s and the covariate vectors ϕ_i's are not standardized to have mean 0. However, this discrepancy can be easily remedied as follows. The key observation is that LARS only depend on geometric information. More specifically, the result depends only on $\langle \phi_i, s \rangle$, $i = 1, 2, ..., m$, and $\langle \phi_i, \phi_j \rangle$, $1 \leq i, j \leq m$. For example, an orthogonal transform of both s and ϕ_i's will retain the results in LARS. We state this without a proof.

Lemma 4: *After a simultaneously orthogonal transform on both response and covariates, the results of LARS from the transformed data is the same orthogonal transform of the LARS results from the original data.*

Hence, if we can find another set of standardized vectors, which retain the inner products and are the orthogonal transforms of ϕ_i's and s in the previous example, the same results can be predicted for LARS.

The standardization can be incorporated according to the following. The main idea is that an n-dimensional linear space can be treated as a subspace of $\mathbb{R}^{n+1}$, which is orthogonal to vector $(1, 1, ..., 1)$. Let $\{b_0, b_1, ..., b_n\}$ denote an orthonormal basis of $\mathbb{R}^{n+1}$, with $b_0 = \frac{1}{\sqrt{n+1}}(1, 1, ..., 1)^T$. Denote the unit-norm vectors $s = (s_1, s_2, ..., s_n)^T$ and $\phi_i = (\phi_{i1}, \phi_{i2}, ..., \phi_{in})^T$, $i = 1, 2, ..., m$. Define $s' = \sum_{j=1}^n s_j b_j$, $\phi_i' = \sum_{j=1}^n \phi_{ij} b_j$, $i = 1, 2, ..., m$. One can easily verify that $\langle s', \phi_i' \rangle = \langle s, \phi_i \rangle$ for $1 \leq i \leq m$, and $\langle \phi_i', \phi_j' \rangle = \langle \phi_i, \phi_j \rangle$ for $1 \leq i, j \leq m$. Hence, applying LARS to s' and ϕ_i''s will produce the same result as in the first case study. It is not hard to verify that s' and ϕ_i''s are standardized. Therefore, the conclusions in our case study can be extended to the case with standardized response and covariates.

Theorem 5: There exists an orthogonal transform that can be applied to the previous example to create a case in which all the covariates and the response are standardized, and LARS select all the covariates outside the optimal subset before it chooses any covariate inside the optimal subset.

4.1.2. *To Create a Dramatic Presentation*

The foregoing example is developed in a fairly general form, without specifying the controlling parameters: A and m. To see how dramatic an example can be, let us consider the case where $A = 10$ and $m = 1,000,000$. Based on the previous analysis, LARS will select the first $999,990$ covariates before it selects any of the last ten covariates. At the same time, the optimal subset is formed by the last ten covariates.

4.2. *Variable Selection with Orthogonal Model Matrix*

In order to gain more insights, a case in which Φ is orthogonal is considered. This example has been studied in the original LARS paper[14]. The purpose of restating it here is to illustrate that there is a case in which LARS find the type-I optimal subset. I.e., **(P0)** and **(P1)** coincide.

Theorem 6: Let $\tilde{x}_0$ and $\tilde{x}_1$ denote the solutions to **(P0)** and **(P1)**, respectively. When Φ is orthogonal, we have

$$\tilde{x}_{0,i} = \begin{cases} 0, & \text{if } |z_i| \leq \sqrt{\lambda_0}, \\ z_i, & \text{if } |z_i| > \sqrt{\lambda_0}, \end{cases}$$

and

$$\widetilde{x}_{1,i} = \begin{cases} 0, & \text{if } |z_i| \le \lambda_1/2, \\ \text{sign}(z_i)(|z_i| - \frac{\lambda_1}{2}), & \text{if } |z_i| > \lambda_1/2. \end{cases}$$

Here, $\widetilde{x}_{0,i}$ and $\widetilde{x}_{1,i}$ denote the ith entry of $\widetilde{x}_0$ and $\widetilde{x}_1$, respectively, and z_i is the ith entry of $z = \Phi^T y$.

For readers who are familiar with soft-thresholding and hard-thresholding[12], the above is not a surprise. Proof is omitted.

From the above, verifying the following becomes an easy task. Let $\text{supp}(x)$ denote the set of indices of the nonzero entries in vector x.

Corollary 7: *When $\sqrt{\lambda_0} = \lambda_1/2$, one has $supp(\widetilde{x}_0) = supp(\widetilde{x}_1)$, i.e., there is a concurrent optimal subset. Moreover,*

$$\widetilde{x}_{0,i} - \widetilde{x}_{1,i} = \begin{cases} 0, & \text{if } i \notin supp(\widetilde{x}_0), \\ \frac{\lambda_1}{2} \cdot sign(z_i), & \text{if } i \in supp(\widetilde{x}_0). \end{cases}$$

The proof is obvious and is omitted.

Now there are two opposing examples. On one hand, if Φ is orthogonal, both LARS and Lasso discover the optimal subset in **(P0)**. On the other hand, we found an example in which a version of LARS would choose all the covariates outside the optimal subset before choosing anything inside. These inconsistencies encourage us to analyze the solutions of **(P0)** and **(P1)**, and the conditions for a subset to be the concurrent optimal subset. This is the place where more results are anticipated. Readers may see details in more technical papers thereafter.

5. Other Topics

We must admit that this article presents a somewhat unique aspect of the model selection problem. In the following, we discuss other works and possibly their relation with the theme of this article.

5.1. *Computing Versus Statistical Properties*

As mentioned earlier, the question that we addressed in this paper is quite different from many other statistical works. In the present paper, we identify easy-to-verify (polynomial time) conditions for the type-I optimal subset. Our direct motivation is that certain greedy algorithm can find a path of type-II optimal subsets. If one of these type-II optimal subset is confirmed to be type-I optimal, then a concurrent optimal subset is obtained. In the above sense, our question is more statistical computing than prediction.

In traditional approaches of subset selection, researchers try to answer the questions regarding the consistency of variable selection, as well as the optimal accuracy rate in submodel prediction. There is a large scope of existing efforts. It is impossible and unnecessary for us to give a comprehensive survey here. We will just list some publications that have been informative and inspiring to us. Papers[14,50,13,45,54], and the references therein give some interesting results in model estimation, integrating the prediction accuracy. Consistency of variable selection has been studied in Zheng and Loh[53].

Nowadays, due to the rapid rising of data sizes, it becomes increasingly important to develop statistical principles that can be realized in computationally efficient ways. Our idea of finding efficient sufficient conditions for otherwise unsolvable (i.e., NP-hard) subset selection principle is an incarnation of this ideology.

5.2. *Other Works in Variable Selection*

Despite their generality, the formulations of **(P0)** and **(P1)** do not cover all the existing works in statistical model selection. We review some recent works that have attracted our attention.

Fan and Li[15] propose a family of new variable selection methods based on a nonconcave penalized likelihood approach. The criterion is to minimize

$$\text{Fan\&Li} = RSS(x) + 2n \cdot \sum_{j=1}^{\|x\|_0} p_\lambda(|\theta_j|),$$

where $p_\lambda(\cdot)$ is a penalty function which is symmetric, nonconcave on $(0, \infty)$ and has singularities at origin. With proper choice of λ, Fan and Li show that the estimators would have good statistical properties, such as sparsity and asymptotic normality. The oracle property that they established is very interesting.

Shen and Ye[46] suggest an adaptive model selection procedure to estimate the algorithmic parameter λ from the data. In detail, the optimal value of λ is obtained by minimizing

$$\text{Shen\&Ye} = RSS(x) + \hat{g}_0(\lambda_0) \cdot \sigma^2,$$

which is derived from the optimal estimator of the loss $l(\theta, \hat{\theta})$. Quantity $\hat{g}_0(\lambda_0)$ is the estimator of $g_0(\lambda_0)$, which is independent of the unknown parameter θ. Value $g_0(\lambda_0)/2$ is called the generalized degrees of freedom in Ye[52].

The above two are merely the representative examples of many interesting approaches.

5.3. *Back Elimination*

Subset selections include at least three basic approaches: forward selection, backward elimination, and all subset selection. Problem **(P0)** is an all subset selection method. The greedy algorithms that have been discussed in this chapter are assumed to be forward selection algorithms.

In Couvreur and Bresler[8], a very interesting result is proved for the backward elimination. It is shown that under certain conditions, back elimination finds the solution of **(P0)**. Such a result reveals the properties of problem **(P0)** from another angle.

5.4. *Other Greedy Algorithms and Absolutely Optimal Subset in Variable Selection*

We have treated LARS as a stepwise algorithm. Other greedy algorithms have made significant impact in other fields (e.g., signal processing). Two representative ones are matching pursuit (MP)[9,34] and its improved version – orthogonal matching pursuit (OMP)[41]. MP and OMP do not generate the regularized solution path, while a version of LARS does. However, the intensive research effort following MP and OMP will provide researchers powerful tools.

Researchers have studied on the subsets that are unconditionally concurrent optimal, i.e., its concurrent optimality depends on neither the coefficients nor the corresponding residuals. The representative works include [10, 49], and [48]. The concept of exact recovery coefficient (ERC)[48] has inspired many recent works.

Note that in our sufficient conditions, both coefficient and residuals are taken into account. This is due to the different emphasis of the problems. Compared with our works, the results mentioned in the last paragraph can be considered as an analysis of the worst cases.

5.5. *Model Selection versus Variable Selection*

We may think that *model selection* and *variable selection* are interchangeable. It is pointed out in [30] that there are differences between the two problems. Model selection is to choose a statistical model that is based on a subset of variables, such that the chosen model has optimal predictive power; while variable selection is to determine the subset of variables that have predictive effect. Conceptually, the model selection may take a subset of the variables from the variable selection to create a model.

It is interesting to read the model-free variable selection approach in Li, et al.[30]. They adopt the framework that is the same as the one for "central subspace." Their proposed procedure is like back elimination, where step-wise statistical hypothesis testings are used to guide the variable selection. We believe that more results along this line will come out in a near future. Some potential research problems include: what is the statistical properties of these methods?

5.6. *Beyond Model Selection*

The model selection considered here is just one stage of statistical inference. Other researchers have considered the statistical properties of the outcomes from these model selection methods. As an example, Shen et al.[44,45] consider the bias of model selection, and suggest methods to correct it. Efron[13] studied the relation between the outcomes and prediction power via their covariance structure. These works require mathematical formulations that are very different from the one that is considered here. We choose not to explore further in this direction.

5.7. *Beyond Ordinary Linear Regression*

In the contemporary statistics, ordinary linear regression is a classical however small fraction. Many other models have been created and studied in statistical practice. We notice some recent works on model selection in longitudinal data analysis[3,17] and survival analysis[16].

5.8. *Bayesian Approach*

Due to the difficulty in solving the model selection problem — as mentioned earlier, they are NP-hard in general — researchers have explored random sampling approaches. Some computational experiments are described in [21], and later on, more thorough Bayesian approaches are developed in [7, 20]. An interesting Monte Carlo strategy is introduced in [31] too.

Although interesting results are obtained in experiments, a major problem associating with this approach is the lack of theoretical justification.

For example, given an estimate from random sampling, can we determine how good this estimator is? Recent works have started to address the problems of this kind. This is another area where we anticipate to see many new results in a near future.

5.9. *Other Related Topics*

Variable selection is a critical problem in supersaturated design. A citation search of Wu[51] will provide most of existing literature. A numerically efficient condition on the optimality of subsets has the potential to identify a good design.

Acknowledgments

The first author would like to thank a start-up fund from the Department of Statistics, University of California at Riverside.

References

1. H. Akaike, Information theory and the maximum likelihood principle. In *International Symposium on Information Theory* (V. Petrov and F. Csáki, Eds.), Budapest, Akademiai Kiádo, 1973.
2. A. C. Atkinson, M. Riani, and A. Cerioli, *Exploring multivariate data with the forward search*, Springer-Verlag, New York, 2004.
3. R. Azari, L. Li, and C.-L. Tsai, Longitudinal data model selection, *Computational Statistics & Data Analysis*, **50** (2005), 3053-3066.
4. J. Chen and X. Huo, Theoretical results on sparse representations of Multiple Measurement Vectors, *IEEE Trans. Signal Processing*, **54** (2006), 4634-4643.
5. J. Chen and X. Huo, Sparse representations for multiple measurement vectors (MMV) in an over-complete dictionary, In *International Conference on Acoustic, Speech, and Signal Processing (ICASSP)*, 2005.
6. S. S. Chen, D. L. Donoho, and M. A. Saunders, Atomic decomposition by basis pursuit, *SIAM J. Sci. Comput.*, 20(1):33–61, 1998. Reprinted at SIAM Rev. 43 (2001), 129-159.
7. M. Clyde and E. I. George, Model uncertainty, *Statist. Sci.*, 19 (2004), 81-94.
8. C. Couvreur and Y. Bresler, On the optimality of the backward greedy algorithm for the subset selection problem, *SIAM J. Matrix Anal. Appl.*, 21 (2000), 797-808.
9. G. Davis, S. Mallat, and Z. Zhang, Adaptive time-frequency decompositions, *Optical Engrg.*, 33 (1994), 2183-2191.
10. D. L. Donoho, M. Elad, and V. Temlyakov, Stable recovery of sparse overcomplete representations in the presence of noise, *IEEE Trans. Information Theory*, 52 (2006), 6-18.
11. D. L. Donoho and X. Huo, Uncertainty principles and ideal atomic decomposition, *IEEE Transactions on Information Theory*, 47 (2001), 2845-2862.

12. D. L. Donoho and I. M. Johnstone, Adapting to unknown smoothness via wavelet shrinkage, *J. Amer. Statist. Assoc.*, 90 (1995), 1200-1224.
13. B. Efron, The estimation of prediction error: Covariance penalties and cross-validation, *Journal of the American Statistical Association*, 99 (2004), 619-632.
14. B. Efron, T. Hastie, I. Johnstone, and R. Tibshirani, Least angle regression, *Ann. Statist.*, 32 (2004), 407-499.
15. J. Fan and R. Li, Variable selection via nonconvave penalized likelihood and its oracle properties, *Journal of the American Statistical Association*, 96 (2001), 1348-1360.
16. J. Fan and R. Li, Variable selection for Cox's proportional hazards model and frailty model, *Ann. Statist.*, 30 (2002), 74-99.
17. J. Fan and R. Li, New estimation and model selection procedures for semiparametric modeling in longitudinal data analysis, *J. Amer. Statist. Assoc.*, 99 (2004), 710-723.
18. G. Furnival and R. Wilson, Regression by leaps and bounds, *Technometrics*, 16 (1974), 499-511.
19. E. I. George and D. P. Foster, The risk inflation criterion for multiple regression, *The Annals of Statistics*, 22 (1994), 1947-1975.
20. E. I. George and D. P. Foster, Calibration and empirical Bayes variable selection, *Biometrika*, 87 (2000), 731–747.
21. E. I. George and R. E. McCulloch, Approaches for Bayesian variable selection, *Statistica Sinica*, 7 (1997), 339-373.
22. E. L. George, The variable selection problem, *Journal of the American Statistical Association*, 95 (2000), 1304-1308.
23. A. C. Gilbert, M. Muthukrishnan, and M. J. Strauss, Approximation of functions over redundant dictionaries using coherence, In *The 14th Annual ACM-SIAM Symposium on Discrete Algorithms*, January 2003.
24. S. G. Gilmour, The interpretation of Mallows's C_p-statistic, *Statistician*, 45 (1996), 49-56.
25. R. Gribonval and M. Nielsen, Sparse representations in unions of bases, *IEEE Trans. Inform. Theory*, 49 (2003), 3320-3325.
26. T. Hastie, S. Rosset, R. Tibshirani, and J. Zhu, The entire regularization path for the support vector machine, *Journal of Machine Learning Research*, 5 (2004), 1391-1415, 2004. [*Also show in Neural Information Processing Systems (NIPS 2004).*]
27. T. Hastie, R. Tibshirani, and J. Friedman, *The elements of statistical learning: data mining, inference, and prediction*, Springer, New York, 2001.
28. X. Huo and X. S. Ni, When do stepwise algorithms meet subset selection criteria? *The Annals of Statistics*, 35 (2007), to appear.
29. J. B. Kadane and N. A. Lazar, Methods and criteria for model selection, *J. Amer. Statist. Assoc.*, 99 (2004), 279-290.
30. L. Li, R. D. Cook, and C. J. Nachtsheim, Model-free variable selection, *J. R. Stat. Soc. Ser. B Stat. Methodol.*, 67 (2005), 285-299.
31. F. Liang and W. H. Wong, Evolutionary Monte Carlo: applications to C_p model sampling and change point problem, *Statistica Sinica*, 10 (2000), 317-

342.

32. D. M. Malioutov, M. Cetin, and A. S. Willsky, Homotopy continuation for sparse signal representation, In *IEEE International Conference on Acoustics, Speech, and Signal Processing*, **5**, pp. 733-736, Philadelphia, PA, March 2005.

33. S. Mallat, *A wavelet tour of signal processing*, Academic Press, Inc., San Diego, CA, 1998.

34. S. Mallat and Z. Zhang, Matching pursuit in a time-frequency dictionary. *IEEE Trans. Signal Proc.*, 41 (1993), 3397-3415.

35. C. L. Mallows, Some comments on C_p, *Technometrics*, 15 (1973), 661-675.

36. A. J. Miller, *Subset selection in regression*, Chapman and Hall, New York, 1990.

37. B. K. Natarajan, Sparse approximate solutions to linear systems, *SIAM Journal on Computing*, 24 (1995), 227-234.

38. X. S. Ni and X. Huo, Regression by enhanced leaps-and-bounds methods via additional optimality tests (LBOT), Working paper, available in http://www.isye.gatech.edu/statistics/papers/, August 2005.

39. M. R. Osborne, B. Presnell, and B. Turlach, On the Lasso and its dual, *Journal of Computational and Graphical Statistics*, 9 (2000), 319–337.

40. M. R. Osborne, B. Presnell, and B. A. Turlach, A new approach to variable selection in least squares problems, *IMA J. Numer. Anal.*, 20 (2000), 389–403.

41. Y. C. Pati, R. Rezaiifar, and P. S. Krishnaprasad, Orthogonal matching pursuit: Recursive function approximation with applications to wavelet decomposition, In *Proc. 27th Asilomar Conference on Signals, Systems and Computers* (A. Singh, Editor), IEEE Comput. Soc. Press, Los Alamitos, CA, 1993.

42. R. T. Rockafellar, *Convex analysis*, Princeton University Press, Princeton, NJ, 1970.

43. G. Schwarz, Estimating the dimension of a model, *The Annals of Statistics*, 6 (1978), 461-464.

44. X. Shen and H.-C. Huang, Optimal model assessment, selection and combination, *Journal of the American Statistical Association*, 101 (2006), 554-568.

45. X. Shen, H.-C. Huang, and J. Ye, Inference after model selection, *Journal of the American Statistical Association*, 99 (2004), 751-762.

46. X. Shen and J. M. Ye, Adaptive model selection, *Journal of the American Statistical Association*, 97 (2002), 210-221.

47. R. Tibshirani, Regression shrinkage and selection via the Lasso, *J. Roy. Statist. Soc. Ser. B*, 58 (1996), 267-288.

48. J. A. Tropp, Just relax: Convex programming methods for subset selection and sparse approximation, *IEEE Trans. Inform. Theory*, 52 (2006), 1030-1051.

49. J. A. Tropp, Greed is good: Algorithmic results for sparse approximation, *IEEE Trans. Inform. Theory*, 50 (2004), 2231–2242.

50. S. Weisberg, Discussion of [14], *The Annals of Statistics*, 32 (2004), 490-494.

51. C. F. J. Wu, Construction of supersaturated designs through partially aliased interactions, *Biometrika*, 80 (1993), 661-669.

52. J. M. Ye, On measuring and correcting the effects of data mining and model selection, *Journal of the American Statistical Association*, 93 (1998), 120-131.
53. X. D. Zheng and W. Y. Loh, Consistent variable selection in linear models, *Journal of the American Statistical Association*, 90 (1995), 151-156.
54. H. Zou, T. Hastie, and R. Tibshirani, On the "degrees of freedom" of the Lasso. Submitted manuscript, Available at http://www-stat.stanford.edu/~hastie/Papers/, 2004.

CHAPTER 3

SOME STATE SPACE MODELS OF AIDS EPIDEMIOLOGY IN HOMOSEXUAL POPULATIONS

Wai Y. Tan

Department of Mathematical Sciences,
The University of Memphis, Memphis, TN 38152-6429, USA
E-mail: Waitan@memphis.edu

This article illustrates how to develop state space models for AIDS epidemic in homosexual populations. A generalized Bayesian procedure is proposed to estimate the unknown parameters and the state variables. As an application, the model and the method are applied to the AIDS incidence data of homosexual and bisexual men of Switzerland. The analysis of these data clearly indicates that the model and methods can solve many difficult problems which are not possible by other currently available models and approaches.

1. Introduction

As shown by Tan[9], the AIDS epidemics are very complicated biologically involving very complex stochastic processes. In these cases, it is very difficult to estimate the unknown parameters and to predict the state variables, especially in cases where not many data are available. To ease the problems of estimation and prediction and to extract more information from the system, in this article we propose a state space modelling approach by combining stochastic models with statistical models. Then one can readily apply the Gibbs sampling method and the Markov Chain and Monte Carlo approach (MCMC) to estimate the unknown parameters and to predict the state variables. By using these estimates, one can validate the model and extract more information from the system which are not possible by using stochastic model alone or statistical model alone. We will illustrate the model and the method by using some data of the AIDS epidemic in homosexual population of Switzerland.

2. The State Space Models and the Generalized Bayesian Approach

To illustrate, consider an infectious disease such as AIDS. Let $\mathbf{X(t)}$ be the vector of stochastic state variables for key responses of the disease. Then, $\mathbf{X(t)}$ is the stochastic model (stochastic process) for this disease. For this process one can derive stochastic equations for the state variables of the system by using basic biological mechanism of the disease; by using these stochastic equations, one may also derive the probability distributions for the state variables. If some observed data are available from this system, one may also derive some statistical models to relate the data to the system. Combining the stochastic model of the system with the statistical model, one has a state space model for the system. That is, the state space model of a system is a stochastic model consisting of two sub-models: The stochastic system model which is the stochastic model of the system and the observation model which is a statistical model relating some available data to the system. It extracts biological information from the system via its stochastic system model and integrates this information with those from the data through its observation model.

2.1. Some Advantages of the State Space Models

The state space model of the system is advantageous over the stochastic model of the system alone or the statistical model of the system alone in several aspects. The following are some specific advantages:

(1) The statistical model alone or the stochastic model alone very often are not identifiable and can not provide information regarding some of the parameters and variables. These problems usually do not exist in state space models (see [2, 9, 15, 17]).

(2) State space model provides an optimal procedure to updating the model by new data which may become available in the future. This is the smoothing step of the state space models (see [3, 6]).

(3) The state space model provides an optimal procedure via Gibbs sampling and the generalized Bayesian approach to estimate simultaneously the unknown parameters and the state variables of interest; see Tan[10], Tan and Ye [15], Tan, Zhang and Xiong[17]. It is optimal in the sense that the estimates are posterior mean values which minimize the Bayesian risk under squared loss function.

(4) The state space model provides an avenue to combine information from various sources (see [10]).

The `state space model` was originally proposed by Kalman and his associates in the early 1960's for engineering control and communication[7]. Since then it has been successfully used as a powerful tool in aero-space research, satellite research and military missile research. It has also been used by economists in econometrics research and time series research[5] for solving many difficult problems which appear to be extremely difficult from other approaches. It was first proposed by Tan and his associates for AIDS research and for cancer research (see [9, 10, 15, 13, 14, 16, 17, 18]). Apparently state space models can be extended to other diseases as well, including heart disease and tuberculosis[11].

2.2. *A General Bayesian Procedure for Estimating Unknown Parameters and State Variables via State Space Models*

Applying the state space models, Tan and his associates[9,10,11,15,16,17] have developed a general Bayesian procedure to estimate simultaneously the unknown parameters and the state variables. These procedures would combine information from three sources: (1) previous information and experiences about the parameters in terms of the prior distribution of the parameters, (2) biological information via the stochastic system equations of the stochastic system, and (3) information from observed data via the statistical model from the system.

The general Bayesian procedure is given and illustrated in detail in Tan[10], Chapter 9 and will be used to derive estimates of the unknown parameters and the state variables in state space models, see Section 4.3.

3. Stochastic Models of AIDS Epidemic in Homosexual and Bisexual Populations

In US and Western countries such as Europe and Australia, the CDC (Center of Disease Control and Prevention, Atlanta, Georgia, USA) had reported that most of the AIDS cases were observed in homosexual and bisexual men (about 60%) and IV drug users (about 30%); other avenues such as heterosexual transmission were not common in these countries.

To illustrate how to develop state space models for the AIDS epidemic, we will thus consider a large population of homosexual and bisexual men who are at risk for AIDS. In this population, under risk for AIDS, then one can identify three types of people in the population: S people (susceptible people), I people (infective people) and AIDS patients (A people).

S people are healthy people but can contract HIV to become I people through sexual contact and/or IV drug contact with I people or A people (AIDS patients) or through contact with HIV-contaminated blood. I people are people who have contracted HIV and can pass the HIV to S people through sexual contact or IV drug contact with S people. According to the 1993 AIDS case definition[4] by the Center of Disease Control (CDC) at Atlanta, GA, an I person will be classified as a clinical AIDS patient when this person develops AIDS symptoms and/or when his/her CD4$^+$ T-cell counts fall below $200/mm^3$. In this section we will illustrate how to develop a discrete time stochastic model for the HIV epidemic with variable infection duration in these populations. (With no loss of generality we will let month be the time unit unless otherwise stated.)

To start the AIDS epidemic, we assume that at time $t_0 = 0$, a few HIV were introduced into the population to start the HIV epidemic so that with probability one, $I(0,0) > 0$ and $I(u,0) = 0$ if $u > 0$.

Let $S(t)$ denote the number of S people at time t, $A(t)$ the number of new AIDS cases during the month $[t, t+1)$ and $I(u,t)$ the number of I people who have contracted HIV at time $t - u$ ($t \geq u$). (We refer u as the infection duration of I people and denote by $I(u)$ infective people with infection duration in $[u, u+1)$.) When time is discrete, we are then entertaining a multi-dimensional stochastic process $\{S(t), I(u,t), u = 0, 1, \ldots, t, A(t)\}$ with discrete time and discrete state space. This is basically a Markov process with discrete state space and with discrete time; however, the number of state variables increases as time increases. For this stochastic process, the traditional approaches from most texts are too complicated and can hardly lead to useful results. For deriving useful results, we will thus use an alternative approach through stochastic difference equations.

3.1. The Stochastic Difference Equations for the State Variables

To develop a stochastic model for the above stochastic process, let $p_S(t)$ be the probability that a S person will contract HIV to become an $I(0)$ person during $[t, t+1)$ and $\gamma(u,t)$ the probability that an $I(u)$ person will develop AIDS symptoms to become a clinical AIDS patient during $[t, t+1)$. Let $d_S(t)$ be the probability that a S person will die during $[t, t+1)$ and $d_I(u,t)$ the probability that an $I(u)$ person will die during $[t, t+1)$. Further, we make the following assumptions:

(1) We may assume that $p_S(t)$ and $\gamma(u,t)$ are deterministic functions[12].

As in the literature [2, 9], we further assume that $\{d_s(t) = d_s, \gamma(u,t) = \gamma(u), d_I(u,t) = d_I(u)\}$.

(2) As in the literature 2, 9], we assume that there are no reverse transition from I to S and from AIDS cases to I.

(3) Because of the awareness of AIDS, we assume that there are no immigration and recruitment of A people and that there are no sexual and IV contacts between S people and AIDS patients.

Let $R_S(t)$ denote the number of immigrants and recruitment of S people during $[t, t+1)$ and $R_I(u,t)$ the number of immigrants and recruitment of $I(u)$ people during $[t, t+1)$. For dealing with immigration and recruitment, in what follows we will assume that the $R_S(t)$ given $S(t)$ and the $R_I(u,t)$ given $I(u,t)$ are negative binomial random variables with parameters $\{S(t), \omega\}$ $(0 < \omega < 1)$ and $\{I(u,t), \omega\}$, respectively, unless otherwise stated. (We note that different distributions with the same mean numbers give similar estimates of the state variables and the HIV infection, the HIV incubation distributions and the death rates.) Then the conditional means and the conditional variances of these variables are given by $\mathrm{E}[R_S(t)|S(t)] = \Lambda_S(t) = S(t)\omega/(1-\omega)$, $\mathrm{E}[R_I(u,t)|I(u,t)] = \Lambda_I(u,t) = I(u,t)\omega/(1-\omega)$, $\mathrm{Var}[R_S(t)|S(t)] = \sigma^2(t) = S(t)\omega/(1-\omega)^2$ and $\mathrm{Var}R_I(u,t) = \sigma_I^2(u,t) = I(u,t)\omega/(1-\omega)^2$.

To derive stochastic equations for the state variables, denote by:

$I(0, t+1) = F_S(t) = $ Number of $S \longrightarrow I(0)$ during $[t, t+1)$,

$F_I(u,t) = $ Number of $I(u) \longrightarrow A$ during $[t, t+1)$,

$D_S(t) = $ Number of death of S people during $[t, t+1)$,

$D_I(u,t) = $ Number of death of $I(u)$ people during $[t, t+1)$.

Assume that $R_S(t)$ and $R_I(u,t)$ are independently distributed of each other and of the other random variables. Then, the conditional distribution of $[F_S(t), D_S(t)]$ given S(t) is multinomial with parameters $\{S(t), p_S(t), d_S\}$ (i.e. $F_S(t)|S(t) \sim ML\{S(t), p_S(t), d_S\}$) independently of the immigration and recruitment process. Similarly, $[F_I(u,t), D_I(u,t)]|I(u,t) \sim ML\{I(u,t), \gamma(u), d_I(u)\}$ independently of the other state variables and the immigration and recruitment processes. Then, under assumptions (1)-(3) given above, we have the following **stochastic equations** for the state variables:

$$S(t+1) = S(t) + R_S(t) - F_S(t) - D_S(t),$$
$$= \Lambda_S(t) + S(t)\{1 - [p_S(t) + d_S(t)]\} + \varepsilon_S(t+1), \quad (1)$$
$$I(0, t+1) = F_S(t) = S(t)p_S(t) + \varepsilon_I(0, t+1), \quad (2)$$
$$I(u+1, t+1) = I(u, t) + R_I(u, t) - F_I(u, t) - D_I(u, t)$$
$$= \Lambda_I(u, t) + I(u, t)\{1 - [\gamma(u) + d_I(u, t)]\}$$
$$+ \varepsilon_I(u+1, t+1), \quad u = 0, \dots, t, \quad (3)$$
$$A(t+1) = \sum_{u=0}^{t} F_I(u, t) = \sum_{u=0}^{t} I(u, t)\gamma(u) + \varepsilon_A(t+1), \quad (4)$$

where the random noises $\varepsilon(t+1) = [\varepsilon_S(t+1), \varepsilon_I(u, t+1), u = 0, 1, \dots, t + 1, \varepsilon_A(t+1)]^T$ are derived by subtracting the conditional means from the respective random variables in the above equations and are given by:

$$\varepsilon_S(t) = [R_S(t) - \Lambda_S(t)] - [F_S(t) - S(t)p_S(t)]$$
$$- [D_S(t) - S(t)d_S],$$
$$\varepsilon_I(0, t+1) = [F_S(t) - S(t)p_S(t)],$$
$$\varepsilon_I(u+1, t+1) = [R_I(u, t) - \Lambda_I(u, t)] - [F_I(u, t) - I(u, t)\gamma(u)]$$
$$- [D_I(u, t) - I(u, t)d_I(u)], u = 0, 1, \dots, t$$
$$\varepsilon_A(t+1) = \sum_{u=1}^{t} [F_I(u, t) - I(u, t)\gamma(u)].$$

In equations (1)-(4), given $\mathbf{X}(\mathbf{t})$ the random noises $\varepsilon(t)$ have expectation zero. It follows that the expected value of these random noises is $\mathbf{0}$. Using the basic formulae $\mathrm{Cov}(X, Y) = \mathrm{E}\{\mathrm{Cov}[(X, Y)|Z]\} + \mathrm{Cov}[\mathrm{E}(X|Z), \mathrm{E}(Y|Z)]$, it is also obvious that elements of $\varepsilon(t)$ are uncorrelated with elements of $\mathbf{X}(\mathbf{t})$ as well as with elements of $\varepsilon(\tau)$ for all $t \neq \tau$. Further, these random noises are linear combinations of negative binomial, binomial and multinomial random variables. Hence one may readily derive variances, covariances and higher moments and cumulants of these random noises.

3.2. The Probability Distributions of $\mathbf{X}(t) = \{S(t), I(r, t), r = 0, 1, \dots, t\}$

Let $\boldsymbol{X} = \{\mathbf{X}(1), \dots, \mathbf{X}(t_M)\}$, where t_M is the last time point and $\Theta = \{\Theta_1, \Theta_2, \Theta_3\}$, where $\Theta_1 = \{p_S(t), \gamma(t), t = 0, 1, \dots, t_M\}$, $\Theta_2 = \{d_S, d_I(u), u = 0, \dots, t_M\}$ and $\Theta_3 = \omega$. Then $\boldsymbol{X}$ is the collection of all the state variables, Θ_1 the collection of all incidence of HIV infection and HIV incubation, Θ_2 the collection of all the death probabilities and Θ_3 the parameter for immigration and recruitment. Let $f_S(j;t)$ be the probability of $(R_S(t) = j)$ and $f_I(j;u,t)$ the probability of $(R_I(u,t) = j)$. Let $Pr\{\mathbf{X}(t+1)|\mathbf{X}(t),\Theta\}$ denote the conditional probability density function of $\mathbf{X}(t+1)$ given $\mathbf{X}(t)$. Using results in Section (2.1), the conditional probability distribution $Pr\{\boldsymbol{X}|\mathbf{X}(0)\}$ of $\boldsymbol{X}$ given $\mathbf{X}(0)$ is

$$Pr\{\boldsymbol{X}|\mathbf{X}(0)\} = \prod_{j=0}^{t_M-1} Pr\{\mathbf{X}(j+1)|\mathbf{X}(j),\Theta\} \tag{5}$$

and

$$Pr\{\mathbf{X}(t+1)|\mathbf{X}(t),\Theta\} = \{\sum_{i=0}^{S(t)} \binom{S(t)}{i} d_S{}^i (1-d_S)^{S(t)-i} \binom{S(t)-i}{I(0,t+1)}$$
$$\times \left[\frac{p_S(t)}{1-d_S}\right]^{I(0,t+1)} \left[1 - \frac{p_S(t)}{1-d_S}\right]^{S(t)-i-I(0,t+1)}$$
$$\times f_S[a_i(t),t] H(i;I(u,t),u=0,\ldots,t)\}, \tag{6}$$

where

$$H(i:I(u,t),u=0,\ldots,t) = \prod_{u=0}^{t} \{\sum_{j_1=0}^{I(u,t)} \sum_{j_2=0}^{I(u,t)-j_1} \binom{I(u,t)}{j_1,j_2} [\gamma(u)]^{j_1}$$
$$\times [d_I(u)]^{j_2} [1 - \gamma(u) - d_I(u)]^{I(u,t)-j_1-j_2}$$
$$\times f_I(b_j(u,t);u,t)\}, \tag{7}$$

where $a_i(t) = \text{Max}(0, S(t+1) - S(t) + I(0,t+1) + i)$, $b_j(u,t) = \text{Max}(0, I(u+1,t+1) - I(u,t) + j_1 + j_2)$.

4. A State Space Model of AIDS Epidemic in Homosexual Populations

Given AIDS incidence data of homosexual and bisexual men, in this section we develop a `state space model` for `AIDS epidemic` in this population. In the state space model, the state variables are $\mathbf{X}(t) = \{S(t), I(u,t), u = 0, 1, \ldots, t\}$ and the stochastic system model is given by the stochastic difference equations (1)-(4) and the probability distribution of these state variables in (3.2). The observation model is a statistical model based on AIDS incidence data which relate the observed AIDS incidence to $A(t)$.

4.1. The Stochastic System Model, the Augmented State Variables and Probability Distributions

The probability distribution of the state variables in equation (6) is quite complicated and not manageable. To implement the multi-level Gibbs sampling procedure to estimate unknown parameters and state variables, we thus expand the model by augmenting some un-observable dummy state variables $\mathbf{U}(t) = \{F_S(t), D_S(t), F_I(u,t), D_I(u,t), u = 0, 1, \ldots, t\}'$. By the distribution results in Section (3.1), it is easily seen that the conditional density of $\mathbf{U}(t)$ given $\mathbf{X}(t)$ is

$$P\{\mathbf{U}(t)|\mathbf{X}(t)\} = \binom{S(t)}{D_S(t), F_S(t)} d_S{}^{D_S(t)} p_S(t)^{F_S(t)} (1 - d_S$$

$$- p_S(t))^{S(t) - D_S(t) - F_S(t)} \prod_{u=0}^{t} \{ \binom{I(u,t)}{F_I(u,t), D_I(u,t)} \gamma(u)^{F_I(u,t)}$$

$$\times [d_I(u)]^{D_I(u,t)} (1 - \gamma(u) - d_I(u))^{I(u,t) - F_I(u,t) - D_I(u,t)} \}. \quad (8)$$

From the model and distribution results in Section (3.1), the conditional density of $\mathbf{X}(t+1)$ given $\{\mathbf{X}(t), \mathbf{U}(t)\}$ is

$$P\{\mathbf{X}(t+1)|\mathbf{X}(t), \mathbf{U}(t)\} = f_S(c_S(t), t) \prod_{u=0}^{t} f_I(c_I(u,t); u, t), \quad (9)$$

where $c_S(t) = \text{Max}(0, S(t+1) - S(t) + I(0, t+1) + F_S(t) + D_S(t))$ and $c_I(u,t) = \text{Max}(0, I(u+1, t+1) - I(u,t) + F_I(u,t) + D_I(u,t))$.

Put $U = \{\mathbf{U}(t), t = 0, 1, \ldots, t_M - 1\}$. Then, the joint density of $\{X, U\}$ is

$$P\{X, U|\Theta\} = P\{\mathbf{X}(0)\} \prod_{i=0}^{t_M - 1} P\{\mathbf{X}(i+1)|\mathbf{X}(i), \mathbf{U}(i)\} P\{\mathbf{U}(i)|\mathbf{X}(i)\}. \quad (10)$$

Notice that the equation in (10) is a product of densities of negative binomials, multinomials and binomial variables so that the above distribution is referred to as a chain negative binomial-multinomial distribution.

4.2. The Observation Model

Let $Y(j)$ be the observed number of new AIDS cases during the time period $[t_{j-1}, t_j)$ $j = 1, \ldots, n$. Then, the equation for the observation model of the state space model is given by the equation:

$$Y(j) = A_j + e(j) = \sum_{t=t_{j-1}}^{t_j-1} A(t) + e(j) = \sum_{t=t_{j-1}}^{t_j} \sum_{u=0}^{t} F_I(u,t) + e(j)$$

where $e(j)$ is the measurement error (reporting error for reporting AIDS incidence) for observing $Y(j)$ and $A_j = \sum_{t=t_{j-1}}^{t_j-1} A(t)$.

After correcting for reporting delay and under reporting for the AIDS incidence data, one may assume that the $e(j)$'s are independently distributed as normal random variables with mean zero and with variance σ_j^2 depending on A_j. Since AIDS may be assumed as an inflated Poisson process (variance is much greater than the mean), one may assume that $W_j = \{Y(j) - A_j\}/\sqrt{A_j}$ as normal with mean 0 and variance σ^2 so that $\sigma_j^2 = A_j\sigma^2$. It follows that the conditional density of $\boldsymbol{Y} = (Y(j), j = 1, \dots, n)$ given $\{\boldsymbol{X}, \boldsymbol{U}\}$ is $P\{\boldsymbol{Y}|\boldsymbol{X}, \boldsymbol{U}\} = \prod_{j=1}^{n} g\{Y(j)|\boldsymbol{X}, \boldsymbol{U}\}$, where

$$g\{Y(j)|\boldsymbol{X}, \boldsymbol{U}\} = g\{Y(j)|A_j\} = (2\pi A_j\sigma^2)^{-\frac{1}{2}}$$
$$\times \exp\{-\frac{1}{2A_j\sigma^2}[Y(j) - A_j]^2\}. \tag{11}$$

The the joint density of $\{\boldsymbol{X}, \boldsymbol{U}, \boldsymbol{Y}\}$ is

$$Pr\{\boldsymbol{X}, \boldsymbol{U}, \boldsymbol{Y}\} = = P\{\boldsymbol{X}(0)\} \prod_{j=1}^{n} g\{Y(j)|A_j\}$$
$$\times \prod_{t=t_{j-1}}^{t_j-1} P\{\boldsymbol{X}(t+1)|\boldsymbol{X}(t), \boldsymbol{U}(t)\} P\{\boldsymbol{U}(t)|\boldsymbol{X}(t)\}. \tag{12}$$

The above distribution will be used to derive the conditional posterior distribution of the unknown parameters $\Omega = \{\Theta, \sigma^2\}$ given $\{\boldsymbol{X}, \boldsymbol{U}, \boldsymbol{Y}\}$. Notice that because the number of parameters is very large, the classical sampling theory approach by using the likelihood function $P\{\boldsymbol{Y}|\boldsymbol{X}, \boldsymbol{U}\}$ is not possible without making assumptions about the parameters; however, this problem can easily be avoided by new information from the stochastic system model and the prior distribution of the parameters.

4.3. *The Posterior Distribution of the Unknown Parameters and State Variables*

Let $P\{\Omega\}$ be the prior distribution of $\Omega = \{\Theta, \sigma^2\}$. From equations (11)-(12), the conditional posterior distribution $P\{\Omega|\boldsymbol{X}, \boldsymbol{U}, \boldsymbol{Y}\}$ of Ω given

$\{X, U, Y\}$ is:

$$P\{\Omega | X, U, Y\} \propto P\{\Omega\} \{(\sigma^2)^{-\frac{n}{2}} exp\left(-\frac{(n-1)\hat{\sigma}^2}{2\sigma^2}\right) d_S^{\{\sum_{t=1}^{t_M} D_S(t)\}}$$

$$\times (1 - d_S)^{\{\sum_{t=1}^{t_M} [S(t) - D_S(t)]\}}$$

$$\times \omega^{\{\sum_{t=0}^{t_M} [R_S(t) + \sum_{u=0}^{t} R_I(u,t)]\}}$$

$$\times (1 - \omega)^{\{\sum_{t=0}^{t_M} [S(t) + \sum_{u=0}^{t} I(u,t)]\}}$$

$$\times \prod_{t=0}^{t_M - 1} [\frac{p_S(t)}{1 - d_S}]^{I(0,t+1)} [1 - \frac{p_S(t)}{1 - d_S}]^{S(t) - D_S(t) - I(0,t+1)}$$

$$\times \gamma(t)^{\sum_{r=t+1}^{t_M} F_I(t,r)} [d_I(t)]^{\sum_{r=t+1}^{t_M} D_I(t,r)}$$

$$\times (1 - \gamma(t) - d_I(t))^{\sum_{r=t+1}^{t_M} [I(t,r) - F_I(t,r) - D_I(t,r)]}\}, \qquad (13)$$

where $\hat{\sigma}^2 = \frac{1}{n-1} \sum_{j=1}^{n} \frac{1}{A_j} [Y(j) - A_j]^2$.

For the prior distribution of the unknown parameters, we will assume that **a priori** $\sigma^2, \Theta_i, i = 1, 2, 3$ are independently distributed of one another. Furthermore, we will follow Box and Tiao[1] to assume $P(\sigma^2) \propto (\sigma^2)^{-1}$ and assume natural conjugate priors for the other parameters. That is, we assume:

$$P\{\Theta_i, i = 1, 2, 3\} \propto d_S^{a_S - 1} (1 - d_S)^{b_S - 1} \omega^{a_0 - 1} (1 - \omega)^{b_0 - 1}$$

$$\times \prod_{t=0}^{t_M - 1} [\frac{p_S(t)}{1 - d_S}]^{u_S(t) - 1} [1 - \frac{p_S(t)}{1 - d_S}]^{v_S(t) - 1}$$

$$\times [\gamma(t)]^{a_G(t) - 1} [d_I(t)]^{b_G(t) - 1}$$

$$\times (1 - \gamma(t) - d_I(t))^{v_G(t) - 1}, \qquad (14)$$

where the hyperparameters $\{a_S, b_S, a_0, b_0, u_S(t), v_S(t), a_G(t), b_G(t), v_G(t)\}$ are positive real numbers. These hyperparameters can be estimated from previous studies. In the event that prior studies and information are not available, we will assume all these parameters to be 1 to reflect the fact that our prior information are vague and imprecise.

4.4. The Generalized Bayesian Method for Estimating Unknown Parameters and State Variables

Using the above distribution results, the multi-level Gibbs sampling procedures for estimating the unknown parameters (Θ, σ^2) and the state variables X are given by the following loop:

(1) Given the parameter values, we will use the stochastic equations (1)-(3) and the associated probability distributions to generate a large sample of $\{X, U\}$. Then, by combining this large sample with $P\{Y|X, U\}$, we select $\{X, U\}$ from this sample through the weighted Bootstrap method due to Smith and Gelfant[8]. This selected $\{X, U\}$ is then a sample generated from $P\{X, U|\Omega, Y\}$ although the latter density is unknown (for proof, see Tan[10], Chapter 3). Call the generated sample $\{X^{(*)}, U^{(*)}\}$.

(2) On substituting $\{U^{(*)}, X^{(*)}\}$ which are generated numbers from the above step, generate $\{\Theta, \sigma^2\}$ from the conditional density $P\{\Theta, \sigma^2|X^{(*)}.U^{(*)}, Y\}$ given by equation (13).

(3) With $\{\Theta, \sigma^2\}$ being generated from Step 2 above, go back to Step 1 and repeat the above (1)-(2) loop until convergence.

The convergence of the above algorithm has been proved in Tan[10], Chapter 3. At convergence, one then generates a random sample of $\{X, U\}$ from the conditional distribution $P\{X, U|Y\}$ of $\{X, U\}$ given Y, independent of Ω and a random sample of Ω from the posterior distribution $P\{\Omega|Y\}$ of Ω given Y, independent of $\{X, U\}$. Repeat these procedures one then generates a random sample of size N of $\{X, U\}$ and a random sample of size M of Ω. One may then use the sample means to derive the estimates of $\{X, U\}$ and Ω and use the sample variances as the variances of these estimates.

5. Some Illustrative Examples

To illustrate the usefulness of state space models of AIDS epidemic given in Section 4, in this section we apply the model and method to the Swiss AIDS data sets of homosexual men. To assess the AIDS epidemic in this population we will estimate simultaneously the death rates, the immigration rate, the HIV infection distribution, the HIV incubation distribution and the numbers of S people, I people and AIDS cases in these populations. Given in Table 1 are the AIDS incidence data from 1981 until 1995 for the homosexual population in Switzerland. (To avoid the problem of reporting delay, we have used the data only up to December 1995.)

Table 1. Some AIDS Incidence Data from the SWISS Population of
Homosexual and Bisexual Men

Year	J	F	M	A	M	J	J	A	S	O	N	D
80	.	.	.	.	.	.	.	.	.	.	1	.
81	.	.	.	.	.	.	.	.	.	1	.	1
82	.	.	.	.	.	.	.	.	.	.	.	.
83	.	.	.	2	.	.	1	1	2	.	1	.
84	2	2	1	2	2	.	4	.	.	3	4	1
85	6	.	5	4	4	2	13	1	6	6	4	3
86	4	6	5	5	9	6	27	4	6	9	4	15
87	13	4	4	12	7	11	15	9	7	14	15	14
88	17	18	15	14	18	15	30	18	16	5	6	19
89	18	18	15	14	20	14	18	15	21	20	23	15
90	15	21	22	13	20	20	37	21	12	20	17	9
91	17	16	22	18	14	15	23	27	14	21	15	14
92	15	22	20	18	27	22	35	22	26	16	27	23
93	24	24	15	20	17	25	44	16	11	10	13	22
94	22	17	19	24	17	24	23	21	15	15	24	21
95	17	14	15	18	14	23	13	11	13	15	26	13

5.1. The Initial Size

Since the average AIDS incubation period is around 10 years and since the
first AIDS case was reported in 1981, to derive the estimates from the state
space model we thus assume January 1, 1970 as $t_0 = 0$. Tan and Xiang[13,14]
have shown that the estimates were very insensitive to the choice of the
time origin t_0.) It is also assumed that at time 0 there are no AIDS cases
and no HIV infected people with infection duration $u > 0$ but to start the
HIV epidemic, some HIV were introduced into the population at time 0 so
that $I(0,0) > 0$.

To specify the initial numbers of S people and $I(0,0)$ people at time 0,
we proceed as follows: (1) We take $I(0,0)$ as $I(0,0) = 3$ for the homosexual
since this is the observed number of AIDS incidence in this population in
1981 and since the average incubation period is about 10 years. (2) We
assume $S(0)$ as $S(0) = 25,000$ for the Swiss homosexual population by
comparing the observed AIDS incidence with that of the San Francisco
homosexual population and by noting that the estimate of $S(0)$ in the
latter population is roughly 40,000 in January 1970. We have also tried

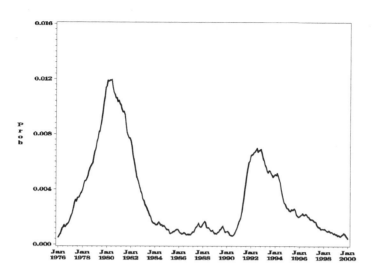

Figure 1. Plots of the estimates of the HIV infection denities in the SWISS populations

other initial size for $S(0)$ and did not notice significant differences of results between them.

5.2. *The Prior Distributions of $p_S(t)$ and $\gamma(u)$*

For the prior distributions, because we have very little information about the Swiss populations, we will assume uniform prior for Θ and will follow Box and Tiao[1] to assume $P(\sigma^2) \propto (\sigma^2)^{-1}$. For assessing effects of different prior distributions and because we believe that behaviors of homosexual populations in the western countries are quite similar, we will also assume natural conjugate priors with hyper-parameters being estimated using estimates from by Tan and Xiang[13,14] for HIV infection and incubation in the San Francisco homosexual population.

Given the above prior distributions and given $\{S(0), I(0,0) = I(0)\}$, by using procedures given in Section 3, we have derived simultaneously the estimates of the HIV infection distribution, the HIV incubation distribution, the death rates, the immigration rate as well as the number of AIDS cases over the time span in the Swiss homosexual and bisexual population. The estimates of the HIV infection, HIV incubation distributions and the numbers of the predicted AIDS cases are plotted in Figures 1-3. Given below we summarize our basic findings:

(a) The estimates of $(d_S, d_I(u) = d_I)$ are given by $(8.35 \times 10^{-7} \pm 4.49 \times 10^{-7}, 3 \times 10^{-4} \pm 1.62 \times 10^{-4})$ per month respectively. These results indicate that the death and retirement rate of I people is much greater (at least 100 times greater) than that of S people in the Swiss population of homosexual and bisexual men. This suggests that HIV infection may have increased the death rates of HIV infected people.

(b) The estimate of the proportion of immigration and recruitment rate are $2.48 \times 10^{-3} \pm 6.094 \times 10^{-4}$ per month for the population of homosexual and bisexual men. This estimates is about 10 times greater than that of the estimates of the death and retirement rates of the I people. These results indicate that the size of the Swiss population of homosexual and bisexual men is increasing with time.

(c) From Figure 1, the estimated density of the HIV infection distributions showed a mixture of distributions with two obvious peaks in the Swiss population of homosexual and bisexual men. The first peak occurs around May of 1980. The second peak occurs around August of 1992 and is considerably lower than that of the first peak. Comparing the estimated density of the HIV infection in Figure 1 with the estimated density from the San Francisco homosexual population by Tan and Xiang[14], one may notice that the two curves are quite similar to each other but the Swiss population appears about 6 months earlier for the first peak and about 2 years earlier for the second peak.

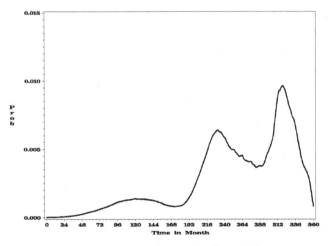

Figure 2. Plots of the estimates of the HIV incubation denities in the SWISS populations

(d) From Figure 2, the estimated density of the HIV incubation distribution also appeared to be a mixture of distributions with two obvious peaks. The higher peak occurs at around 320 months after infection and the lower peak occurs around 232 months after infection in the homosexual population. These results seem to suggest a staged model for HIV incubation as used by many statisticians (see 9, Chapter 4).

(e) From Figure 3, we observe that the estimates of the AIDS incidence by the Gibbs sampler are almost identical to the corresponding observed AIDS incidence, suggesting the usefulness of the method. These results indicate that the estimates by the Gibbs sampler can trace the observed values very closely if observed values are available.

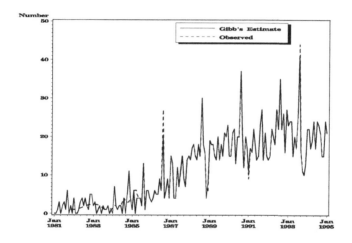

Figure 3. Plots showing the estimates of the number of AIDScases in the SWISS populations of homosexual and bisexual men

(f) From results not shown here, it appears that the prior distributions seem to have little effects on both the HIV infection distribution and the HIV incubation distribution.

(g) To start the procedure, one needs some initial parameter values for $p_S(t)$ and $\gamma(u)$. In this chapter, we first assumed a Weibull distribution for the initial incubation distribution with a mean of 10 years and derive estimates of the infection distribution by using the standard backcalculation method[2]. This assumed incubation distribution and the associated estimate of the infection distribution will then be used to give initial values for the parameters $p_S(t)$ and $\gamma(u)$. To check effects of the initial incubation distribution and to monitor convergence of the multi-level Gibbs sampling method, we have assumed many other different incubation distributions as the initial assumed distribution. These assumed distributions include uniform distribution, exponential distribution, Gamma distribution, Weibull distribution and the generalized Gamma distributions with the same mean value of 10 years. We are elated to find out that all initial distributions gave almost identical estimates.

6. Conclusions

In this article, we have developed a state space model for the AIDS epidemic in homosexual and bisexual populations. We have developed a generalized Bayesian method to estimate the unknown parameters and the state variables. The numerical examples indicate that the methods are useful and promising. Of course, more studies are needed to further confirm the usefulness of the method and to check the efficiency of the method.

References

1. G.E.P. Box and G.C. Tiao, *Bayesian Inferences in Statistical Analysis*, Addison-Wesley, Reading, MA, 1973.
2. R. Brookmeyer and M.H. Gail, *AIDS Epidemiology: A Quantitative Approach*, Oxford University Press, Oxford, England, 1994.
3. D.E. Catlin, *Estimation, Control and Discrete Kalman Filter*, Spring-Verlag, New York, 1989.
4. CDC, *Revised classification system for HIV infection and expanded surveillance case definition for AIDS among adolescents and adults, MMWR*, **41**, No RR17-1992, 1993.
5. J. Durbin and K.J. Koopman, *Time Series Analysis by State Space Models*, Oxford University Press, Oxford, England, 2005.
6. A. Gelb, *Applied Optimal Estimation*, MIT Press, Cambridge, MA, 1974.
7. R.E. Kalman, A new approach to linear filter and prediction problems, *J. Basic Eng.*, **82** (1960), 35-45.
8. A.F.M. Smith and A.E. Gelfand, Bayesian statistics without tears: A sampling-resampling perspective, *American Statistician*, **46** (1992), 84-88.
9. W.Y. Tan, *Stochastic Modeling of AIDS Epidemiology and HIV Pathogenesis*, World Scientific, Singapore and River Edge, New Jersey, 2000.
10. W.Y. Tan, *Stochastic Models With Applications to Genetics, Cancers, AIDS and Other Biomedical Systems*, World Scientific, Singapore and River Edge, New Jersey, 2002.
11. W.Y. Tan and W.M. Ke, State space models in survival analysis, In: *Handbook of Survival Analysis*, (C.R. Rao and N. Balakrishnan Eds.), Chapter 29, North Holland, Netherland, 2004.

12. W.Y. Tan, S.C. Tang, and S.R. Lee, Effects of Randomness of Risk Factors on the HIV Epidemic in Homosexual Populations, *SIAM Jour. Appl. Math.*, **55** (1995), 1697-1723.

13. W.Y. Tan and Z.H. Xiang, State space models of the HIV epidemic in homosexual populations and some applications, *Math. Biosciences*, **152** (1998), 29-61.

14. W.Y. Tan and Z.H. Xiang, Modeling the HIV epidemic with variable infection in homosexual populations by state space models, *J. Statist. Inference and Planning*, **78** (1999), 71-87.

15. W.Y. Tan and Z.Z. Ye, Estimation of HIV infection and HIV incubation via state space models, *Math. Biosciences*, **167** (2000), 31-50.

16. W.Y. Tan, P. Zhang, and C.W. Chen, Stochastic modeling of carcinogenesis: State space models and estimation of parameters, *Discrete and Continuous Dynamic Systems*, **B4** (2004), 297-322.

17. W.Y. Tan, P. Zhang, and X. Xiong, A State Space Model for HIV Pathogenesis Under Anti-Viral Drugs and Applications, In: *Deterministic and Stochastic Models of AIDS Epidemics and HIV Intervention*, (W.Y. Tan and H. Wu Eds.), World Scientific, Singapore and River Edge, New Jersey, 2005.

18. H. Wu and W.Y. Tan, Modeling the HIV epidemic: A state space approach, *Math. Computer Modelling* **32** (2000), 197-215.

CHAPTER 4

STOCHASTIC AND STATE SPACE MODELS OF CARCINOGENESIS: SOME NEW MODELING APPROACHES

W. Y. Tan[a] and L. J. Zhang

Department of Mathematical Sciences,
The University of Memphis, Memphis, TN 38152-6429, USA
E-mail: [a] waitan@memphis.edu

By surveying recent studies by molecular biologists and cancer geneticists, in this chapter we have proposed general stochastic models of carcinogenesis and provided biological evidences for these models. Because most of these models are quite complicated far beyond the scope of the MVK two-stage model, the traditional Markov theory approach becomes too complicated to obtain analytical results. To develop these stochastic models, in this chapter we thus propose an alternative approach through stochastic differential equations. Given observed cancer incidence data, we further combine these stochastic models with statistical models to develop state space models for carcinogenesis. By using these state space models, we then develop a generalized Bayesian procedure to estimate the unknown parameters and to predict state variables via multi-level Gibbs sampling procedures. In this chapter we have used the multi-event model as an example to illustrate our modeling approach and some basic theories.

Keywords: Generalized Bayesian procedures, Observation model, Multi-event model of carcinogenesis, Multi-level Gibbs sampling procedures, Multiple pathway model of carcinogenesis, State space model, Stochastic differential equations, Stochastic system model.

1. Introduction

It is now universally recognized that `carcinogenesis` is a multi-stage random process involving genetic changes, epigenetic changes and stochastic proliferation and differentiation of normal stem cells and genetically altered stem cells (see [41, 55] and **Remark 1**). Specifically, studies in molecular biology have confirmed that each cancer tumor develops through stochastic proliferation and differentiation from a single stem cell which has sustained a series of irreversible genetic changes. Furthermore, the number of stages and the number of pathways of the carcinogenesis process are significantly influenced by environmental factors underlying the individual[41,55]. Recently, it has been demonstrated that carcinogenesis is an evolution process in cell populations referred to as a micro-evolution process; and each cancer tumor is the outcome of growth of a most fitted genetically altered stem cell[8,28].

In this chapter we will summarize recent results from cancer biology and propose general stochastic models of carcinogenesis. For these models, mathematical results by the classical methods are very difficult even under some simplifying assumptions which may not be realistic in the real world; see **Remark 2**. It follows that except possibly for the simplest two stage model, analytical mathematical results remain to be developed and published. In order to derive analytical mathematical results and to relax some unrealistic assumptions, in this chapter we will provide new approaches through **stochastic differential equations** to analyze these models. For combining information from different sources and for easing problems of identifiability, we will combine these stochastic models with statistical models to develop state space models for carcinogenesis. By using these state space models, we will develop generalized Bayesian method and predictive inference procedures to estimate the unknown parameters and to predict the state variables.

In Section 2, we will summarize recent results from cancer biology. Based on these cancer biology, in Section 3, we will propose general stochastic models of carcinogenesis. To derive analytical results and to extend the models, in Section 4, we will propose an alternative approach to analyze these stochastic models through stochastic differential equations. For combining information from stochastic models and statistical models and for fitting the models to cancer data, in Section 5, we will proceed to develop **state space models** for the process of carcinogenesis. In Section 6, we will illustrate the application of the models and methods by analyzing the British data from physician's lung cancer and smoking. Finally in Section 6, we will discuss some possible applications of these models and methods.

Remark 1: The number of cells increases through somatic cell division by entering into cell division cycle and complete the cell division cycle giving rise to daughter cells. This has been referred to as cell proliferation. When a cell enters into cell division cycle, there is also a chance that this cell would differentiate to become a differentiated cell without completing the cell division cycle. This is referred to as cell differentiation. In terms of the stochastic birth-death process, proliferation is equivalent to birth and differentiation to death in general terms in the stochastic birth-death process. Notice that cell differentiation is not death but simply a process to remove cells from the cell population.

Remark 2: In the `multi-stage stochastic models`, as illustrated in many publications[36,38,39,55,58], to apply the classical method to derive analytical results, one need to make several assumptions. These assumptions include: (a) The last stage initiated cell (ie. I_k cells in the k-stage model) grow instantaneously into malignant tumors, (b) the mutation rates, birth rates, death rates are independent of time (i.e., time homogeneous), (c) all mutation rates before the (k-1)-stage in the k-stage model are equal[39]. (d) the number of normal stem cells is a deterministic function of time and hence grows deterministically with no random disturbances. Obviously, many of these assumptions do not hold in many practical situations[68]. For example, assumptions (b) and (c) may not hold in many cases and if assumption (a) is violated, the process involving cancer tumors is no longer Markov (see [58]). Hanin and Yakovlev[24] have also shown that even for the simplest 2-stage homogeneous model, using the classical approach the model is not identifiable in the sense that one can only estimate 3 parametric functions; in particular, one can not estimate the birth rate and death rate of the initiated cell, only the difference of birth rate and death rate.

2. Some Recent Cancer Biology for Modeling Carcinogenesis

Using tissue culture method, biologists have shown that all organs consist of two types of cells: The differentiated cells which are major components of the organ proper and the stem cells from which cancer tumors develop (see [1, 4]). Only stem cells can divide giving rise to new stem cells and new differentiated cells to replace old differentiated cells; the differentiated cells do not divide and are end cells to serve as components of the tissue and to perform specific functions of the tissue. That is, stem cells are subject to stochastic proliferation and differentiation with differentiated cells replacing old cells of the organ.

To understand cancer, notice that in normal individuals, there is a balance between proliferation and differentiation in stem cells and there are devices such as the DNA repair system and apoptosis in the body to protect against possible errors in the metabolism process. Thus, in normal individuals, the proliferation rate of stem cells equals to the differentiation rate of stem cells so that the size of organ is normally not changed. If some genetic changes have occurred in a stem cell to increase the proliferation rate of the cell; then the proliferation rate is greater than the differentiation rate in this genetically altered cell so that this type of genetically altered cells will accumulate; however, with high probability these genetically altered cells will be eliminated by apoptosis or other protection devices unless more genetic changes have occurred in these cells to abrogate apoptosis and to overcome other existing protection devices. Furthermore, it requires at least one round of cell proliferation for a genetic change to be fixed (see [15, 33]). Also, since genetic changes are rare events, further genetic changes will occur in at least one of the genetically altered cells only if the number of these cells is very large. These steps have clearly been demonstrated by cell culture experiments by Barrett and coworkers[42] using rat tracheal epithelial cells and on Syrian hamster embryo fibroblasts; for more detail and some more specific examples, see Chapter 1 in Tan[55].

These results as well as cancer biology studies[41] indicate that carcinogenesis in humans and animals is a multi-step random process and that these steps reflect genetic changes and/or epigenetic changes that drive the progressive transformation of normal stem cells into highly malignant ones. The age-dependent cancer incidence data for many human cancers imply four to seven rate-limiting stages from normal stem cells to malignant cancer tumors[48].

The above discussion and studies in cancer biology[41] illustrate that cancer is initiated by some genetic changes or epigenetic changes to increase cell proliferation while decreasing differentiation and death. Further genetic changes or epigenetic changes are required to overcome existing protection devises in the body resulting in abrogation of apoptosis, telomere protection (immortalization) and uncontrolled growth as well as angiogenesis and metastasis. Because somatic cell division occurs through cell division cycle whereas gene mutation and genetic changes occur only during cell division, most of the genetic changes affect carcinogenesis through the control of cell division cycle. By articulating these findings, Hanahan and Weinberg[23] have proposed six basic acquired capabilities which each normal stem cell must require to become a malignant cancer tumor. These six capabilities are: (1) Self-sufficiency of growth factor signals via genetic changes and/or epigenetic changes. This follows from the observation that cells can be induced to enter cell division cycle to start cell division only by growth factor signals[23]. (2) Insensitivity to anti-growth signals via silencing or inactivation of some tumor suppressor genes to abrogate cell differentiation. (3)

Evading apoptosis. (4) Unlimited replicative potential (immortalization). (5) Sustained angiogenesis, and (6) Tissue invasion and metastasis. The first 4 capabilities are required to establish uncontrollable growth of stem cells (avacular carcinogenesis) whereas the last two are for the development of cancer spread and metastasis of cancer cells (vascular carcinogenesis). Each of the above capabilities involves at least one or many genetic and/or epigenetic changes although in some cases some genetic changes may invoke more than one capabilities. To understand carcinogenesis, in what follows we further discuss some important items in carcinogenesis.

2.1. *The Multi-Staging and Sequential Nature of Carcinogenesis*

The discussion above and studies in cancer biology[41] also indicate that for a normal stem cell to develop into a malignant cancer tumor cell, it must accumulate many gene mutations or genetic changes. Because gene mutations and genetic changes are rare events and can occur only during cell division, it is a statistical near-impossibility that all mutation and genetic changes can occur simultaneously during a single cell division. It follows that different gene mutations or genetic changes must occur in different cell division at different times. This also leads to the observation that all steps in the carcinogenesis process must occur in sequence. Furthermore, while any genetic changes can take place at any time, only certain sequence or order of genetic changes can lead to a successful completion of the cascade of carcinogenesis to generate cancer tumors. For example, in FAP (Familial Adenomatous Polys) and in most sporadic human colon cancer, the first event leading to the cancer phenotype is the mutation or loss of the APC gene at 5q, followed by loss or inactivation or mutation of the Smad4 gene in chromosome 18q and p53 in chromosome 17p (see [29, 31, 35, 47, 53, 10, 18]). The mutation or activation of the oncogenes ras and src, and the mutation or inactivation of the suppressor p53 appear to be relatively late. In human lung cancer, as reported by Fong and Sekido[20], Osada and Takahashi[44], and Wistuba et al.[67], the loss of the suppressor genes (i.e. FHIT and VHL) in 3p through Loss of Heterozygosity (LOH) are the early event, followed by the loss of the gene $p16^{INK4}$ in 9p through LOH, the loss of p53 in 17p through LOH and the mutation of the oncogene ras.

2.2. *The Genetic Changes and Cancer Genes*

Carcinogenesis is initiated either by genetic changes (see [23, 27, 37, 41, 46, 52, 55, 66]) or by epigenetic change through activation of oncogene product or silencing effects of suppressor genes (see [2, 3, 7, 14, 17, 30, 32, 40, 43, 49, 64]). The genetic change may either be as small as point gene mutation, or as large as some chromosomal aberrations such as deletion of chromosomal segments, chromosome inversion and chromosomes translocation leading to mutation or deletion of some cancer genes, or activation of some dominant cancer genes, or inactivation of some recessive cancer genes. The cancer genes which contribute to the creation of cancer phenotype are the oncogenes (dominant cancer genes), the suppressor genes (recessive cancer genes) and the mis-match repair genes (MMR) which are involved in DNA synthesis and repair and/or chromosomal segregation. (As the suppressor genes, MMR genes are recessive genes.) The oncogenes, the suppressor genes and the MMR genes are the major genes for the creation of the cancer phenotype although some other modifying genes may also contribute to cancer through its interaction with proteins of oncogenes and/or suppressor genes or its interference with some cancer pathways. To date, about 200 oncogenes and about 50 suppressor genes have been identified.

Oncogenes are highly preserved dominant genes which regulate development and cell division. When these genes are activated or mutated, normal control of cell growth is unleashed, leading to the cascade of carcinogenesis. Specifically, some of the oncogenes such as the Ras oncogene induces $G_0 \to G_1$ by functioning as a signal propagator from signal receptor at the cell membrane to the transcription factors in the cell nucleus in the signal transduction process. Some of the oncogenes serve as transcription factors (e.g., myc, jun and fos, etn) to affect DNA synthesis during the S stage while some other oncogenes serve as anti-apoptosis (e.g. bcl-2) agents.

Suppressor genes are recessive genes whose inactivation or mutation lead to uncontrolled growth. Mutation or deletion of MMR genes (suppressor genes) lead to microsatellite repeats and create a mutator phenotype, predisposing the affected cells to genetic instability and to increase mutation rates of many relevant cancer genes. Many of the suppressor genes either function to control the gap stages (G_1 and G_2) or by abrogating the apoptosis process or function to control the activation of an oncogene such as myc. For example, the protein of the suppressor gene RB forms a complex with E2F and some poked proteins to block transition from $G_1 \to S$; when the RB gene protein is phosphorylated or the RB gene inactivated or mutated, $E2F$ is unleashed to push the cell cycle from the G_1 phase to the S phase. The protein products of the suppressor gene $p16^{INK4}$ at 9p21 inhibit the function of cyclin D1 and CDk4 proteins which phosphorylate the RB gene product to release E2F. The inactivation of many suppressor genes such as the p53 gene abrogates or suppresses the apoptosis process. In colon cancer, the mutation or deletion of both copies of the suppressor gene APC at 5q lead to increased expression level of the myc gene and D1 gene in the nucleus. Recent studies have shown that the APC gene may also affect the G_2 checking point dominantly by interfering with the microtube and hence centrosome causing aberrant chromosomal segregation and hence aneuploidy and polyploidy daughter cells[19,21]. (In this sense, the APC gene in chromosome 5q act both as a recessive gene and a dominant gene.)

2.3. *Epigenetic and Cancer*

Cancer initiation and progression are achieved and controlled by gene mutations and genetic changes. However, these genetic effects can also be achieved by changes of functions of these gene products through non-genetic avenues without affecting the nucleotide sequences in DNA molecules (see [2, 3, 7, 14, 17, 30, 32, 40, 43, 49, 64]). These are called epigenetic changes which mainly involve activation of oncogenes products or silencing of suppressor genes proteins through DNA methylation of cytosine at C_pG base pair islands (see [2, 3, 7, 14, 17, 30, 32, 40, 43, 49, 64]) or histone acetylation[43], or loss of imprinting (LOI)[49], or tissue disorganization and gap junction disruption[40,43]. For example, Ferreira et al[16] have showed that besides genetic inactivation or mutation of the RB gene, the process that the RB gene represses E2F-regulated genes in differentiated cells can also be achieved by an epigenetic mechanism linked to heterochromatin and involving histone H3 and promoter DNA methylation. In human colon cancer, Breivik and Gaudernack[7] showed that either methylating carcinogens or hypermethylation at C_pG islands would lead to G/T mismatch which in turn leads to Mis-match Repair (MMR) gene deficiency or epigenetic silencing of the MMR genes and hence MSI (Microsatellite Instability); alternatively, either hypo-methylation, or bulky-adduct forming (BAF) carcinogens such as alkylating agents, UV radiation and oxygen species promote chromosomal rearrangement via activation of mitotic check points (MCP), thus promoting CIS (Chromosomal Instability). These data clearly suggest that the epigenetic changes and/or interaction between genetic and epigenetic changes cancer phenotype are equally important as genetic changes in generating the cancer phenotype.

2.4. *Telomere, Immortalization and Cancer*

It is well-documented that normal stem cells have finite life span and can divide only a finite number of times whereas cancer tumor cells can proliferate indefinitely (i.e. immortalized)[5,25,50]. Biological studies have shown that this is related to telomeres which make up the ends of chromosomes to protect it from recombination and degradation activities. Telomeres are special chromatin structures and are composed of tandem repeats of TTAGGG sequences and single stranded overhang of the G-rich strand. When each normal stem cell divides, telomeres shorten by 50-200 bp, due to the fact that the lagging strand of DNA synthesis is unable to replicate the extreme $3'$ end of the chromosome. When telomeres are sufficiently shortened, cells enter an irreversible growth arrest called cellular senescence; when the length of the telomeres have shortened below some critical points resulting in loss of telomere protection of the chromosomes, then the cells will die or lead to chromosomal instability. In cancer cells, the telomerase helps to stabilize telomere length so that cancer cells become immortalized and can divide indefinitely.

Telomerase is a reverse transcriptase and is encoded by the TERT (Telomerase Reverse Transcriptase) gene. This gene recognizes the $3'$-OH group of the end of the G-strand overhang of telomere. It elongates telomeres by extending from this group using the RNA, which is encoded by the TERT, as a template. Blasco[5] has shown that besides being substrate for telomerase and the telomere repeat-binding factors, the telomeres are also bound and regulated by many chromatin regulators and related proteins, including TRF1, TRF2, TERT, TERC, DKC1, SUV39H1, SUV39H2, SUV20H1, HP1α, HP1β, HP1γ and the retinoblastoma family of proteins (RB1, RBL1, RBL2). This implies that the telomere length and function are also regulated by many chromatin and regulator proteins as given above. For example, if the retinoblastoma gene has been inactivated so that the RB1 function is lost, then trimethylation of H4-K20 is down, leading to abnormally long telomeres; as shown by Blasco[5], this telomere length elongation can also be achieved by epigenetic regulation of telomeric chromatin. Henson et al.[26] have shown that lengthening of telomere and hence immortalization can also be achieved by telomerase-independent mechanisms.

2.5. *Single Pathway Versus Multiple Pathways of Carcinogenesis*

In some type of cancers such as retinoblastoma, cancer tumor is derived by a single pathway[9,34,55]. In many other cancers, however, the same cancer may arise from different carcinogenic pathways. This include skin cancers, liver cancers and mammary gland in animals, the melanoma development in skin cancer in human beings, breast cancer, colon cancer, liver cancer and lung cancer in human beings.

To serve as an example, consider the colon cancer of human beings. For this cancer, genetic studies have indicated that there are two major avenues by means of which colon cancer is developed (see [29, 31, 35, 39, 47, 53, 10, 18, 22, 45, 65]): The Chromosomal Instability (CIN) and the Micro-Satellite Instability (MSI). The CIN pathway involves loss or mutation of the suppressor genes- the APC gene in chromosome 5q, the Smad4/DCC gene in chromosome 18q and the p53 gene in chromosome 17p. This pathway accounts for about 75-80% of all colon cancers and has been referred to as the LOH (Loss Of Heterozygosity) pathway because it is often characterized by aneuploidy /or loss of chromosome segments (chromosomal instability); it has also been referred to as the APC-$\beta - catenin - Tcf - myc$ pathway because it involves β- catenin, Tcf (T-cell factor) and the myc oncogene; see **Remark 3**. The MSI pathway involves microsatellite mis-match repair genes (MMR gene), hMLH1, hMSH2, hPMS1, hPMS2, hMSH6 and hMSH3. (Mostly hMLH1 and hMSH2.) This pathway accounts for about 10-15% of all colon cancers and appears mostly in the right colon. It has been referred to as the MSI (Micro-Satellite Instability) pathway or the mutator phenotype pathway because it is often characterized by the loss or mutations in the mis-match repair genes creating a mutator phenotype to significantly increase the mutations rate of many critical genes.

Remark 3: In the APC-$\beta - catenin - Tcf - myc$ pathway, the APC gene forms a complex with β-catenin and $GSK - 3\beta$ (Glycogen Synthase Kinases 3-β) to degrade the $\beta - catenin$ protein. When both copies of APC gene is lost or mutated, the β-catenin protein then accumulates to form a complex with Tcf to promote cell proliferation, usually via the elevated level of the myc gene and /or cyclin D1.

3. Some Stochastic Models of Carcinogenesis

Based on the above biological mechanisms of carcinogenesis, we now propose some general stochastic models of carcinogenesis.

3.1. *The Extended Multi-Event Model of Carcinogenesis*

The most general model for a single pathway is the extended k-stage $(k \geq 2)$ `multi-event model` proposed by Tan and co-workers[58,63]. This is an extension of the multi-event model first proposed by Chu[11] and studied by Tan[55] and Little[36]. It views carcinogenesis as the end point of k $(k \geq 2)$ discrete, heritable and irreversible events (mutations, genetic changes or epigenetic changes) with intermediate cells subjected to stochastic proliferation and differentiation. It takes into account cancer progression by following Yang and Chen[69] to postulate that cancer tumors develop from primary I_k cells by clonal expansion (i.e. stochastic birth-death process), where a primary I_k cell is an I_k cell which arise directly from an I_{k-1} cell.

Let N denote normal stem cells, T the cancer tumors and I_j the j–th stage initiated cells arising from the $(j - 1)$–th stage initiated cells $(j = 1, \ldots, k)$ by mutation or some genetic changes. Then the model assumes $N \rightarrow I_1 \rightarrow I_2 \rightarrow \cdots \rightarrow I_k$ with the N cells and the I_j cells subject to stochastic proliferation and differentiation. The cancer tumors develop from primary I_k cells by clonal expansion.

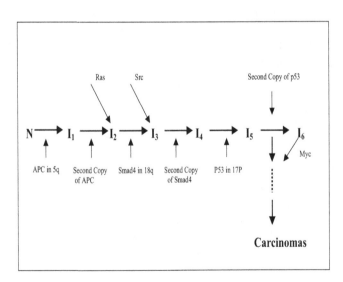

Fig. 1.   The APC-β-Catenin-TCF-Myc Pathway of Human Colon Cancer. Here, **N** = Normal stem cell, $\mathbf{I}_j$ = The jth-stage initiated cell in the LOH pathway, $\downarrow$ denotes mutation, inactivation or loss of suppressor genes (APC, Smad, p53), and $\searrow$ denotes mutation or activation of oncogenes (Ras, Src, Myc).

As an example, consider the $APC - \beta - Catenin - Tcf$ pathway for human colon cancer. This is a `multi-stage model` involving the suppressor genes in chromosomes 5q, 17p and 18q (see [29, 31, 35, 39, 47, 53, 10, 18]). A schematic presentation of this pathway is given in Figure 1. This is only one of the pathways for the colon cancer although it is the major pathway which accounts for 80% of all colon cancers (see [29, 31, 35, 39, 47, 53, 10, 18]). In Figure 2, we present another multistage model for human colon cancer involving mis-match repair genes (mostly hMLH1 and hMSH2) and the Bax gene in chromosome 19q and the $TGF\beta R_I I$ gene in chromosome 3p. This pathway accounts for about 15% of all human colon cancer.

The above example and studies in cancer biology[41] illustrate that carcinogenesis may involve a large number of cancer genes but only a few are stage limiting genes whereas other cancer genes may be dispensed with although these genes can enhance the cascade of carcinogenesis. As shown by Renan[48], it has been noted that while mutation of a single gene may initiate the cascade of carcinogenesis in some cases such as retinoblastoma, the process of carcinogenesis would usually involve 5 to 10 genes.

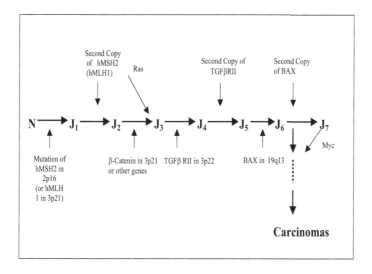

Fig. 2. The MSI-BAX-TGFβ RII Pathway of Human Colon Cancer. Here, **N** = Normal stem cell, $\mathbf{J}_i$ = The ith-stage initiated cell in the MSI pathway, $\downarrow$ denotes mutation, inactivation or loss of suppressor genes (hMSH2, hMLH1, BAX, TGFβ RII), $\searrow$ denotes mutation or activation of oncogenes (Ras, Myc).

3.2. *The Mixed Models of Carcinogenesis*

In the population, for the same type of cancer, different individual may involve different pathways or different number of stages (see [41, 54, 55, 56, 57, 59, 60, 61, 62]). These models have been referred by Tan[54,55] and Tan and Singh[62] as mixed models of carcinogenesis. These models are basic consequences of the observations: (1) Different individuals are subject to different environmental conditions, (2) the mutation of critical cancer genes can occur in either germline cells or in somatic cells, and (3) As shown in the previous section, the same cancer can be derived by several different pathways, referred to as multiple pathways.

To serve as an example, consider again the human colon cancer. The multiple pathways for human colon cancer as described in the previous section then leads to the following 5 different pathways: The sporadic LOH (about 70%, see Figure 1), the familial LOH (FLOH, about 10-15%), the FAP (Familial Adenomatous Polys, about 1%), the sporadic MSI (about 10-15%, see Figure 2) and the HNPCC (Hereditary Non-Polyposis Colon Cancer, about 4-5%). For sporadic pathways, the individuals at birth are normal individuals and do not carry any mutated or inactivated suppressor genes. For FAP, the individual has inherited a mutated APC gene in chromosome 5 at birth. For HNPCC, the individuals has inherited a mutated mis-match gene hMLH1 or hMSH2. For the familial colon cancer, the individuals have inherited a low penetrance mutated gene such as APCI1307K at birth. Hence, FAP and FLOH are special cases of the APC-$\beta - catenin - Tcf - myc$ pathway and HNPCC a special case of the MSI pathway.

The above indicates that from the population perspective, the human colon cancer can best be described by a mixture of five pathways. Let Y_j be the number of people who develop colon cancer during the $j-$th age group $[t_{j-1}, t_j)$. The above then indicates that the probability density of Y_j is:

$$P(Y_j) = \sum_{i=1}^{5} \omega_i(j) f_i(Y_j; \Theta_i),$$

where $f_i(Y_j; \theta_i)$ is the probability that the individual develops colon cancer during the $j-$th age group $[t_{j-1}, t_j)$ by the $i-$th pathway and where $\omega_i(j)$ is the proportion for the $i-$th pathway during the $j-$th age group; see **Remark 4**

Remark 4: Notice that $\omega_i(j)$ is a function of j (the age group). For the earlier age group, one may expect that most of the colon cancer cases are derived by the FAP and/or the HNPCC pathways while for the age groups after 50 years old, most of the colon cancer cases would derive from the LOH pathway. To reflect the real situation, we will thus assume that $\omega_i(j) = \omega_i P_i(j) / \{\sum_{u=1}^{5} \omega_u P_u(j)\}$, where $P_i(j)$ is the conditional probability that the individual will develop colon cancer during the j-th age group given that this person develops colon cancer by following the i-th pathway.

4. Some New Approaches for Analyzing Stochastic Models of Carcinogenesis

To develop mathematical theories for the **stochastic models** of carcinogenesis, the traditional approach in the literature[55] is by way of Markov theories. The basic approach along this line consists of the following four basic steps: (a) Deriving the probability generating function (PGF) of the number of cancer tumors, (b) deriving the incidence function of cancer tumors, (c) deriving the probability distribution of time to tumor onset, and (d) deriving the probabilities of the number of cancer tumors. This approach has been described and illustrated in detail in [55].

Using the above approach, theoretically one may derive some useful information for stochastic models of carcinogenesis. However, a careful scrutiny would reveal that the above approach suffers from several drawbacks: (1) The process may not be Markov so that the above approach is not applicable. For example, if one can not ignore cancer progression, then the number of cancer tumors is not Markov since it depends on the time when the last stage initiated cell is generated (see [54, 58, 60, 61, 63]) ; see also **Remark 2**. (2) As illustrated in [55], it is mathematically manageable only for a two stage model under very restrictive assumptions as described in **Remark 2**; further many of these assumptions have significant impacts on cancer incidence (see [54, 55, 58, 60, 61, 63, 68]). (3) It is extremely difficult, if not impossible, to fit and to adapt to cancer data, especially beyond the simplest MVK two stage model. (4) The cancer stages and many of the parameters are not identifiable when three or more stages are involved. In fact, as shown by Hanin and Yakovlev[24], even for the simple homogeneous two-stage MVK model, it is not possible to estimate $\{b_1, d_1, \lambda_0\}$ and α_1 separately; hence, not all parameters are estimable by using the above Markov approach unless some other data and some further external information about the parameters is available.

Because of the above difficulties, we have developed an alternative approach to developed stochastic models of carcinogenesis. As shown by Tan and Chen[58] through pgf (probability generation function) method, this alternative approach is equivalent to the above approach but is more powerful and can get more information. In this section we illustrate how to derive some basic results by using an extended k-stage multi-event model of carcinogenesis with ($k \geq 2$) carcinogenesis as an example.

4.1. Stochastic Differential Equations

For the extended k-stage multi-event model, it is assumed that the number $N_0(t) = I_0(t)$ of normal stem cells are deterministic functions of time since these numbers are usually very large. Hence, for this model, the state variables are ($I_i(t), i = 1, \ldots, k-1, T(t)$), where $I_i(t)$ = number of I_i cells at time t, and $T(t)$ =number of cancer tumors at time t.

To derive stochastic differential equations for $I_j(t), j = 1, \ldots, k-1$, note: (i) The numbers of $\{I_j, j = 1, \ldots, k-1\}$ cells at time $t + \Delta t$ derive from the numbers of $\{I_j, j = 0, 1, \ldots, k-1\}$ cells at time t through stochastic birth and death processes and mutation processes. (ii) The birth-death-mutation processes during the small interval with length Δt is equivalent to multinomial distributions.

Define for $j = 1, \ldots, k-1$:

- $B_j(t)$ =Number of new I_j cells generated by stochastic cell proliferation (birth) of I_j cells during $(t, t + \Delta t]$,
- $D_j(t)$ =Number of death of I_j cells during $(t, t + dt]$,
- $M_j(t)$ =Number of new I_j cells arising from I_{j-1} cells by mutation or some genetic changes during $(t, t + \Delta t], j = 1, 2, \ldots, k$.

Then, for $j = 0, 1, \ldots, k-1$, the above principle leads to:

$$M_1(t) \sim Poisson\{\lambda_0(t)\Delta t\},$$

where $\lambda_0(t) = I_0(t)\alpha_0(t)$, and for $j = 1, \ldots, k-1$,

$$[B_j(t), D_j(t), M_{j+1}(t)]|I_j(t) \sim ML[I_j(t); b_j(t)\Delta t, d_j(t)\Delta t, \alpha_j(t)\Delta t].$$

It follows that $EM_1(t) = \lambda_0(t)\Delta t$ and for $j = 1, \ldots, k-1$,

$$E\{B_j(t)|I_j(t)\} = I_j(t)b_j(t)\Delta t,$$
$$E\{D_j(t)|I_j(t)\} = I_j(t)d_j(t)\Delta t,$$
$$E\{M_{j+1}(t)|I_j(t)\} = I_j(t)\alpha_j(t)\Delta t,$$

By the conservation law,we have then for $i = 1, \ldots, k-1$,

$$I_i(t + \Delta t) = I_i(t) + M_i(t) + B_i(t) - D_i(t).$$

The stochastic differential equations for the state variables are:

$$\Delta I_j(t) = I_j(t + \Delta t) - I_j(t) = M_j(t) + B_j(t) - D_j(t)$$
$$= \{I_{j-1}(t)\alpha_{j-1}(t) + I_j(t)\gamma_j(t)\}\Delta t + \epsilon_j(t)\Delta t,$$
$$j = 1, \ldots, k - 1, \tag{1}$$

where $\gamma_j(t) = b_j(t) - d_j(t)$, $j = 0, 1, \ldots, k - 1$ and for $j = 1, \ldots, k - 1$,
$e_j(t)\Delta t = [M_j(t) - I_{j-1}(t)\alpha_{j-1}(t)\Delta t] + [B_j(t) - I_j(t)b_j(t)\Delta t] - [D_j(t) - I_j(t)d_j(t)\Delta t]$.

4.2. The Probability Distribution of $T(t)$

To develop probability distribution for $T(t)$, observe that cancer tumors develop from primary I_k cells by following a stochastic birth-death process with birth rate $b_T(s,t)$ and death rate $d_T(s,t)$, where s is the time the primary tumor cell was generated. Hence we can derive the probability distribution for number of detectable cancer tumors at time t (i.e. $T(t)$).

Then as shown in Tan[56], Chapter 8, the conditional distribution of $T(t)$ given $\{I_{k-1}(s), s \le t\}$ is:

$$T(t)|\{I_{k-1}(s), s \le t\} \sim Poisson(\Lambda_T(t)), \tag{2}$$

where $\Lambda_T(t) = \int_{t_0}^t I_1(x)\alpha_{k-1}(x)P_T(x,t)dx$, and the $P_T(s,t)$ is given by:

$$P_T(s,t) = \frac{1}{h_T(s,t) + g_T(s,t)} \left(\frac{g_T(s,t)}{h_T(s,t) + g_T(s,t)}\right)^{N_T - 1}, \tag{3}$$

where N_T is the number of tumor cells for the tumor to be detectable,

$$h_T(s,t) = \exp\{-\int_s^t [b_T(s,y) - d_T(s,y)]dy\}$$

and

$$g_T(s,t) = \int_s^t b_T(s,y)h_T(y,t)dy.$$

4.3. Probability Distribution of the State Variables

Chose some fixed small interval for Δt as 1 time unit (i.e. $\Delta t \sim 1$) and denote by $\underset{\sim}{X}(t) = \{I_i(t), i = 1, \ldots, k - 1\}$. Let $g_0\{j; \lambda_0(t)\}$ denote the probability $M_1(t) = j$ from the Poisson distribution $M_1(t) \sim$

$Poisson\{\lambda_0(t)\}$; for $r = 1, \ldots, k - 1$, let $f_r\{i, j | I_r(t)\}$ denote the probability $\{B_r(t) = i, D_r(t) = j\}$ from the multinomial distribution $\{B_r(t), D_r(t)\} \sim ML[I_r(t); b_r(t), d_r(t)]$ and let $h_r\{j | i_r, j_r, I_r(t)\}$ be the probability of $(M_r(t) = j)$ from the binomial distribution $M_r(t) \sim Binomial\{I_r(t) - i_r - j_r; \frac{\alpha_r(t)}{1 - b_r(t) - d_r(t)}\}$. Then, from results in Section (4.1), the probability density function of $\boldsymbol{X} = \{\underset{\sim}{X}(1), \ldots, \underset{\sim}{X}(t_M)\}$ is

$$P(\boldsymbol{X}) = \prod_{t=1}^{t_M} \{P[\underset{\sim}{X}(t) | \underset{\sim}{X}(t-1)]\}$$

and for $t = 0, 1, \ldots, t_M - 1$,

$$P\{\underset{\sim}{X}(t+1) | \underset{\sim}{X}(t)\} = \sum_{i_1=0}^{I_1(t)} \sum_{j_1=0}^{I_1(t) - i_1} f_1\{i_1, j_1 | I_1(t)\} g_0\{a_1(t), \lambda_0(t)\}$$

$$\times \sum_{i_2=0}^{I_2(t)} \sum_{j_2=0}^{I_2(t) - i_2} f_2\{i_2, j_2 | I_2(t)\} h_1\{a_2(t) | i_2, j_2, I_2(t)\}$$

$$\times \cdots \times \sum_{i_{k-1}=0}^{I_{k-1}(t)} \sum_{j_{k-1}=0}^{I_{k-1}(t) - i_{k-1}} f_{k-1}\{i_{k-1}, j_{k-1} | I_{k-1}(t)\}$$

$$\times h_{k-2}\{a_{k-1}(t) | i_{k-1}, j_{k-1}, I_{k-1}(t)\}, \tag{4}$$

where $a_r(t) = Max(0, I_{r+1}(t) - I_r(t) - i_r + j_r)$.

5. A State Space Model for the Extended Multi-Event Model of Carcinogenesis

State space model is a stochastic models which consists of two sub-models: The stochastic system model which is the stochastic model of the system and the observation model which is a statistical model based on available observed data from the system. Hence it takes into account the basic mechanisms of the system and the random variation of the system through its stochastic system model and incorporate all these into the observed data from the system; furthermore, it validates and upgrades the stochastic model through its observation model and the observed data of the system. Thus the state space model adds one more dimension to the stochastic model and to the statistical model by combining both of these models into one model. As illustrated in [56], Chapters 8-9, the state space model has many advantages over both the stochastic model and the statistical model when used alone since it combines information and advantages from both of these models.

As an example, in this section we will illustrate how to develop a state space model for the extended multi-event model given in Section (3.1) with the observation model being based on the observed number of cancer incidence over time. For this state space model, the stochastic system model is specified by the stochastic equations given by (1) with the probability distribution of state variables being given in Section (4.3). The observation model is a statistical model based on the number of cancer cases $(y_i(j), i = 1, \ldots, m, j = 1, \ldots, n)$ over n different age groups and m different exposure levels.

5.1. *The Stochastic System Model, the Augmented State Variables and Probability Distribution*

The probability distribution for the state variables in equation (4) is extremely complicated involving many summations. For implementing the Gibbs sampling procedures to estimate the unknown parameters and the state variables, we thus expand the model by augmenting the dummy un-observable variables $\underset{\sim}{U}(t) = \{B_r(t), D_r(t), r = 1, \ldots, k - 1\}$ and put $\underset{\sim}{U} = \{\underset{\sim}{U}(t), t = 0, \ldots, t_M - 1\}$. Then, from the distribution results in Section (4.3), we have:

$$P\{\underset{\sim}{U}(t)|\underset{\sim}{X}(t)\} = \prod_{i=1}^{k-1} f_i\{B_i(t), D_i(t)|I_i(t)\};$$

$$P\{\underset{\sim}{X}(t+1)|\underset{\sim}{U}(t), \underset{\sim}{X}(t)\} = g_0\{b_0(t), \lambda_0(t)\} \prod_{i=2}^{k-1} h_{i-1}\{b_i(t)|B_i(t), D_i(t)\},$$

where for $i = 1, \ldots, k - 1$, $b_{i-1}(t) = I_i(t+1) - I_i(t) - B_i(t) + D_i(t)$.

The joint density of $\{X, U\}$ is

$$P\{X, U\} = \prod_{t=1}^{t_M} P\{\underset{\sim}{X}(t)|\underset{\sim}{X}(t-1), \underset{\sim}{U}(t-1)\}P\{\underset{\sim}{U}(t-1)|\underset{\sim}{X}(t-1)\}. \quad (5)$$

5.2. *The Observation Model and the Probability Distribution of Cancer Incidence*

The observation model is based on y_{ij}, where y_{ij} is the observed number of new cancer cases in the j−th age group $[t_{j-1}, t_j)$ under exposure to the carcinogen with dose level s_i. Let $n_i(j)$ be the number of normal people from whom the y_{ij} are generated. To derive the probability distribution of

y_{ij} given $n_i(j)$ and given the state variables, let $\{I_{k-1}(t;i,r)$ be the number of $I_{k-1}(t)$ cells in the r−th individual who was exposed to the carcinogen with dose level s_i and let $\alpha_{k-1}(i)$ be the rate of the transition $I_{k-1} \to I_k$ under exposure to the carcinogen with dose level s_i. Among people who have been exposed to the carcinogen with dose level s_i, let $P_r(i,j)$ denote the conditional probability given the state variables that the r−th individual would develop cancer during the j-th age group. Then, as shown in Tan[56], Chapter 8, $P_r(i,j)$ is given by:

$$P_r(i,j) = exp\{- \sum_{t=0}^{t_{j-1}-1} I_{k-1}(t;i,r)\alpha_{k-1}(i)\}(1 - e^{-R(i,j,r)\alpha_{k-1}(i)}),$$

where $R(i,j,r) = \sum_{t=t_{j-1}}^{t_j-1} I_{k-1}(t;i,r)$.

From the above it follows that the conditional probability density of y_{ij} given $n_i(j)$ and given the state variables $\underset{\sim}{I}_{k-1}(i,j) = \{I_{k-1}(t;i,r), t \leq t_j, r = 1, \ldots, n_i(j)\}$ is

$$P\{y_{ij}|n_i(j), \underset{\sim}{I}_{k-1}(i,j)\} = \binom{n_i(j)}{y_{ij}} \prod_{r=1}^{y_{ij}} P_r(i,j) \prod_{u=y_{ij}+1}^{n_i(j)} [1 - P_u(i,j)]. \quad (6)$$

Let $I_{k-1}(t;i)$ denote the number of I_{k-1} cells at time t under dose level s_i. When $n_i(j)$ and $n_i(j) - y_i(j)$ are very large and when $n_i(j)P_r(i,j)$ are finite for all r, the above probability is closely approximated by:

$$P\{y_{ij}|n_i(j), \underset{\sim}{I}_{k-1}(i,j)\} = \frac{1}{y_{ij}!}exp\{-\lambda_i(j)\} \prod_{r=1}^{y_{ij}}[n_i(j)P_r(i,j)], \quad (7)$$

where $\lambda_i(j) = n_i(j)EP_T(i,j) = n_i(j)EP_r(i,j), r = 1, \ldots, n_i(j)$ and where

$$P_T(i,j) = exp\{- \sum_{t=0}^{t_{j-1}-1} I_{k-1}(t;i)\alpha_{k-1}(i) + \log(1 - e^{\{-R(i,j)\alpha_{k-1}(i)\}})\},$$

with $R(i,j) = \sum_{t=t_{j-1}}^{t_j-1} I_{k-1}(t;i)$. (For Proof, see [63])

From equation (7), the conditional likelihood of the parameters given data $Y = \{y_{ij}, i = 1, \ldots, m, j = 1, \ldots, n\}$ and given the state variables is

$$L\{\Theta|Y, \underset{\sim}{I}_{k-1}\} = \prod_{i=1}^{m} \prod_{j=1}^{n} P\{y_{ij}|n_i(j), \underset{\sim}{I}_{k-1}(i,j)\}, \quad (8)$$

Also, since $\alpha_{k-1}(i)$ is very small, it can be shown[63] that with $\bar{\alpha}_{k-1}(i) = 10^6\alpha_{k-1}(i)$,

$$E[P_T(i,j)] = \exp\{-\frac{1}{10^6}\sum_{t=0}^{t_{j-1}-1} EI_{k-1}(t;i)\bar{\alpha}_{k-1}(i)$$

$$+ E\log(1 - e^{-\frac{1}{10^6}R(i,j)\bar{\alpha}_{k-1}(i)})\}$$

$$\approx B_i(j)\bar{\alpha}_{k-1}(i)exp\{-A_i(j)\bar{\alpha}_{k-1}(i)\},$$

where $A_i(j) = \frac{1}{10^6}\{\sum_{t=0}^{t_j-1} EI_{k-1}(t;i) - \frac{1}{2}ER(i,j)\}$ and $B_i(j) = \frac{1}{10^6}ER(i,j)$.

From the above distribution results, it is obvious that the joint density of $\{\boldsymbol{X}, \boldsymbol{U}, \boldsymbol{Y}\}$ is

$$P\{\boldsymbol{X}, \boldsymbol{U}, \boldsymbol{Y}\} = \prod_{i=1}^{m}\prod_{j=1}^{n} P\{y_{ij}|n_i(j), \underset{\sim}{I}_{k-1}(i,j)\}$$

$$\times \prod_{t=t_{j-1}+1}^{t_j} P\{\underset{\sim}{X}(t)|\underset{\sim}{X}(t-1), \underset{\sim}{U}(t-1)\}$$

$$\times P\{\underset{\sim}{U}(t-1)|\underset{\sim}{X}(t-1)\}. \qquad (9)$$

Notice that in the above equation, the birth rates, death rates and mutation rates $\{\lambda_0(t), b_r(t), d_r(t), \alpha_r(t), r = 1, \ldots, k-1\}$ are functions of the dose level s_i.

The above distribution will be used to derive the conditional posterior distribution of the unknown parameters Θ given $\{\boldsymbol{X}, \boldsymbol{U}, \boldsymbol{Y}\}$. Notice that because the number of parameters is very large, the classical sampling theory approach by using the likelihood function $P\{\boldsymbol{Y}|\boldsymbol{X}, \boldsymbol{U}\}$ is not possible without making assumptions about the parameters; however, this problem can easily be avoided by new information from the stochastic system model and the prior distribution of the parameters.

5.3. *The Posterior Distribution of the Unknown Parameters and State Variables*

In many practical situations, one may assume that the birth rates, death rates and mutation rates are time homogeneous. For the *i-th* dose level, denote these rates by $\{\lambda_i, \alpha_{ji}, b_{ji}, d_{ji}, j = 1, \ldots, k-1\}$. Then the set of unknown parameters are $\Theta = \{\lambda_i, \alpha_{ji}, b_{ji}, d_{ji}, j = 1, \ldots, k-1, i = 1, \ldots, m\}$. To derive the posterior distribution of Θ given $\{\boldsymbol{X}, \boldsymbol{U}, \boldsymbol{Y}\}$, let $P\{\Theta\}$ be the prior distribution of Θ and for the i-th dose level, denote the $\{\underset{\sim}{X}(t), \underset{\sim}{U}(t)\}$ by $\underset{\sim}{X}^{(i)}(t) = \{I_j^{(i)}(t), j = 1, \ldots, k-1\}$ and $\underset{\sim}{U}^{(i)}(t) = \{B_j^{(i)}(t), D_j^{(i)}(t), j = $

$1, \ldots, k-1\}$. From equations (7)-(9), the conditional posterior distribution $P\{\Theta|X,U,Y\}$ of Θ given $\{X,U,Y\}$ is:

$$P\{\Theta|X,U,Y\} \propto P\{\Theta\} \prod_{i=1}^{m} \lambda_i^{\{\sum_{t=0}^{t_M-1} M_1(t)\}} e^{\{-t_M \lambda_i\}} \prod_{j=1}^{k-1} [b_{ji}]^{\{\sum_{t=0}^{t_M-1} B_j^{(i)}(t)\}}$$

$$\times [d_{ji}]^{\{\sum_{t=0}^{t_M-1} D_j^{(i)}(t)\}} \alpha_{ji}^{\{\sum_{t=0}^{t_M-1} R_j^{(i)}(t)\}}$$

$$\times (1 - b_{ji} - d_{ji} - \alpha_{ji})^{\{\sum_{t=1}^{t_M} [I_j(t) - B_j^{(i)}(t) - D_j^{(i)}(t) - R_j^{(i)}(t)]\}},$$

(10)

where $R_j^{(i)}(t) = I_j^{(i)}(t+1) - I_j^{(i)}(t) - B_j^{(i)}(t) + D_j^{(i)}(t)$.

For the prior distribution of the unknown parameters, we will assume that **a priori** the parameters in Θ are independently distributed of one another. Furthermore, we will assume natural conjugate priors for all the parameters. That is, we assume:

$$P\{\Theta\} \propto \prod_{i=1}^{m} \lambda_i^{p_i-1} exp\{-\lambda_i q_i\} \prod_{j=1}^{k-1} [b_{ji}]^{u_{ji}-1} [d_{ji}]^{v_{ji}-1} \alpha_{ji}^{r_{ji}-1}$$

$$\times (1 - b_{ji} - d_{ji} - \alpha_{ji})^{w_{ji}-1},$$

(11)

where the hyperparameters $\{p_i, q_i, u_{ji}, v_{ji}, w_{ji}, r_{ji}\}$ are positive real numbers. These hyperparameters can be estimated from previous studies. In the event that prior studies and information are not available, we will follow Box and Tiao[6] to assume that $P\{\lambda_i, i = 1, \ldots, m\} \propto \prod_{i=1}^{m}(\lambda_i)^{-1}$ and that all other parameters are uniformly distributed to reflect the fact that our prior information are vague and imprecise.

5.4. The Generalized Bayesian Method for Estimating Unknown Parameters and State Variables

Using the above distribution results, the multi-level Gibbs sampling procedures for estimating the unknown parameters Θ and the state variables X are given by the following loop:

(i) Given the parameter values, we will use the stochastic equation (1) and the associated probability distributions to generate a large sample of $\{X,U\}$. Then, by combining this large sample with $P\{Y|X,U\}$, we select $\{X,U\}$ from this sample through the weighted Bootstrap method due to Smith and Gelfand[51]. This selected $\{X,U\}$ is then a sample generated from $P\{X,U|\Theta,Y\}$ although the latter density is unknown (for proof, see Tan[56], Chapter 3). Call the generated sample $\{X^{(*)}, U^{(*)}\}$.

(ii) On substituting $\{U^{(*)}, X^{(*)}\}$ which are generated numbers from the above step, generate Θ from the conditional density $P\{\Theta | X^{(*)}.U^{(*)}, Y\}$ given by equation (10).

(iii) With Θ being generated from Step (ii) above, go back to Step (i) and repeat the above [i]-[ii] loop until convergence.

The convergence of the above algorithm has been proved in Tan[56], Chapter 3. At convergence, one then generates a random sample of $\{X, U\}$ from the conditional distribution $P\{X, U | Y\}$ of $\{X, U\}$ given Y, independent of Θ and a random sample of Θ from the posterior distribution $P\{\Theta | Y\}$ of Θ given Y, independent of $\{X, U\}$. Repeat these procedures one then generates a random sample of size N of $\{X, U\}$ and a random sample of size M of Θ. One may then use the sample means to derive the estimates of $\{X, U\}$ and Θ and use the sample variances as the variances of these estimates. Alternatively, one may also use Efron's bootstrap method[13] to derive estimates of the standard errors of the estimates.

6. Analysis of British Physician Data of Lung Cancer and Smoking

It has long been recognized that smoking can cause lung cancer[20,44,67] in most cases. To reveal the basic mechanisms of how tobacco nicotine cause lung cancer, in this section we will apply the above state space model to analyze the British physician smoking data given in Doll and Peto[12]. Given in Table 1 is the British physician data extracted from the paper by Doll and Peto[12]. In this data set, we have included only the age groups between 40 years old and 80 years old because in this data set, lung cancer incidence are non-existent before 40 years old and are also rare among people who are older than 80 years old.

From data in Table 1, observe that there are 8 dose levels represented by the number of cigarettes smoked per day and there are 8 age groups each with a period of 5 years. Because lung cancer incidence were reported for a 5 years period, as in [36, 38, 39, 55] we will assume that the initiated cells in the last stage grow instantaneously into malignant tumors, unless otherwise stated. To implement the procedures in Sections 5, we let $\Delta t \sim 1$ correspond to a period of 3 months.

To analyze data given in Table 1, we will use the state space model with the observation model being given by the number (y_{ij}) of total lung cancer incidence. For the stochastic system model we will entertain four extended k-stage multi-event models: (a) A time non-homogeneous 2-stage model, (b) a time homogeneous 2-stage model, (c) a time homogeneous 3-stage model, (d) a time homogeneous 4-stage model, and (e) a time homogeneous 5-stage model. In models (b)-(e), the mutation rates, the birth rates and the death rates are assumed to be independent of time. In model (a), while the mutation rates are independent of time, we assume the birth rate and the death rate on initiated cells are 2-step piece-wise non-homogeneous with $t_1 = 60$ years old as the cut-off time point.

To assess effects of dose level, we let $x_i = \log(1 + u_i)$, where u_i is the mean dose of the i-th dose level. Then, based on some preliminary analysis[63] we assume a Cox regression model for the mutation rates and assume linear regression models for the birth rates and the death rates. Thus, we let $\lambda_0(i, t) = a_{00}(t)e^{a_{01}(t)x_i}$, $\alpha_j(i) = a_{j0}e^{a_{j1}x_i}$ for all models; but let $\{b_j(i) = b_{j0} + b_{j1}x_i, d_j(i) = d_{j0} + d_{j1}(i)x_i\}$ for the time homogeneous models and let $\{b_1(i, s) = b_{10}(s) + b_{11}(s)x_i, d_1(i) = d_{10}(s) + d_{11}(s)x_i\}$ with $s = 1$ for $t \leq t_1$ and $s = 2$ for $t > t_1$ for the two-stage time nonhomogeneous model.

Applying the procedures in Section 5, we have estimated the parameters and fitted the data in Table 1. The AIC and BIC values of all models as well as the p-values for testing goodness of fit of the models are given in Table 2. The p-values are computed using the approximate probability distribution results $\sum_{i=1}^{m} \sum_{j=1}^{n} (y_{ij} - \hat{\lambda}_{ij})^2 / \hat{\lambda}_{ij} \sim \chi^2(mn - k)$, for large mn, where k is the number of parameters estimated under the model. The estimates for the unknown parameters given the 4-stage model are given in Table 3. From the p-values of the models, apparently that all models except the 5-stage model fit the data well, but the values of AIC and BIC suggested that the 4-stage model is more appropriate for the data. This 4-stage model seems to fit the following molecular biological model for squamous cell lung carcinoma proposed recently by Wistuba et al.[67]: Normal epithelium → Hyperplasia (3p/9p LOH, Genomic Instability) → Dysplasia (Telomerase dysregulation) → In situ Carcinoma (8p LOH, FHIT gene inactivation, gene methylation) → Invasive Carcinoma (p53 gene inactivation, k-ras mutation).

From results given in Tables 3, we observe the following interesting results:

(1) The estimates of $\lambda_0(i)$ increases as the dose level increases. This indicates the tobacco nicotine is an initiator. From molecular biological studies, this initiation process may either be associated with the LOH (loss of heterozygosity) of some suppressor genes from chromosomes 3p or silencing of these genes by epigenetic actions

(see [2, 3, 7, 14, 17, 30, 32, 40, 43, 49, 64]).

(2). The estimates of the mutation rates $\alpha_j(i) = \alpha_j$ for $j = 1, 2, 3$ are in general independent of the dose level x_i. These estimates are of order 10^{-5} and do not differ significantly from one another.

(3). The results in Table 3 indicate that for non-smokers, the death rates $d_j(0)$ ($j = 1, 2, 3$) are slightly greater than the birth rates $b_j(0)$ so that the proliferation rates $\gamma_j(0) = b_j(0) - d_j(0)$ are negative. For smokers, however, the proliferation rates $\gamma_j(i) = b_j(i) - d_j(i)(i > 0)$ are positive and increases as dose level increases (the only exception is $\gamma_2(3)$). This is not surprising since most of the genes are tumor suppressor genes which are involved in cell differentiation and cell proliferation and apoptosis (e.g., p53) (see [20, 44, 67]).

(4). From Table 3, we observed that the estimates of $\gamma_3(i)$ are of order 10^{-2} which are considerably greater that the estimates of $\gamma_1(i)$ respectively. The estimates of $\gamma_1(i)$ are of order 10^{-3} and are considerably greater than the estimates of $\gamma_2(i)$ respectively. The estimates of $\gamma_2(i)$ are of order 10^{-4} and $\gamma_2(3)$ assumed negative value. One may explain these observations by noting the results: (1) Significant cell proliferation may trickle apoptosis leading to increased cell death unless the apoptosis gene (p53) has been inactivated and (2) the inactivation of the apoptosis gene (p53) occurred in the very last stage; see [67].

7. Conclusions and Summary

Based on most recent biological studies, in this chapter we have presented some stochastic models for carcinogenesis. To develop mathematical analysis for these models, the traditional approach based on theories of Markov process is extremely difficult and has some serious drawbacks. To get around these difficulties, in this chapter we have proposed an alternative approach through stochastic differential equations and state space models for carcinogenesis. This provides an unique approach to combine information from both stochastic models and statistical models of carcinogenesis. By using state space models, we have developed a general procedure via multiple Gibbs sampling method to estimate the unknown parameters. In this paper we have used the multi-event model as an example to illustrate the basic approach and our new modeling ideas.

To illustrate some applications of results of this chapter, we have applied the model and method to the British physician data on lung cancer and smoking. Our analysis has shown that a 4-stage homogeneous stochastic model fits the data well. This model appears to be consistent with the molecular biological model of squamous cell lung carcinoma proposed by Wistuba[67]. By assuming a 4-stage model for the data we have obtained the following results:

(1) The tobacco nicotine is both an initiator and promoter.

(2) The mutation rates can best be described by the Cox regression model so that $\alpha_j(i, t) = \alpha_{j0}(t) \exp\{\alpha_{j1}(t)x_i\}, j = 0, 1$; similarly, the birth rates $b_j(i, t)$ and the death rates $d_j(i, t)$ can best be described by linear regression models.

(3) The estimates of the mutation rates and proliferation rates appear to be consistent with biological observations.

8. Acknowledgments

The research of this paper is supported by a research grant from NCI/NIH, grant number R15113347-01.

References

1. M. Al-Hajj and M.F. Clarke, Self-renewal and solid tumor stem cells, *Oncogene* **23** (2004), 7274-7288.
2. S.B. Baylin, DNA methylation and gene silencing in cancer, *Nature Clinical Practice Oncology*, **2** (2005), S4-S11.
3. S.A. Belinsky, Gene-promoter hypermethylation as a biomarker in lung cancer, *Nature Rev. Cancer*, **4** (2004), 707-717.
4. D.R. Bell and G.V. Zant, Stem cells, aging, and cancer:Inevitabilities and outcomes, *Oncogene*, **23** (2004), 7290-7296.
5. M.A. Blasco, Telemeres and human diseases: Aging, cancer and beyond, *Nature Rev. Genetics*, **6** (2005), 611-622.
6. G.E.P. Box and G.C. Tiao, *Bayesian Inferences in Statistical Analysis*, Addison-Wesley, Reading, MA, 1973.
7. J. Breivik and G. Gaudernack, Genomic instability, DNA methylation, and natural selection in colorectal carcinogenesis, *Semi. Cancer Biol.*, **9** (1999), 245-254.
8. D.P. Cahill, K.W. Kinzler, B. Vogelstein, and C. Lengauer, Genetic instability and Darwinian selection in tumors, *Trends Cell Biol.*, **9** (1999), M57-60.
9. W.E. Cavenee, et al., Genetic origin of mutations predisposing to retinoblastoma, *Science*, **228** (1985), 501-503.
10. A. de la Chapelle, Genetic predisposition to colorectal cancer, *Nature Review Cancer*, **4** (2004), 769-780.
11. K.C. Chu, Multi-event model for carcinogenesis: A model for cancer causation and prevention. In: *Carcinogenesis: A Comprehensive Survey Volume*

8: *Cancer of the Respiratory Tract-Predisposing Factors*, (M.J. Mass, D.G. Ksufman, J.M. Siegfied, V.E. Steel, and S. Nesnow, Eds.), pp. 411-421, Raven Press, New York, 1985.

12. R. Doll and R. Peto, Cigarette smoking and bronchial carcinoma: Dose and time relationships among regular smokers lifelong non-smokers. *Journal of Epidemiology and Community Health*, **32** (1978), 303-313.

13. B. Efron, *The Jackknife, the Bootstrap and Other Resampling Plans*, SIAM, Philadelphia, PA, 1982.

14. M. Esteller, Epigenetic lesions causing genetic lesions in human cancer: Promoter hypermethylation of DNA repair genes, *Eur. J. Cancer*, **36** (2000), 2294-2300.

15. E. Farber, Experimental industion of hepatocellular carcinoma as a paradigm for carcinogenesis, *Clin. Physiol. Biochem.*, **5** (1987), 152-159.

16. R. Ferreira, I. Naguibneva, L.L. Pritchard, S. Ait-Si-Ali, and A. Harel-Bellan, The Rb/chromatin connection and epigenetic control: Opinion, *Genes and Oncogene*, **20** (2001), 3128-3133.

17. L. Flintoft, Silent transmission, *Nature Rev. Genetics*, **5** (2005), 720-721.

18. R. Fodde, R. Smit, and H. Clevers, APC, signal transduction and genetic instability in colorectal cancer, *Nature Review Cancer*, **1** (2001), 55-67.

19. R. Fodde, J. Kuipers, C. Rosenberg, et al., Mutations in the APC tumor suppressor gene cause chromosomal instability, *Nature Cell Biology*, **3** (2001), 433-438.

20. K.M. Fong and Y. Sekido, The molecular biology of lung carcinogenesis. In: *The Molecular Basis of Human Cancer*, (W.B. Coleman and G.J. Tsongalis, Eds.), pp.379-405, Humana Press, Totowa, NJ, 2002.

21. R.A. Green and K.B. Kaplan, Chromosomal instability in colorectal tumor cells is associated with defects in microtubule plus-end attachments caused by a dominant mutation in APC, *The Journal of Cell Biology*, **163** (2003), 949-961.

22. N.J. Hawkins and R.L. Ward, Sporadic colorectal cancers with microsatellite instability and their possible origin in hyperplastic polyps and serrated adenomas, *J. Natl. Cancer Institute*, **93** (2001), 1307-1313.

23. D. Hanahan and R.A. Weinberg, The hallmarks of cancer, *Cell*, **100** (2000), 57-70.

24. L.G. Hanin and A.Y. Yakovlev, A nonidentifiability aspect of the two-stage model of carcinogenesis, *Risk Analysis*, **16** (1996), 711-715.

25. W.C. Hahn and M. Meyerson, Telomere activation, cellular immortalization and cancer, *Ann. Med.*, **33** (2001), 123-129.

26. J.D. Henson, A.A. Neumann, T.R. Yeager, and R.R. Reddel, Alternative lengthening of telomeres in mammalian cells, *Oncogene*, **21** (2002), 589-610.

27. R. Hesketh, *The Oncogene and Tumor Suppressor Gene Facts Book*, (Second Edition), Academic Press, San Diego, 1997.

28. K. Hopkin, Tumor evolution: Survival of the fittest cells, *J. NIH Research*, **8** (1996), 37-41.

29. M. Ilyas, J. Straub, I.P.M. Tomlinson, and W.F. Bodmer, Genetic pathways in colorrectal and other cancers, *Eur. J Cancer*, **35** (1999), 335-351.

30. L.F. Jaffe, Epigenetic theory of cancer initiation, *Advances in Cancer Research*, Elsevier Inc. USA, 2003.
31. J.M. Jessup, G.G. Gallic, and B. Liu, The molecular biology of colorectal carcinoma: Importance of the Wg/Wnt signal transduction pathway, In: *The Molecular Basis of Human Cancer*, (W.B. Coleman and G.J. Tsongalis, Eds.), pp. 251-268, Humana Press, Totowa, NJ, 2002.
32. P.A. Jones and S.B. Baylin, The fundamental role of epigenetic events in cancer, *Nat. Rev. Genet.*, **3** (2002), 415-428.
33. T. Kalunaga, Requirement for cell replication in the fixation and expression of the transformed state in mouse cells treated with 4-nitroquinoline-1-oxide, *Int. J. Cancer*, **14** (1974), 736-742.
34. A.G. Knudson, Genetics and etiology of human cancer, *Advances in Human Genetics*, **8** (1977), 1-66.
35. P. Laurent-Puig, H. Blons, and P.-H. Cugnenc, Sequence of molecular genetic events in colorectal tumorigenesis, *European J. Cancer Prevention*, **8** (1999), S39-S47.
36. M.P. Little, Are two mutations sufficient to cause cancer? Some generalizations of the two-mutation model of carcinogenesis of Moolgavkar, Venson and Knudson, and of the multistage model of Armitage and Doll, *Biometrics*, **51** (1995), 1278-1291.
37. K.R. Loeb and L.A. Loeb, Significance of multiple mutations in cancer, *Carcinogenesis*, **21** (2000), 379-385.
38. E.G. Luebeck, W.F. Heidenreich, W.D. Hazelton, and S.H. Moolgavkar, Analysis of a cohort of Chinese tin miners with arsenic, radon, cigarette and pipe smoke exposures using the biologically-based two stage clonal expansion model, *Radiation Research*, **156** (2001), 78-94.
39. E.G. Luebeck and S.H. Moolgavkar, Multistage carcinogenesis and colorectal cancer incidence in SEER, *Proc. Natl. Acad. Sci. USA*, **99** (2002), 15095-15100.
40. A.H. Lund and van M. Lohuizen, Epigenetics and cancer, *Genes and Development*, **18** (2004), 2315-2335.
41. F. MacDonald, C.H.J. Ford, and A.G. Casson *Molecular Biology of Cancer*, (Second Edition), Taylor and Francis, Florence, KY, 2004.
42. P. Nettesheim and J.C. Barrett, In ivtro transformation of rat tracheal epithelial cells as a model for the study of multistage carcinogenesis. In: *Carcinogenesis*, (J.C. Barrett and R.W. Tennant, Eds.), **Vol. 9**, pp. 283-292, Raven Press, NY, 1985.
43. R. Ohlsson, C. Kanduri, J. Whitehead, et al., Epigenetic variability and evolution of human cancer, *Advances in Cancer Research*, Elsevier Inc, USA, 2003.
44. H. Osada and T. Takahashi, Genetic alterations of multiple tumor suppressors and oncogenes in the carcinogenesis and progression of lung cancer, *Oncogene*, **21** (2002), 7421-7434.
45. P. Peltomaki, Deficient DNA mismatch repair: A common etiologic factor for colon cancer, *Human Molecular Genetics* **10** (2001), 735-740.
46. P.D.P. Pharoah, A.M. Dunning, B.A.J. Ponder, and D.F. Easton, Associa-

tion studies for finding cancer-susceptaibility genetic variants, *Nature Rev. Cancer,* **4** (2004), 850-860.

47. J.D. Potter, Colorectal cancer: molecules and population. *J. Natl. Cancer Institute* , **91** (1999), 916-932.

48. M.J. Renan, How many mutations are required for tumorigenesis? Implications from human cancer data, *Mol. Carcinog.,* **7** (1993), 139-146.

49. T. Robertson, DNA methylation and human diseases, *Nature Rev. Genetics,* **6** (2005), 597-610.

50. J.W. Shay, Y. Zou, E. Hiyama, and W.E. Wright, Telomerase and cancer, *Mol. Genet.,* **10** (2001), 677-685.

51. A.F.M. Smith and A.E. Gelfand, Bayesian statistics without tears: A sampling-resampling perspective, *American Statistician,* **46** (1992), 84-88.

52. K.N. Smolinski and S.J. Meltzer, Inactivation of negative regulators during neoplastic transformation, In: *The Molecular Basis of Human Cancer,* (W.B. Coleman and G.J. Tsongalis, Eds.), pp.81-111, Humana Press, Totowa, NJ, 2002.

53. A.B. Sparks, P.J. Morin, B. Vogelstein, and K.W. Kinzler, Mutational analysis of the APC/beta-catenin/Tcf pathway in colorectal cancer, *Cancer Res.,* **58** (1998), 1130-1134.

54. W.Y. Tan, Some mixed models of carcinogenesis, *Math. Computer Modelling,* **10** (1988), 765-773.

55. W.Y. Tan, *Stochastic Models of Carcinogenesis,* Marcel Dekker, New York, 1991.

56. W.Y. Tan, *Stochastic Models With Applications to Genetics, Cancers, AIDS and Other Biomedical Systems,* World Scientific, New Jersey, 2002.

57. W.Y. Tan and C.W. Chen, A multiple pathway model of carcinogenesis involving one stage models and two-stage models. In: *Math. Population Dynamics,* pp. 469-482 (O. Arino, David E. Axelrod and M. Kimmel, Eds.), Marcel Dekker, New York, 1991.

58. W.Y. Tan and C.W. Chen, Stochastic Modeling of Carcinogenesis: Some New Insight. *Math. Computer Modeling* **28** (1998), 49-71.

59. W.Y. Tan and C.W. Chen, Assessing effects of changing environment by a multiple pathway model of carcinogenesis, *Math. Computer Modelling,* **32** (2000), 229-250.

60. W.Y. Tan and C.W. Chen, Cancer stochastic models, In: *Encyclopedia of Statistical Sciences,* (Revised edition), John Wiley and Sons, New York, 2005.

61. W.Y. Tan, C.W. Chen, and W. Wang, Stochastic modelling of carcinogenesis by state space models: A new approach, *Math. Computer Modelling,* **33** (2001), 1323-1345.

62. W.Y. Tan K.P. Singh, A mixed model of carcinogenesis - With applications to retinoblastoma, *Math. Biosciences,* **98** (1990), 201-211.

63. Tan W.Y., Zhang, L.J. and Chen C.W. (2004). Stochastic modeling of carcinogenesis: State space models and estimation of parameters, *Discrete and Continuous Dynamical Systems, Series B,* 4, 297-322.

64. T. Ushijima, Detection and interpretation of altered methylation patterns in cancer cells, *Nature Rev. Genetics,* **5** (2005), 223-231.

65. R. Ward, A. Meagher, I. Tomlinson, T. O'Connor, et al., Microsatellite instability and the clinicopathological features of sporadic colorectal cancer, *Gut* **48** (2001), 821-829.

66. J.N. Welch and S.A. Chrysogelos, Positive mediators of cell proliferation in neoplastic transformation, In: *The Molecular Basis of Human Cancer*, (W.B. Coleman and G.J. Tsongalis, Eds.), pp. 65-79, Humana Press, Totowa, NJ, 2002.

67. I.I. Wistuba, L. Mao, and A.F. Gazdar, Smoking molecular damage in bronchial epithelium, *Oncogene*, **21** (2002), 7298-7306.

68. A.Y. Yakovlev and A.D. Tsodikov, *Stochastic Models of Tumor Latency and Their Biostatistical Applications*, World Scientific, Singapore and River Edge, NJ, 1996.

69. G.L. Yang and C.W. Chen, A stochastic two-stage carcinogenesis model: a new approach to computing the probability of observing tumor in animal bioassays, *Math. Biosciences* **104** (1991), 247-258.

Table 1. British Physician Lung Cancer Data with Smoking Information

Age Group (years)	CIGARETTES/DAY(RANGE AND MEAN)								
	0 / 0	1-4 / 2.7	5-9 / 6.6	10-14 / 11.3	15-19 / 16	20-24 / 20.4	25-29 / 25.4	30-34 / 30.2	35-40 / 38
40-44	17846.5^1 0^2 0^3	1216 0 0	2041.5 0 0	3795.5 1 0	4824 0 0	7046 1 1	2523 0 0	1715.5 1 1	892.5 0 0
45-49	15832.5 0 0	1000.5 0 0	1745 0 0	3205 1 1	3995 1 1	6460.5 1 2	2565.5 2 1	2123 2 2	1150 0 1
50-54	12226 1 1	853.5 0 0	1562.5 0 0	2727 2 1	3278.5 4 2	5583 6 4	2620 3 3	2226.5 3 3	1281 3 2
55-59	8905.5 2 1	625 1 0	1355 0 0	2288 1 2	2466.5 0 2	4357.5 8 6	2108.5 5 4	1923 6 5	1063 4 4
60-64	6248 0 0	509.5 1 0	1068 1 0	1714 1 2	1829.5 2 2	2863.5 13 9	1508.5 4 5	1362 11 7	826 7 6
65-69	4351 0 0	392.5 0 0	843.5 1 0	1214 2 3	1237 2 2	1930 12 10	974.5 5 6	763.5 9 7	515 9 7
70-74	2723.5 1 1	242 1 0	696.5 2 0	862 4 4	683.5 4 2	1055 10 8	527 7 7	317.5 2 4	233 5 5
75-79	1772 2 0	208.5 0 0	517.5 0 0	547 4 4	370.5 5 2	512 7 7	209.5 4 4	130 2 3	88.5 2 3

Notes: [1] population, [2] observed lung cancer incidence, [3] predicted lung cancer incidence based on 4 stage homogeneous model.

Table 2. BIC, AIC and Loglikelihood Values for 2, 3 and 4 Stages Models

Model	BIC	AIC	Log of Likelihood Values $= \log L(\hat{\Theta}|Y)$	P-value for Goodness of fit
Homogeneous 2-stage	188.93	182.07	-87.04	0.10
None-Homogeneous 2-stage	177.48	167.20	-77.60	0.42
Homogeneous 3-stage	151.42	139.42	-62.71	0.98
Homogeneous 4-stage	150.76	133.61	-56.81	0.99
Homogeneous 5-stage	211.67	189.38	-81.69	0.06

Notes: (1)The p-value is based on $\sum_{i=1}^{m} \sum_{j=1}^{n} \{y_{ij} - \hat{\lambda}_{ij}\}^2 / \hat{\lambda}_{ij} \sim \chi^2(72 - k)$,
(k = the number of parameters under the model)
(2) $\log L(\hat{\Theta}|Y) = \sum_{i=1}^{m} \sum_{j=1}^{n} \{-\hat{\lambda}_{ij} + y_{ij} \log \hat{\lambda}_{ij} - \log(y_{ij}!)\}, \hat{\lambda}_{ij} = n_{ij} p_i(j)$

Table 3. Estimates of Parameters for the 4 Stage Homogeneous Model
with Predictive

	CIGARETTES/DAY(RANGE AND MEAN)				
Parameters	0 0	1-4 2.7	5-9 6.6	10-14 11.3	15-19 16
$\lambda_0(i)$	218.03 ± 12.81	247.95 ± 15.79	286.41 ± 16.79	285.07 ± 16.04	295.57 ± 16.73
$b_1(i)$	$5.93E-02$ $\pm 8.77E-05$	$6.72E-02$ $\pm 5.40E-05$	$7.17E-02$ $\pm 3.43E-05$	$7.47E-02$ $\pm 1.46E-05$	$7.66E-02$ $1.16E-05$
$d_1(i)$	$6.18E-02$ $\pm 9.68E-05$	$6.02E-02$ $\pm 4.78E-05$	$5.99E-02$ $\pm 2.90E-05$	$5.95E-02$ $\pm 1.06E-05$	$5.93E-02$ $1.50E-05$
$b_1(i) - d_1(i)$	$-1.31E-03$ $\pm 5.60E-05$	$1.78E-03$ $\pm 6.07E-05$	$3.95E-03$ $\pm 6.64E-05$	$5.21E-03$ $\pm 4.12E-05$	$6.21E-03$ $3.17E-05$
$\alpha_1(i)$	$5.29E-05$ $\pm 2.67E-06$	$6.74E-05$ $\pm 1.67E-06$	$5.48E-05$ $\pm 1.12E-06$	$5.68E-05$ $\pm 3.96E-07$	$5.52E-05$ $\pm 3.65E-07$
$b_2(i)$	$8.08E-02$ $\pm 1.59E-03$	$8.92E-02$ $\pm 7.34E-04$	$8.97E-02$ $\pm 5.04E-04$	$9.14E-02$ $\pm 2.10E-04$	$9.34E-02$ $2.62E-04$
$d_2(i)$	$8.84E-02$ $\pm 1.99E-03$	$8.63E-02$ $\pm 6.82E-04$	$9.00E-02$ $\pm 5.52E-04$	$9.19E-02$ $\pm 2.15E-04$	$9.37E-02$ $2.15E-04$
$b_2(i) - d_2(i)$	$-7.60E-03$ $\pm 2.55E-03$	$2.90E-03$ $\pm 1.00E-03$	$-3.00E-04$ $\pm 7.47E-03$	$-5.00E-04$ $\pm 3.01E-04$	$-3.00E-04$ $3.39E-04$
$\alpha_2(i)$	$4.01E-05$ $\pm 3.86E-05$	$5.55E-06$ $\pm 4.99E-06$	$3.28E-06$ $\pm 3.70E-06$	$3.84E-05$ $\pm 4.75E-06$	$1.61E-05$ $\pm 3.37E-06$
$b_3(i)$	$1.08E-02$ $\pm 1.07E-02$	$9.32E-02$ $\pm 2.53E-04$	$4.79E-02$ $\pm 1.65E-02$	$9.84E-02$ $\pm 7.63E-04$	$1.01E-01$ $4.89E-04$
$d_3(i)$	$7.18E-02$ $\pm 2.45E-02$	$6.27E-02$ $\pm 1.68E-04$	$1.10E-01$ $\pm 2.45E-02$	$8.59E-02$ $\pm 5.60E-04$	$8.16E-02$ $4.49E-04$
$b_3(i) - d_3(i)$	$-2.21E-03$ $\pm 2.42E-03$	$7.88E-03$ $\pm 2.71E-03$	$1.46E-02$ $\pm 1.84E-03$	$1.97E-02$ $\pm 4.78E-04$	$2.11E-02$ $5.79E-04$
$\alpha_3(i) = \alpha_3$		$9.54E-06 \pm 2.51E-08$			

(Table 3 continued)

	CIGARETTES/DAY(RANGE AND MEAN)			
Parameters	20-24 20.4	25-29 25.4	30-34 30.2	35-40 38
$\lambda_0(i)$	313.02 ± 16.86	318.24 ± 16.40	330.79 ± 18.61	341.41 ± 19.33
$b_1(i)$	$7.81E-02$ $\pm 7.85E-06$	$7.94E-02$ $\pm 8.83E-06$	$8.04E-02$ $\pm 9.26E-06$	$8.18E-02$ $\pm 7.29E-06$
$d_1(i)$	$5.92E-02$ $\pm 7.83E-06$	$5.91E-02$ $\pm 7.30E-06$	$5.90E-02$ $\pm 7.99E-06$	$5.89E-02$ $\pm 6.56E-06$
$b_1(i)-d_1(i)$	$6.79E-03$ $\pm 2.09E-05$	$7.30E-03$ $\pm 2.66E-05$	$7.86E-03$ $\pm 2.15E-05$	$8.30E-03$ $\pm 3.21E-05$
$\alpha_1(i)$	$5.52E-05$ $\pm 2.03E-07$	$5.44E-05$ $\pm 2.24E-07$	$5.56E-05$ $\pm 2.28E-07$	$5.51E-05$ $\pm 1.85E-07$
$b_2(i)$	$9.49E-02$ $\pm 1.49E-04$	$9.61E-02$ $\pm 1.34E-04$	$9.70E-02$ $\pm 1.30E-04$	$9.80E-02$ $\pm 1.26E-04$
$d_2(i)$	$9.42E-02$ $\pm 1.54E-04$	$9.40E-02$ $\pm 1.42E-04$	$9.46E-02$ $\pm 1.67E-04$	$9.53E-02$ $\pm 1.24E-04$
$b_2(i)-d_2(i)$	$7.00E-04$ $\pm 2.13E-04$	$2.10E-03$ $\pm 1.95E-04$	$2.40E-03$ $\pm 2.12E-04$	$2.70E-03$ $\pm 1.77E-04$
$\alpha_2(i)$	$1.42E-05$ $\pm 2.12E-06$	$7.39E-06$ $\pm 1.16E-06$	$1.48E-05$ $\pm 2.11E-06$	$1.20E-05$ $\pm 1.50E-06$
$b_3(i)$	$1.01E-01$ $\pm 9.55E-04$	$1.05E-01$ $\pm 4.39E-04$	$1.04E-01$ $\pm 6.81E-04$	$1.07E-01$ $\pm 2.70E-04$
$d_3(i)$	$8.16E-02$ $\pm 8.36E-04$	$7.90E-02$ $\pm 4.00E-04$	$7.99E-02$ $\pm 6.56E-04$	$8.02E-02$ $\pm 2.06E-04$
$b_3(i)-d_3(i)$	$2.48E-02$ $\pm 2.58E-04$	$2.69E-02$ $\pm 2.98E-04$	$2.74E-02$ $\pm 1.85E-04$	$2.98E-02$ $\pm 3.85E-04$
$\alpha_3(i)=\alpha_3$		$9.54E-06 \pm 2.51E-08$		

Notes:
$\lambda_{00} = 215.17 \pm 4.90$ $\qquad \lambda_{01} = 0.12 \pm 7.90E\text{-}03$
$b_{10} = 0.0592 \pm 0.0001$ $\qquad b_{11} = 0.0062 \pm 0.0001$
$d_{10} = 0.0615 \pm 0.0002$ $\qquad d_{11} = -0.0008 \pm 0.0001$
$\alpha_{10} = 5.82E\text{-}05 \pm 3.63E\text{-}06$ $\qquad \alpha_{11} = -0.01 \pm 0.02$
$b_{20} = 0.0814 \pm 0.0008$ $\qquad b_{21} = 0.0044 \pm 0.0003$
$d_{20} = 0.0862 \pm 0.0012$ $\qquad d_{21} = 0.0024 \pm 0.0005$
$\alpha_{20} = 3.30E\text{-}05 \pm 1.16E\text{-}05$ $\qquad \alpha_{21} = -0.30 \pm 0.18$
$b_{30} = 0.0265 \pm 0.0153$ $\qquad b_{31} = 0.0239 \pm 0.0057$
$d_{30} = 0.0752 \pm 0.0107$ $\qquad d_{31} = 0.0025 \pm 0.0040$

CHAPTER 5

SEMIPARAMETRIC METHODS FOR DATA FROM AN OUTCOME-DEPENDENT SAMPLING SCHEME

Haibo Zhou[a] and Jinhong You

Department of Biostatistics,
University of North Carolina at Chapel Hill,
Chapel Hill, NC 27599-7400, USA
E-mail: [a]zhou@bios.unc.edu

Outcome-dependent sampling (ODS) is a cost effective way to enhance study efficiency. The case-control design for binary outcomes is a mainstay of epidemiology research. As the field of epidemiology expanding and evolving, an increasing number of studies are conducted using the ODS design with a "continuous" outcome. In an ODS design, observations made on a judiciously chosen subset of the base population can provide nearly the same statistical efficiency as observing the entire base population. Different statistical inference procedures are needed in order to reap the benefits of such sampling. We review recently developed methods that account for the ODS design. These methods are all semiparametric approaches.

1. Introduction

Observational epidemiologic studies are to evaluate the relationship between an exposure and a disease, taking into account the effects of additional covariates such as age and sex. Cohort and `case-control` designs are the two most commonly used designs in such studies. In a cohort study, subjects are randomly selected from the population. The selection may or may not depend on covariates, but is independent of the response. In a case-control study, sampling is conditional on the response. Both designs allow one to evaluate the association between risk factors and disease. Some large cohort studies cost hundreds of millions of dollars to conduct. Case-control studies, on the other hand, are often preferred for rare diseases because they can yield an equal number of diseased individuals in a much smaller study. Since the work by Cornfield[1], the case-control method has become a fundamental statistical tool in epidemiologic studies because of its efficiency relative to the cohort study. An `outcome-dependent sampling` (ODS) scheme is a retrospective sampling scheme like the case-control study where one observes the exposure/covariates with a probability, maybe unknown, that depends on the outcome variable. The principal idea of an ODS design is to concentrate resources where there is the greatest amount of information. By allowing the selection probability of each individual in the ODS sample to depend on the outcome, the investigators attempt to enhance the efficiency and reduce the cost of the study.

Although the case-control design for binary outcomes is a mainstay of epidemiology research, an increasing number of studies are conducted using the ODS design with a "continuous" outcomes as the field of epidemiology expanding and evolving. In particular, analytical epidemiology investigations are often designed to characterize the study population, such as with respect to disease prevalence, and investigate the potential effect of an exposure on various health outcomes. Without a more appropriate method for handling the ODS with a continuous outcome, many investigators have chosen to analyze data using a dichotomized outcome that is defined based on whether the measurement is above or below a certain cutoff point (e.g. hypertension and neuro development abnormality). Drawbacks of dichotomizing or categorizing a continuous outcome include a loss of efficiency, an increased risk of misclassification bias, and a decrease in the external validity of the analysis since the results may be sensitive to the choice of cut point.

An example of using ODS design is a study from the Collaborative Perinatal Project (CPP) to access the relationship between maternal polychlorinated biphenyls (PCB) level and children's health development. The CPP is a propespectively designed study to provide precise data for studies of a wide variety of neurological outcome and birth detects[2]. Subjects were enrolled through 12 university affiliated medical clinics, with the centers contributing unequal numbers of subjects. In all, 55,908 pregnancies were registered, representing the experience of about 44,000 women. The study subjects are children who were born into the CPP. Eligible children met the following criteria: a) live born singleton, b) availability of a 3 ml third trimester maternal serum specimen, and c) non missing data for at least one of 8 specified study outcomes. Of the CPP children, 44,075 met all of the eligibility criteria. Since it was too expensive to assay the PCB exposure for the entire study population of 44,075 subjects, the investigators decided to obtain exposure measurements for an ODS from the population. In particular, in addition to taking an SRS from the entire population, they decided to oversample from the tails of the distributions about the children's health development indices such as the Weschler Intelligence Scale(IQ), hearing level, vision and birth defect, etc.

Likelihood based inference for data from an ODS scheme inevitably involves the distribution of covariates. Parametric modeling of a covariate distribution is not robust to model misspecification. Methods that do not require parametric modeling of the underlying distribution of covariates are desirable.

We discuss the recently developed methods that deal with various forms of data sets from ODS schemes. In particular, we consider (i) an overall SRS sample and several supplemental samples with continuous outcome (Section 2); (ii) an overall SRS sample, several supplemental samples and some information for the underlying population with continuous outcome (Section 3); (iii) an overall SRS sample, several supplemental samples with ordinal outcome and auxiliary covariate (Section 4); and (iv) an overall SRS sample, several supplemental samples and additional information for the underlying population with ordinal outcome (Section 5). These methods are all semiparametric in nature and include semiparametric empirical likelihood, semiparametric estimated likelihood, and semiparametric penalized spline estimated likelihood methods.

In Section 2, we discuss a semi-parametric approach for data from an ODS design with a continuous outcome. In Section 3, we discuss an estimated likelihood method when in addition to the ODS sample, information on the underlying population is available. In Section 4, we discuss application of ODS methods to an ordinal outcome. In Section 5, we review a penalized spine methods to deal with nonlinear problems in ODS design.

2. Semiparametric Empirical Likelihood for ODS with a Continuous Outcome Variable

This section considers semiparametric methods for dealing with ODS data with X observed on an overall SRS sample and several supplemental samples, and the outcome being continuous. In the CPP data structure, complete data are only available for 849 children from the SRS and for 189 children from the two supplemental samples. Specifically, there are 81 children with IQs less than or equal to 82 and 108 children with IQs greater than 110.

Empirical likelihood (EL) in its simplest form is just a nonparametric likelihood. Let $x_1, \ldots, x_n$ be i.i.d. observations from an unknown d-variate distribution F. The nonparametric likelihood is in fact maximized by the empirical CDF, $F_n(x) = \frac{1}{n} \sum_{i=1}^{n} I(X_i \leq x)$. Owen[3,4] introduced an empirical likelihood ratio statistic for nonparametric parameters. He showed that the statistic has a limiting chi-square distribution and how to obtain tests and confidence intervals for a parameter, expressed as functional $\theta(F)$. Many extensions and applications of empirical likelihood have been developed for biased sampling and censored data. See [5] for a comprehensive review. Zhou, *et al.*[15], Wang and Zhou[12] have applied the empirical likelihood to the problem of biased sampling (outcome dependent sampling). Vardi[10,11] and Qin[6] have discussed the biased sampling problem in the case of a completely known the weight function. When the weight function involves unknown parameters, one usually needs methods to combine the empirical likelihood with the parametric likelihood.

2.1. *Data Structure and Likelihood*

Zhou, *et al.*[15] proposed a semiparametric empirical likelihood to deal with the two component outcome dependent data set, in which there is an overall SRS sample and several supplemental samples. These supplemental samples are selected dependent on the outcome. The proposed semiparametric empirical likelihood can deal with the continuous outcome and does not make any assumption for the distribution of covariates.

Let Y denote the continuous outcome variable and X denote the vector of covariates. Assume that the domain of Y is a union of K mutually exclusive intervals: $C_k = (a_{k-1}, a_k], \quad k = 1, \ldots, K$ with $a_k, k = 0, 1, \ldots, K$ being known constants satisfying $a_0 = -\infty < a_1 < a_2 < \ldots < a_K = \infty$. The structure of the two component ODS sample consists an overall simple random sample (the SRS sample) and a simple sample from each of the K intervals of Y (the supplement samples). Let k be the index for intervals of Y and i be the individuals. Then the observed data structure is as follows: one observes the supplement sample $\{Y_{ki}, X_{ki} | Y_{ki} \in C_k\}$ where $k = 1, 2, \ldots, K$ and $i = 1, 2, \ldots, n_k$. The overall SRS sample is denoted by $\{Y_{0i}, X_{0i}\}$ where $i = 1, 2, \ldots, n_0$. For CPP data, in the sampling notation, we have that $a_1 = 82, a_2 = 110, n_0 = 849, n_1 = 81, n_2 = 0$ and $n_3 = 108$.

For the ease of the presentation, let G_X and g_X denote the cumulative distribution and density function of X, respectively. The joint likelihood function of the observed ODS data is

$$\mathcal{L}(\beta, G_X) = \prod_{i=1}^{n_0} f_\beta(Y_{0i}, X_{0i}) \prod_{k=1}^{K} \prod_{i=1}^{n_k} f_\beta(Y_{ki}, X_{ki} | Y_{ki} \in C_k).$$

By the Bayes' law, one can rewrite $\mathcal{L}(\beta, G_X)$ into

$$\mathcal{L}(\beta, G_X) = \left\{ \prod_{i=1}^{n_0} f_\beta(Y_{0i} | X_{0i}) \prod_{k=1}^{K} \prod_{i=1}^{n_k} \frac{f_\beta(Y_{ki} | X_{ki})}{Pr(Y_{ki} \in C_k | X_{ki})} \right\}$$
$$\cdot \left\{ \prod_{k=0}^{K} \prod_{i=1}^{n_k} g_X(X_{ki}) \prod_{k=1}^{K} \prod_{i=1}^{n_k} \frac{Pr(Y_{ki} \in C_k | X_{ki})}{Pr(Y_{ki} \in C_k)} \right\}$$
$$= \mathcal{L}_1(\beta) \times \mathcal{L}_2(\beta, G_X),$$

where

$$Pr(Y_{ki} \in C_k) = \int Pr(Y_{ki} \in C_k | x) g_X(x) dx.$$

Obviously, $\mathcal{L}(\beta)$ is the conditional likelihood function based on the observed ODS data. $\mathcal{L}(\beta, G_X)$ can be viewed as a marginal likelihood based on $(X_{01}, \ldots, X_{0n_0}, \ldots, X_{11}, \ldots, X_{1n_1}, \ldots, X_{Kn_K})$. For fixed β, this is an extension of the biased sampling likelihood as discussed by Vardi[10,11] and Qin[6].

2.2. *Algorithm and Asymptotics*

The semiparametric empirical likelihood estimation for β proposed by Zhou, et al[15] can be obtained as follows.

• First profile $\mathcal{L}_2(\beta, G_X)$ by fixing β and obtaining an empirical likelihood estimator $\hat{G}_X(\cdot)$, over all discrete distributions whose support contains the observed X values. This can be achieved by using the Lagrange multiplier method.

• The resulted profile likelihood function is $\mathcal{L}(\beta, \hat{G}_X)$.

• Use the Newton-Raphason procedure to maximize the resulted likelihood from $\mathcal{L}(\beta, \hat{G}_X)$.

They illustrate the above algorithm with a simple setting corresponding to a real study (the CPP in Zhou, *et al.*[15]).

$K = 3, n_2 = 0, n_1 > 0, n_3 > 0$ which corresponds to the Collaborative Perinatal Project. Denote $\pi_1 = F(a_1)$, $\pi_3 = 1 - F(a_2)$, $p_i = g_X(w_i)$, where $(w_1, \ldots, w_n) = (X_{01}, \ldots, X_{0n_0}, X_{11}, \ldots, X_{1n_1}, X_{31}, \ldots, X_{3n_3})$. Then, for a fixed β, one has

$$\mathcal{L}_2(\beta, \{p_{ki}\}) \infty \prod_{k=0}^{3} \prod_{i=1}^{n_k} p_{ki} \prod_{k=1}^{3} \pi_k^{-n_k}.$$

$\{\hat{p}_{ki}\}, k = 0, \ldots, K, i = 1, \ldots, n_k$ can be searched by maximizing $\mathcal{L}_2$ under the following constraints:

$$\left[\sum_{k=0}^{K} \sum_{i=1}^{n_k} p_{ki} = 1, \quad \sum_{k=0}^{K} \sum_{i=1}^{n_k} p_{ki} \{Pr(Y \in C_s | X_{ki}) - \pi_s\} = 0, s = 1, 3 \right]$$

where $p_{ki} \geq 0$. These constraints reflect the properties of $G_X(x)$ as a discrete distribution with support points at the observed X values. Using the Lagrange multiplier argument to derive the maximum over $\{p_{ki}\}$. Specifically, write

$$\mathcal{H} = \log \mathcal{L}_2(\beta, \{p_{ki}\}) + \rho \left(1 - \sum_{k=0}^{K} \sum_{i=1}^{n_k} p_{ki} \right)$$

$$-n \left[\lambda_1 \sum_{k=0}^{K} \sum_{i=1}^{n_k} p_{ki} \{Pr(Y \in C_1 | X_{ki}) - \pi_1\} \right]$$

$$-n \left[\lambda_3 \sum_{k=0}^{K} \sum_{i=1}^{n_k} p_{ki} \{Pr(Y \in C_3 | X_{ki}) - \pi_3\} \right]$$

where ρ and $(\lambda_1, \lambda_3)'$s are Lagrange multipliers. Take derivatives with respect to p_{ki}, and setting

$$\partial \mathcal{H} / \partial p_{ki} = 0 \quad \text{and} \quad \sum_{k=0}^{K} \sum_{i=1}^{n_k} p_{ki} \partial \mathcal{H} / \partial p_{ki} = 0,$$

one has

$$\rho = n, \, p_{ki} = \frac{1}{n} \cdot \frac{1}{1 + \lambda_1 \{Pr(Y \in C_1 | X_{ki}) - \pi_1\} + \lambda_3 \{Pr(Y \in C_3 | X_{ki}) - \pi_3\}},$$

with restriction

$$\sum_{k=0}^{K} \sum_{i=1}^{n_k} \frac{1}{n} \frac{Pr(Y \in C_j | X_{ki}) - \pi_j}{1 + \sum_{s=1}^{K-1} \lambda_s \{Pr(Y \in C_s | X_{ki}) - \pi_s\}} = 0, \quad \text{for} \quad j = 1, \ldots, K - 1.$$

where $n = n_0 + n_1 + n_3$. Let $\nu_1 = \lambda_1 - k_1/\pi_1$, $\nu_3 = \lambda_3 - k_3/\pi_3$, $k_i = n_i/n$, $i = 0, 1, 3$, $\eta = (\pi_1, \pi_3, \nu_1, \nu_3)$, $\xi' = (\beta', \eta')$. The log transformation of the resulting profile likelihood function has the form

$$l(\xi) = \log \mathcal{L}_1(\beta) + \log \mathcal{L}_2(\beta, \eta) = l_1(\beta) + l_2(\beta, \eta),$$

$$l_2(\beta, \eta) = -\sum_{i=1}^{n} \log\{1 + \nu' h(w_i)\} - \sum_{i=1}^{n} \log\{\Delta(w_i)\} - n_1 \log \pi_1 - n_3 \log \pi_3$$

$$+ \sum_{j=1}^{n_1} \log F(a_1|x_{1j}) + \sum_{k=1}^{n_3} \log\{1 - F(a_2|x_{3k})\}$$

where $h(w) = (h_1(w), h_3(w))$, $h_1 = \{F(a_1|w_i) - \pi_1\}/\Delta(w_i)$, $h_3 = \{1 - F(a_2|w_i) - \pi_3\}/\Delta(w_i)$ and $\Delta(w_i) = k_0 + \frac{k_1}{\pi_1} F(a_1|w_i) + \frac{k_3}{\pi_3}\{1 - F(a_2|w_i)\}$.

Let $\hat{\xi}$ be the maximizer for $l(\xi)$. Define

$$V_1(\beta) = \begin{pmatrix} I_1(\beta) & 0 \\ 0 & 0 \end{pmatrix}, \quad I_1(\beta) = -\frac{1}{n} E\{\partial^2 l_1/\partial \beta \partial \beta'\}$$

$$V_2(\xi) = k_0 Cov(e_0) + k_1 Cov(e_1) + k_3 Cov(e_3), \quad U(\xi) = -\frac{1}{n} E\{\partial^2 l(\xi)/\partial \xi \partial \xi'\},$$

where vectors e_0, e_1, e_3 are

$$e_{0i} = \begin{pmatrix} -\frac{1}{\Delta(x_{0i})} \frac{\partial \Delta(x_{0i})}{\partial \beta} \\ \frac{1}{\Delta(x_{0i})} \frac{k_1}{\pi_1^2} F(a_1|x_{0i}) \\ \frac{1}{\Delta(x_{0i})} \frac{k_3}{\pi_3^2} \bar{F}(a_2|x_{0i}) \\ -h(x_{0i}) \end{pmatrix}, \quad e_{1j} = \begin{pmatrix} \frac{1}{F(a_1|x_{1j})} \frac{\partial F(a_1|x_{1j})}{\partial \beta} - \frac{1}{\Delta(x_{1j})} \frac{\partial \Delta(x_{0j})}{\partial \beta} \\ \frac{1}{\Delta(x_{1j})} \frac{k_1}{\pi_1^2} F(a_1|x_{1j}) - \frac{1}{\pi_1} \\ \frac{1}{\Delta(x_{1j})} \frac{k_3}{\pi_3^2} \bar{F}(a_2|x_{1j}) \\ -h(x_{1j}) \end{pmatrix}$$

and

$$e_{3k} = \begin{pmatrix} \frac{1}{\bar{F}(a_2|x_{3k})} \frac{\partial \bar{F}(a_2|x_{3k})}{\partial \beta} - \frac{1}{\Delta(x_{3k})} \frac{\partial \Delta(x_{3k})}{\partial \beta} \\ \frac{1}{\Delta(x_{3k})} \frac{k_1}{\pi_1^2} F(a_1|x_{3k}) \\ \frac{1}{\Delta(x_{3k})} \frac{k_3}{\pi_3^2} \bar{F}(a_2|x_{3k}) - \frac{1}{\pi_3} \\ -h(x_{3k}) \end{pmatrix}.$$

The following theorem is due to Zhou, *et al.*[15].

Theorem 1: Under general regularity conditions, $n^{1/2}(\hat{\xi} - \xi_0) \to_D N(0, \Sigma(\xi_0))$ in a neighborhood of the true $\xi_0 = (\beta, \pi_1, \pi_2, 0, 0)'$, where $\to_D$ denotes convergence in distribution, $\Sigma(\xi_0) = U^{-1}(\xi_0) V(\xi_0) U^{-1}(\xi_0)$ and $V(\xi_0) = V_1(\xi_0) + V_2(\xi_0)$. A consistent estimator of the variance-covariance matrix is $\hat{U}^{-1}(\hat{\xi}) \hat{V}(\hat{\xi}) \hat{U}^{-1}(\hat{\xi})$, where $\hat{U}$ and $\hat{V}$ are obtained by replacing the large sample quantities in U and V with their corresponding small sample quantities.

3. Semiparametric Estimated Likelihood for Two-Stage ODS with a Continuous Outcome Variable

This section concerns statistical inference for ODS design where in addition to the complete data considered in Section 2, some information about the

rest of study cohort is also available. In CPP study, the additional information about various health outcomes for the 44,075 subjects is known.
Weaver and Zhou[14] considered statistical inference for a two-stage ODS
design where in addition to the ODS data considered by Zhou *et al.*[15] some
information is available for the underlying population. These information
includes IQ, SES (socioeconomic status of the child's family), EDU (the
mother's education), SEX (the gender of the child) and RACE (the race of
the child) (i.e., everything but PCB).

Assume Y partitions the study population into K strata such that for
$k = 1, \ldots, K$ the $\{Y \in C_k\}$ stratum has N_k individuals. The total sample
size in is $N = \sum_{k=1}^{K} N_k$. For each stratum $\{Y \in C_k\}$ of the first stage, one
selects an outcome-dependent validation subsample, denoted as V_k, of size
n_{V_k} such that individuals in V_k will have their true exposure variable X
observed besides their Y, while the remaining $n_{\bar{V}_k} = N_k - n_{V_k}$ individuals,
denoted as $\bar{V}_k$, have only their Y observed. For the $\{Y \in C_k\}$ stratum of
the study population, the date structure of two-stage sampling is

$$\text{The first stage:} \{Y_i\} \quad \text{for } i \in V_k + \bar{V}_k$$
$$\text{The second stage:} \{X_i | Y \in C_k\} \quad \text{for } i \in V_k$$

When data have been obtained through a two-stage design, it is easy
to see that conditional on the observed size $\{n_{\bar{V}_k}\}$, the observations in the
non-validation sample are independent of the observations in the validation
sample.

Using the Bayes formula, Weaver and Zhou[14] showed that the likelihood
for the second stage observations can be shown to be

$$\mathcal{L}_1(\beta) = \prod_{k=1}^{K} \prod_{i \in V_k} f_\beta(Y_i | X_i, Y_i \in C_k) g_X(X_i)$$
$$= \prod_{k=1}^{K} \prod_{i \in V_k} \frac{I(Y_i \in C_k) f_\beta(Y_i | X_i) g_X(X_i)}{E I(Y_i \in C_k)}$$
$$= \prod_{k=1}^{K} \prod_{i \in V_k} f_\beta(Y_i | X_i) g_X(X_i) \prod_{k=1}^{K} \{E I(Y_i \in C_k)\}^{-n_{V_k}}.$$

They derived the likelihood function based on all N observations, both with
complete and incomplete information. Conditional on the component sizes
of the ODS being fixed, the stratum sizes for the nonvalidation sample,

$n_{\bar{V}_k} = N_k - n_k$, $k = 1, \ldots, K$, follow a multinomial law such that

$$Pr(\{n_{\bar{V}_k}\}) = \frac{N}{\prod_{k=1}^{K} N_k!} \prod_{k=1}^{K} \{EI(Y_i \in C_k)\}^{N_k}.$$

Furthermore, the observations in the nonvalidation sample contribute the following terms to the full-information likelihood function,

$$\mathcal{L}_2(\beta) = \prod_{k=1}^{K} \prod_{j \in \bar{V}_k} f_\beta(Y_j) / \{EI(Y_i \in C_k)\}$$

where the quantity $f_\beta(Y_j) = \int f_\beta(Y_j|x) dG_X(x)$ is the contribution from a non-validation set member which involves an unspecified G_X.

Conditional on the observed size $n_{\bar{V}_k}$, the observations in the nonvalidation sample are independent of the observations in the validation sample, which contribute the terms in $\mathcal{L}_2$ to the full-information likelihood. Thus, after combining and simplifying these terms, the joint likelihood of the two-stage study can be written as

$$\mathcal{L}(\beta) = \prod_{k=1}^{K} \prod_{i \in V_k} f_\beta(Y_i|X_i) g_X(X_i) \prod_{k=1}^{K} \prod_{j \in \bar{V}_k} f_\beta(Y_j).$$

Obviously, direct maximization $\mathcal{L}(\beta)$ is not possible since G_X is unknown. Recognizing the distribution of X can be written as

$$G_X(x) = Pr(X \le x) = \sum_{k=1}^{K} Pr(X \le x | Y \in C_k) Pr(Y \in C_k),$$

therefore, a consistent estimator of $G(x)$ has the form

$$\hat{G}_X(x) = \sum_{k=1}^{K} \hat{G}_k(x) \frac{N_k}{N},$$

where $\hat{G}_k(x) = \sum_{i \in V_k} I(X_i \le x)/(n_k + n_{0,k})$. Accordingly, a weighted estimator for $f_\beta(Y_j)$ is

$$\hat{f}_\beta(Y_j) = \int f_\beta(Y_j|x) d\hat{G}_X(x) = \sum_{k=1}^{K} \sum_{i \in V_k} \frac{N_k}{(n_k + n_{0,k})N} f_\beta(Y_j|X_i).$$

Then the estimated log likelihood function has the form

$$\hat{\mathcal{L}}(\beta) = \sum_{i \in V} \log f_\beta(Y_i|X_i) + \sum_{j \in \bar{V}} \log \left\{ \sum_{k=1}^{K} \sum_{i \in V_k} \frac{N_k}{(n_k + n_{0,k})N} f_\beta(Y_j|X_i) \right\}.$$

The proposed estimator $\hat{\beta}$ is the solution to the score equation $\partial \hat{\mathcal{L}}(\beta)/\partial \beta = 0$. Estimates can be obtained by using the Newton-Raphson iterative procedure. The following theorem is due to Weaver and Zhou[14].

Theorem 2: Under some regularity conditions the proposed estimator $\hat{\beta}$ is asymptotic normally distributed. That is

$$\sqrt{N}(\hat{\beta} - \beta) \to_D N(0, \Omega) \quad \text{as } N \to \infty,$$

where

$$\Omega = I^{-1}(\beta) + \sum_{k=1}^{K} \frac{\pi_k^2}{\rho_k \rho_V + \pi_k \rho_0 \rho_V} I^{-1}(\beta) \Sigma_k(\beta) I^{-1}(\beta)$$

where

$$I(\beta) = -\rho_0 \rho_V E\left[\frac{\partial^2 \log f_\beta(Y|X)}{\partial \beta \partial \beta'}\right] - \sum_{k=1}^{K} \rho_k \rho_V E_k\left[\frac{\partial^2 \log f_\beta(Y|X)}{\partial \beta \partial \beta'}\right]$$
$$- \sum_{k=1}^{K} [\pi_k(1 - \rho_0 \rho_V) - \rho_k \rho_V] E_k\left[\frac{\partial^2 \log f_\beta(Y)}{\partial \beta \partial \beta'}\right]$$

$$\Sigma_k(\beta) = \text{Var}_{X|Y \in C_k}\left\{\sum_{k_1=1}^{K} [\pi_{k_1}(1 - \rho_0 \rho_V) - \rho_{k_1} \rho_V] E_{X|Y \in C_k}[\mathbf{M}_X(Y; \beta)]\right\}$$

and

$$\mathbf{M}_X(Y; \beta) = \frac{\partial f_\beta(Y|X)/\partial \beta}{\hat{f}_\beta(Y)} - \frac{\partial f_\beta(Y)/\partial \beta}{(\hat{f}_\beta(Y))^2} \times f_\beta(Y|X).$$

A consistent estimator for Ω can be constructed using sample quantities. Specifically, define

$$\hat{\Omega} = \hat{I}^{-1}(\hat{\beta}) + \sum_{k=1}^{K} \frac{(N_k/N)^2}{(n_k + n_{0,k})/N} \hat{I}^{-1}(\hat{\zeta}) \hat{\Sigma}_k(\hat{\zeta}) \hat{I}^{-1}(\hat{\beta}),$$

where

$$\hat{I}(\beta) = -\frac{1}{N} \frac{\partial^2 \hat{\mathcal{L}}(\beta)}{\partial \beta \partial \beta'}, \quad \hat{\Sigma}_k(\beta) = \hat{\text{Var}}_{(\mathbf{X}_i : i \in V_k)}\left\{\sum_{l=1}^{K} \frac{n_{\bar{V},k}}{N}\right\} \hat{\bar{M}}_{X_i,l}(\beta)$$

with

$$\hat{\bar{M}}_{X_i,l}(\beta) = \sum_{j \in \bar{V}_l}\left\{\frac{\frac{\partial f_\beta(Y_j|X_i)}{\partial \beta}}{\hat{f}_\beta(Y_j)} - \frac{f(Y_j|X_i)\frac{\partial f_\beta(Y_j)}{\partial \beta}}{\left[\hat{f}_\beta(Y_j)\right]^2}\right\} / n_{\bar{V},l}.$$

4. ODS with an Ordinal Outcome Variable and Auxiliary Covariate

In this section, we consider inference for ODS design with ordinal outcomes. For example, in CPP one ordinary outcome variable is preterm birth where preterm is defined as delivery that occurs before 37 completed weeks of gestation.

In this section, we will review some semiparametric methods for the ODS scheme in which the outcome variable is ordinal.

4.1. *Semiparametric Empirical Likelihood*

Wang and Zhou[12] extended the semiparametric empirical likelihood method developed by Zhou, *et al.*[15] to the case that there exists auxiliary covariate information. They focused on the ordinal outcome variable.

Let Y be a categorical disease outcome with possible values $1, \ldots, J$, and X be a vector of covariates, X be a vector of covariates, X can consist of either continuous or discrete variable. $f_\beta(Y|X)$ is the conditional density function of Y given X. Let W be an auxiliary covariate for X with possible values $1, \ldots, K$. Wang and Zhou[12] considered a sampling scheme in which the subsamples in the two-component study are observed from the K strata defined by W. From each of the strata $\{k : W = k\}$ in the study population, one observes a SRS subsample, denoted as V_{0k}, of size n_{0k}. In addition, one observes an ODS subsample from each of the strata $\{j, k : Y = j, W = k\}$ denoted as V_{jk}, having sizes $n_{1,k}, \ldots, n_{jk}$, respectively. Then the likelihood of the two-component study with auxiliary information is

$$\mathcal{L} = \prod_{k=1}^{K} \prod_{i \in V_{0k}} f_\beta(Y_i|X_i) dG(X_i|W_i = k) \prod_{k=1}^{K}$$
$$\cdot \prod_{j=1}^{J} \frac{Pr(Y_i = j|X_i)}{Pr(Y_i = j|W_i = k)} dG(X_i|W_i = k)$$

where $G(x|w)$ is the cumulative distribution of X given W. Because of the constraint $Pr(Y_i = j|w) = \int Pr(Y = j|x) dG(x|w)$, the above likelihood involves $G(x|w)$.

For ease of presentation, Wang and Zhou[12] considered the case of a binary outcome. Let Y be a binary disease outcome with 1 for the positive outcome and 2 for the negative outcome. Without losing generality, let $W = 1, 2 (K = 2)$ be a binary auxiliary covariate. Define $V_k = \cup_{j=0}^{2} V_{jk}$ with size $n_k = \sum_{j=0}^{2} n_{jk}$ and $V = \cup_{k=1}^{2} V_k$ with the total study size $n = \sum_{k=1}^{2} n_k$,

$\pi_{jk} = Pr(Y = j|w = k)$. Then the logarithm transformation of the resulted profile likelihood function has the form

$$l(\xi) = \log \mathcal{L}_1(\beta) + \log \mathcal{L}_2(\beta, \eta) = l_1(\beta) + l_2(\beta, \eta),$$

where

$$\log \mathcal{L}_1(\beta) = \sum_{i \in V} \log f_\beta(Y_i|X_i),$$

$$\mathcal{L}_2(\beta, \eta) = -\sum_{k=1}^{2} \sum_{i \in V_k} \log S_k(X_i) - \sum_{k=1}^{2} \sum_{j=1}^{2} n_{jk} \log \pi_{jk} - \sum_{k=1}^{2} \sum_{i \in V_k} \log\{1 + \nu_k h_k(X_i)\}$$

where

$$S_k(X_i) = \frac{n_{0k}}{n_k} + \frac{n_{1k}/n_k}{\pi_{1k}} Pr(Y = 1|X_i) + \frac{n_{2k}/n_k}{1 - \pi_{1k}} P(Y + 2|X_i),$$

$$h_k(X_i) = \frac{Pr(Y = 1|X_i) - \pi_{1k}}{S_k(X_i)} \quad \text{and} \quad \nu_k = \lambda_k - \frac{n_{1k}/n_k}{\pi_{1k}} + \frac{n_{2k}/n_k}{1 - \pi_{1k}}.$$

Let $\hat{\xi}$ be the maximizer for $l(\xi)$. Denote

$$V(\xi^0) = \sum_{k=1}^{k} \rho_k \sum_{j=1}^{2} \rho_{jk} \left\{ \int m_{jk}(x, y, \xi)^{\otimes 2} w_{jk}(x, \xi) dy dG_k(x) \right.$$

$$\left. - \left(\int m_{jk}(x, y, \xi) w_{jk}(x, xi) dy dG_k(x) \right)^{\otimes 2} \right\}$$

$$U(\xi) = -\frac{1}{n} E\{\partial^2 l(\xi)/\partial \xi \partial \xi'\},$$

where $a^{\otimes 2} = aa'$, $\rho_k = n_k/n$ and $\rho_{jk} = n_{jk}/n_k$ as $n \to \infty$, $w_{0k}(x, \xi) = 1$, $w_{1k}(x, \xi) = Pr(Y = 1|X)/\pi_{1k}$ and $w_{2k} = Pr(Y = 2|X)/(1 - \pi_{1k})$,

$$m_{jk}(x, y, \xi) = \begin{pmatrix} \frac{\partial \log f_\beta(y|x)}{\partial \beta} - \frac{\partial S_k(x)/\partial \beta}{S_k(x)} - \frac{\nu_k \partial h_k(x)/\partial \beta}{1 + \nu_k h_k(x)} \\ d_{jk} - \frac{\partial S_k(x)/\partial \pi_{1k}}{S_k(x)} - \frac{\nu_k \partial h_k(x)/\partial \pi_{1k}}{1 + \nu_k h_k(x)} \\ -\frac{h_k(x)}{1 + \nu_k h_k(x)} \end{pmatrix}$$

with $d_{0k} = 0, d_{1k} = -1/\pi_{1k}$ and $d_{2k} = 1/(1 - \pi_{1k})$.

The following theorem is due to Wang and Zhou[12].

Theorem 3: Under general regularity conditions, $n^{1/2}(\hat{\xi} - \xi_0) \to_D N(0, \Sigma(\xi_0))$ in a neighborhood of the true $\xi_0 = (\beta, \pi_{11}, \pi_{12}, \pi_{21}, \pi_{22}, 0, 0)'$, where $\Sigma(\xi^0) = U^{-1}(\xi^0)V(\xi^0)U^{-1}(\xi^0)$. A consistent estimator of the variance-covariance matrix is $\hat{U}^{-1}(\hat{\xi})\hat{V}(\hat{\xi})\hat{U}^{-1}(\hat{\xi})$, where $\hat{U}$ and $\hat{V}$ are obtained by replacing the large sample quantities in U and V with their corresponding small sample quantities.

4.2. *Semiparametric Estimated Likelihood*

Wang and Zhou[12] extended the semiparametric estimated likelihood method to allow some components of the covariate vector to be observed for each individual in the population and there exists auxiliary information for unobserved exposure variables. Especially, let $\{X, Z\}$ be the vector of modeling covariates, where X is an exposure variable that is observed only when an individual is selected into the second stage and Z is a vector of additional covariates that are always observed. In addition, let W be a discrete or continuous variable, which contains auxiliary information for X. Wang and Zhou[13] considered a two-stage design in which the subsample selection depends on both the outcome Y and a discrete variable C. Let C be a discrete variable with L levels defined on the auxiliary covariate W; $C = h$ if $W \in (c_{l-1}, c_l]$ for $l = 1, \ldots, L$. The lth interval, $(c_{l-1}, c_l]$, is defined by a pair of ordered real values where $c_0 = -\infty$ and $c_L = \infty$. They assumed $Y \times C$ partitions the study cohort into a total $K \times H$ strata such that the stratum $\{Y = k, C = l\}$ contains N_{kl} subjects. The total sample size in is $N = \sum_{k=1}^{K} \sum_{l=1}^{L} N_{kl}$. For each stratum $\{Y = k, C = l\}$ of the first stage, one selects an outcome-dependent validation subsample, denoted as V_{kl}, of size $n_{V_{kl}}$ such that individuals in V_{kl} will have their true exposure variable X observed besides their Y and W, while the remaining $n_{\bar{V}_{kl}} = N_{kl} - n_{V_{kl}}$ individuals, denoted as $\bar{V}_{kl}$, have only their Y and W observed. For the $\{Y = k, C = l\}$ stratum of the study population, the date structure of two-stage sampling is

The first stage: $\{Y_i, Z_i, W_i\}$ for $i \in V_{kl} + \bar{V}_{kl}$

The second stage: $\{X_i, Z_i, W_i | Y = k, C = l\}$ for $i \in V_{kl}$

By the same argument as in last section, after combining and simplifying these terms, the joint likelihood of the two-stage study can be written as

$$\mathcal{L}(\beta) = \prod_{k=1}^{K} \prod_{l=1}^{L} \prod_{i \in V_{kl}} f_\beta(Y_i | X_i, Z_i) g(X_i | Z_i, W_i) \prod_{k=1}^{K} \prod_{l=1}^{L} \prod_{j \in \bar{V}_{kl}} f_\beta(Y_j | Z_j, W_j).$$

Obviously, direct maximization $\mathcal{L}(\beta)$ is not possible. Note that some components of (Z, W) may be uninformative with respect to the distribution of

X. Let S denote the informative components of (W, Z), in the sense that $G(X|Z, W) = G(X|S)$ almost surely. Recognizing

$$G(x|s) = \sum_{k=1}^{K} \sum_{l=1}^{L} \pi_{kl}(s) G_{kl}(x|s),$$

where

$$\pi_{kl}(s) = Pr(Y = k, C = l|s) \quad \text{and} \quad G_{kl}(x|s) = G(x|s, Y = k, C = l).$$

Further, a kernel estimator of $\pi_{kl}(s)$ is given by

$$\hat{\pi}_{kl}(s) = \frac{\sum_{i=1}^{N} I(Y_i = k, C_i = l) K_h(S_i - s)}{\sum_{i=1}^{N} K_h(S_i - s)}$$

and a kernel estimator of $G_{kl}(x|s)$ is given by

$$\hat{G}_{kl}(x|s) = \frac{\sum_{i \in V_{sl}} I(X_i \leq x) K_h(S_i - s)}{\sum_{i \in V_{sl}} K_h(S_i - s)}$$

where $K_h(\cdot) = K(\cdot/h)/h$ and h is the bandwidth. Then one can construct a weighted kernel-based empirical distribution estimator for $G(x|s)$,

$$\hat{G}(x|s) = \sum_{l=1}^{L} \sum_{k=1}^{K} \hat{\pi}_{lk}(s) \hat{G}_{lk}(x|s).$$

Accordingly, a weighted estimator for $f_\beta(Y_j|Z_j, W_j)$ is

$$\hat{f}_\beta(Y_j|Z_j, W_j) = \int f_\beta(Y_j|x, Z_j) d \left\{ \sum_{k=1}^{K} \sum_{l=1}^{L} \hat{\pi}_{kl}(S_j) \hat{G}_{kl}(x|S_j) \right\}.$$

Then the estimated log likelihood function has the form

$$\hat{\mathcal{L}}(\beta) = \sum_{k=1}^{K} \sum_{l=1}^{L} \sum_{i \in V_{kl}} \log f_\beta(Y_i|X_i, Z_i) + \sum_{k=1}^{K} \sum_{l=1}^{L} \sum_{j \in \bar{V}_{kl}} \log \hat{f}_\beta(Y_j|Z_j, W_j).$$

The proposed estimator $\hat{\beta}$ is the solution to the score equation $\partial \hat{\mathcal{L}}(\beta)/\partial \beta = 0$. The following theorem is due to Wang and Zhou[13].

Theorem 4: Under some regularity conditions $\hat{\beta}$ is asymptotically normal, that is $\sqrt{N}(\hat{\beta} - \beta) \to_D N(0, \Omega)$ as $N \to \infty$ where

$$\Omega = I^{-1}(\beta) + \sum_{k=1}^{K} \sum_{l=1}^{L} \frac{\pi_{kl}^2}{\psi_{kl}} I^{-1}(\beta) \Sigma_{kl}(\beta) I^{-1}(\beta),$$

where

$$I(\beta) = -\sum_{k=1}^{K}\sum_{l=1}^{L}\left\{\psi_{kl}E_{kl}\left[\frac{\partial^2 \log f_\beta(Y|X,Z)}{\partial\beta\partial\beta'}\right]\right.$$
$$\left.+(\pi_{kl}-\psi_{kl})E_{kl}\left[\frac{\partial^2 \log f_\beta(Y|Z,W)}{\partial\beta\partial\beta'}\right]\right\}$$

$$\Sigma_{kl}(\beta) = \text{Var}_{X,Z,W|Y\in C_k,W\in B_l}$$
$$\cdot\left\{\sum_{k_1=1}^{K}\sum_{l_1=1}^{L}\left(1-\frac{\psi_{k_1l_1}}{\pi_{k_1l_1}}\right)\pi_{k_1l_1}(W_i)E_{Y|Y\in C_k,W\in B_l}\left\{M_{X,Z,W}(Y)\right\}\right\}$$

and

$$\mathbf{M}_{X,Z,W}(Y) = \frac{\partial f_\beta(Y|X,Z)/\partial\beta}{\hat{f}_\beta(Y|Z,W)} - \frac{\partial f_\beta(Y|Z,W)/\partial\beta}{\{\hat{f}_\beta(Y|Z,W)\}^2}\times f_\beta(Y|X,Z).$$

By the same argument as in last section, one can construct a consistent estimator for Σ.

5. Penalized Spline Estimated Likelihood

In this section, we consider nonlinear covariate effects in the ODS designs. Most of the the results for ODS regression analysis are established in the setting of linear regression. While in some applications, parametric models are adequate to capture the underlying relationships between the response variables and the associated covariates, most of the time they are chosen simply for their convenience. For example, Zhou, You and Longnecker[16] found that the relationship between IQ and EDU may be not linear. In this section, we review the partially linear regression analysis for a two-stage outcome dependent sample in which one allow the relationship between the response and exposure variable to be unspecified[16,7]. By combining the penalized splines[8] and the estimated maximum likelihood[14,16] proposed a penalized spline maximum likelihood estimation (PSMLE) for the parametric and nonparametric components of a partially linear regression model under the population based two component ODS sampling scheme.

Assume that the conditional density of Y_i given $\{X_i, Z_i\}$ belongs to a canonical exponential family, i.e.,

$$f_{\alpha(\cdot),\beta}(Y_i|X_i,Z_i) = \exp\{[Y_i\eta_i - b(\eta_i)]/a(\phi) + c(Y_i,\phi)\},$$

where $a(\cdot)$, $b(\cdot)$ and $c(\cdot,\cdot)$ are all known functions, ϕ is a dispersion parameter and η_i is related to the X_i and Z_i by

$$\eta_i = \alpha(X_i) + \beta'Z_i.$$

where $\alpha(\cdot)$ is an unknown function. Similar to Section 3 we can construct an estimated log likelihood for (Y_i, X_i, Z_i) which has the form:

$$\hat{\mathcal{L}}(\alpha(\cdot), \beta) = \sum_{k=1}^{K} \sum_{i \in V_k} \log f_{\alpha(\cdot), \beta}(Y_i | X_i, Z_i) + \sum_{k=1}^{K} \sum_{j \in \bar{V}_k} \log \hat{f}_{\alpha(\cdot), \beta}(Y_j | Z_j).$$

The unknown univariate function $\alpha(\cdot)$ can be estimated by a penalized spline[8,9]. Assume that

$$\alpha(x) = \delta_0 + \delta_1 x + \ldots + \delta_m x^m + \sum_{k=1}^{\kappa} \delta_{m+k} (x - \vartheta_k)_+^m,$$

where $\{\vartheta_k\}_{k=1}^{\kappa}$ are spline knots. Define the spline coefficient vector $\delta = (\delta_0, \delta_1, \ldots, \delta_{m+\kappa})'$ and spline basis

$$B(z) = (1, z, \ldots, z^m, (z - \vartheta_1)_+^m, \ldots, (z - \vartheta_\kappa)_+^m).$$

the spline model is $\alpha(z) = \delta' B(z)$. The PSMLE of $(\beta', \delta')'$ is defined as $(\hat{\beta}', \hat{\delta}')'$ that minimizes

$$Q_{\lambda, N}(\beta, \delta) = \hat{\mathcal{L}}(\beta, \delta) + \lambda \delta' D \delta$$

where $\lambda \geq 0$ is a penalty parameter, D is an appropriate positive semi-definite symmetric matrix such that

$$\delta' D \delta = \int_{\min(X_i)}^{\max(X_i)} [\alpha''(x)]^2 dx,$$

which yields the usual quadratic integral penalty (Ruppert 2002),

$$\hat{\mathcal{L}}(\beta, \delta) = \sum_{k=1}^{K} \sum_{i \in V_k} \log f_{\delta, \beta}(Y_i | X_i, Z_i) + \sum_{k=1}^{K} \sum_{j \in \bar{V}_k} \log \hat{f}_{\delta, \beta}(Y_j | Z_j).$$

The proposed estimator $\hat{\zeta} = (\hat{\beta}', \hat{\delta}')'$ of $\zeta = (\beta', \delta')'$ is the solution to the score equation $\partial \hat{\mathcal{L}}(\beta, \delta) / \partial \zeta = 0$. Estimates can be obtained by using the Newton-Raphson iterative procedure.

The asymptotic property of the proposed estimator $\hat{\zeta}$ is summarized in the following theorem (see [16]).

Theorem 5: Under some regularity conditions and $\lambda_N = o(N^{-1})$, $\hat{\zeta}$ is asymptotically normal, that is $\sqrt{N}(\hat{\zeta} - \zeta) \to_D N(0, \Omega)$ as $N \to \infty$, where Ω has the same form as in Theorem 3.

6. Concluding

In this paper, we have reviewed several recently developed statistical modeling procedures for data from an ODS scheme. These procedures include semiparametric empirical likelihood and semiparametric estimated likelihood. Semiparametric empirical likelihood can be used to deal with the ODS scheme with an overall SRS sample and several supplemental samples and the semiparametric estimated likelihood can be used to deal with the ODS scheme with an overall SRS sample, several supplemental samples and some information for the underlying population. These are robust methods as they do not require parametric modeling of the underlying distribution of covariates. Generally, an ODS design, coupled with an appropriate analysis, can be a powerful alternative to commonly used sampling scheme.

A complexity in practical studies often involves the cluster- or center-effects of the study subjects. In this situation a random effects model is often used since it allows the investigators to interpret their results beyond the limited participating centers. Zhou, You and Longnecker[16] has extended the semiparametric empirical likelihood method developed by Zhou, *et al.*[15] to the setting with center-effects. However, there are no results for other two semiparametric methods.

Another important case is that the response may be multivariate. An example is the Collaborative Perinatal Project (CPP) about the study of left and right hearing level. When the response is multivariate, extending the above work to multiple responses is still an open problem.

Acknowledgments

This research is supported by a grant from National Institute of Health (CA 79949)

References

1. J. Cornfield, A method of estimating comparative rates from clinical data, Applications to cancer of lung, breast, and cervix, *Journal of National Cancer Institute*, **11** (1951), 1269-1275.
2. M.P. Longnecker, M.A. Klebanoff, H. Zhou, and J.W. Brock, Maternal serum level of the DDT metabolite DDE is associated with premature and small-for-gestational-age birth, *Lancet*, **358** (2001), 110-114.
3. A.B. Owen, Empirical likelihood ratio confidence intervals for a single functional, *Biometrika*, **74** (1988), 237-249.
4. A.B. Owen, Empirical likelihood for confidence regions, *Ann. Statist.*, **18** (1990), 90-120.

5. J.F. Lawless, J.D. Kalbfleisch, and C.J. Wild, Semiparametric Methods for Response-selective and missing data problems in regression, *Journal of the Royal Statistical Society, B*, **61** (1999), 413-438.

6. J. Qin, Empirical likelihood in biased sample problems, *Ann. Statist.*, **21** (1993), 1182-1196.

7. H. Zhou and M. Weaver, Outcome-dependent selection models, *Encyclopedia of Enviornmetrics*, **3** (2001), 1499-1502.

8. D. Ruppert and R. Carroll, Spatially-adaptive penalties for spline fitting, *Austr. and New Zeal. J. Statist.*, **42** (2000), 205-223.

9. D. Ruppert, Selecting the number of knots for penalized splines, *J. Comput. Graph. Statist.*, **11** (2002), 735-757.

10. Y. Vardi, Nonparametric estimation in presence of length bias, *Ann. Statist.*, **10** (1982), 616-620.

11. Y. Vardi, Empirical distribution in selection bias models, *Ann. Statist.*, **13** (1985), 178-203. (With discussion by C. L. Mallows.)

12. X. Wang and H. Zhou, A Semiparametric Empirical Likelihood Method For Biased Sampling Schemes In Epidemiologic Studies With Auxiliary Covariates, *Biometrics*, **62** (2006), 1149-1160.

13. X. Wang and H. Zhou, Analysis of Epidemiologic Studies With Outcome-Dependent Subsample Using A Weighted Estimated Likelihood Method, manuscript, 2006.

14. M.A. Weaver and H. Zhou, An Estimated Likelihood Method for Continuous Outcome Regression Models with Outcome-Dependent Subsampling, *J. Amer. Statist. Assoc.*, **100** (2005), 459-469.

15. H. Zhou, M.A. Weaver, J. Qin, M.P. Longnecker, and M.C. Wang, A semiparametric empirical likelihood method for data from an outcome-dependent sampling design with a continuous outcome, *Biometrics*, **58** (2002), 413-421.

16. H. Zhou, J. You and M. Longnecker, A partially linear regression model for data from an outcome-dependent sampling. *Biometrics*, **x** (2007), to appear.

UNIT II

PROTEOMICS AND GENOMICS

CHAPTER 6

AUTOMATED PEAK IDENTIFICATION IN A TOF-MS SPECTRUM

Haijian Chen[a], Eugene R. Tracy[a], William E. Cooke[a],
O. John Semmes[b], Maciek Sasinowski[c] and Dennis M. Manos[a]

[a] *Department of Physics, College of William and Mary, Williamsburg, VA, USA*
[b] *Department of Microbiology and Molecular Cell Biology,*
Eastern Virginia Medical School, Norfolk, VA, USA
[c] *INCOGEN, Inc., Williamsburg, VA, USA*

The high throughput capabilities of protein mass fingerprints measurements have made mass spectrometry one of the standard tools for proteomic research, such as biomarker discovery. However, the analysis of large raw data sets produced by the time-of-flight (TOF) spectrometers creates a bottleneck in the discovery process. One specific challenge is the preprocessing and identification of mass peaks corresponding to important biological molecules. The accuracy of mass assignment is another limitation when comparing mass fingerprints with databases. Under survey conditions, where the positions of the desired mass peaks are not known beforehand, a TOF instrument requires a peak-picking procedure to distinguish mass peaks from a slowly varying background. We have developed an automated peak identification algorithm based on a maximum likelihood approach that effectively and efficiently detects peaks in a TOF spectrum. This approach produces maximum likelihood estimates of peak positions and intensities, and simultaneously develops estimates of the uncertainties in each of these quantities. Shifts in arrival time of the same peak in different spectra have been observed. Using the quantities from this peak detection procedure, different spectra can be brought into alignment.

1. Introduction

Though great success has been made in genome sequencing, it has been increasingly recognized that the genome, by itself, is not sufficient to understand the behavior and functions of cells, tissues, and biological systems. A current research focus in molecular biology is to test the hypothesis that proteins, instead of DNA, give more complete information related to cell function. Hence, proteins, the final product of genes, are receiving increased attention and a new field, proteomics, which focuses on protein characterization, protein identification and protein function, has emerged.

Although two-dimensional gel electrophoresis and amino acid sequencing, which have been in use for decades, retain their important roles in biochemical analysis, recent developments in **mass spectrometry** (MS) have now made it an additional analytical tool in proteome research[1,2]. Mass spectrometry can give accurate mass "fingerprints" which, in conjunction with protein database searching, can rapidly provide information about protein identification, protein function and protein post-translational modification (*i.e.*, modifications after the polypeptide is synthesized).

In protein identification, matrix assisted laser desorption/ionization mass spectrometry (MALDI-MS) and electrospray ionization mass spectrometry (ESI-MS) are often used because they can ionize large biological molecules 'softly' without breaking most of them into smaller pieces.

To identify proteins, proteins are often digested by a protease such as trypsin into peptides and mass fingerprints of the resulting peptides are often measured by MALDI. The mass fingerprints of these peptides are then compared with tryptic peptide masses that are theoretically generated from protein sequence databases using programs such as Sequest or Mascot. These programs use sophisticated scoring algorithms to evaluate the degree of match between the theoretically predicted mass spectra and the experimentally generated spectra.

The high throughput, high sensitivity and quantitative analysis of mass spectrometry make it possible to analyze hundreds of analytes over a large mass range simultaneously even if the sample volume is small. If a biological fluid, such as blood, is measured, a protein "profile" may be developed. This leads to the potential for finding biomarkers that are overexpressed or underexpressed or modified. Such biomarkers can then be used to differentiate pathological states (disease) from normal states or to assess and guide drug treatments. If desired, the discovered biomarker can be chemically extracted for further analysis. Progress has been made with this line of cancer research as summarized in [3, 4, 5, 6, 7, 8].

All information that mass spectrometry provides is encoded by peaks that occur at different masses with various intensities in the spectrum. The number of peaks present varies with the sample under investigation and the type of mass spectrometer used. If biological or organic samples are investigated, the peak number can easily rise to a few hundred. In blood serum, it is estimated that there may be up to 10,000 proteins with concentrations ranging over at least 9 orders of magnitude[9,10]. However, the dynamic range of MS instruments is only 3∼ 4 orders of magnitude[11], thus careful biochemical sample preparation is critical. As more effort has been devoted to improving the performance of MS instruments to provide more detailed information about the sample, to increase resolving power, and to lower the detection limit, the resulting mass spectra have inevitably become more complicated. Very often, as in the biomarker discovery for disease detection, it is not clear beforehand which peak is important. Thus as many peaks as possible must be detected and characterized. This is also true for protein identification. Compounding the problem of dense data sets, roboticized sample preparation and computerized data collection allow researchers to generate dozens, or hundreds, of such spectra in a few hours.

The analysis of such large raw data sets produced by survey mass spectrometers creates a bottleneck in the research process. To overcome this bottleneck, the first step is to simplify a spectrum that contains thousands, even millions, of data points down to only the essential information about peaks, *i.e.*, positions and intensities. In this way, a spectrum can be reduced to only a few hundreds points that represent peak positions, intensities and uncertainties in the peak positions and intensities.

We should emphasize that not only mass spectrometry faces this peak detection problem. In fact, peak identification is a quite general problem in many analytical instruments. A good automated peak detection procedure should run rapidly, and give repeatable and accurate results. It should find all significant peaks in a spectrum but not report false peaks. For some biological samples, the concentration is very small and the spectrum has a low signal-to-noise ratio, hence finding peaks is difficult. Missing peaks in a spectrum, and reporting false peaks, can both potentially lead to discovery of false "biomarkers." This could lead to wasted further investment, which could potentially be costly and time consuming.

A good peak detector should give accurate peak position assignments and peak intensity estimations. The importance of accuracy in peak position is obvious, it has significant influence on the database searching results. Accurate peak intensity estimations are also important when quantitative analysis is required. For example, when looking for proteins that are associated with disease, it is very possible that the proteins we are looking for are common in both healthy and sick people but are overexpressed or underexpressed. In this case, it is not a "yes or no" problem, but rather a "more or less" problem, and the correct peak intensity estimation is essential.

Another important factor is that the full peak identification procedure should be automated as much as possible for high-throughput data handling. An additional advantage of an automated peak detection algorithm is that it minimizes human interaction and thus eliminates potential bias introduced by investigators. It has been reported that in an inter-laboratory investigation conducted by the NIST, the same samples were analyzed by MALDI in different laboratories. It turned out that when comparing experimental results from different laboratories, the reduced data showed more differences than the raw data in some cases. The differences in the reduced data were traced back to detailed decisions that investigators made when the data were reduced[12,13]. This result highlights the need for adoption of common, well tested and well understood, automated methods to avoid *ad hoc* methods developed in each research group.

During the past few years, various algorithms have been developed for peak detection. For example, Bryant *et al.* find peaks by cross-correlating the spectrum with a predefined peak lineshape[14]; Gras *et al.* find peaks in a spectrum by comparing a segment of the spectrum with a template which describes the peak shape and isotopic pattern[15].

While the above methods require knowledge about the peak lineshape, Wallace *et al.* have developed an algorithm based on iterative segmentation that makes no assumption about peak shape and does not need to smooth the data before peak detection[12]. Another peak detection algorithm that does not depend on the peak shape is due to Jarman *et al.*[16] In their approach, a spectrum is viewed as a histogram. In regions where there is no peak, the spectrum is relatively flat and the intensity varies around a constant. Hence, it can be viewed as a histogram for a noisy uniform distribution. Deviation from this distribution will be considered evidence of peak presence.

Efforts have also been made to smooth the spectrum to increase the signal-to-noise ratio before attempting peak detection. For example, Morris *et al.* developed an algorithm to detect peaks based on the mean spectrum of the spectra from an ensemble of similar samples[17]. By averaging spectra of similar samples, the noise is reduced. The mean spectrum can be further smoothed by wavelet denoising.

Though all of the above peak identification procedures proposed reasonable ways for finding peaks in a spectrum, none of them addresses the confidence level in peak position and intensity assignments. Because of the noise in the spectrum, there are always **uncertainties** associated with the estimates made. These uncertainties represent the confidence level about the peak position and intensity assignments and occur in addition to the instrument precision. A peak detection procedure that leads to a low peak position confidence level would degrade the instrument performance that researchers spent vast amounts of money and effort to improve.

When a peak is detected in a spectrum and compared with a database, it is very rare to find an exact match. It is almost certain that a search will return a list of possible chemical IDs around the detected peak. Knowing the position uncertainty will help us to determine how many possible chemical IDs we should seriously consider. The position uncertainty would also help to determine whether peaks that appear at slightly different positions in different spectra are in fact the same, which is a crucial step in disease associated biomarker discovery where comparison among a large number of spectra is involved.

To summarize, what we want is an automated peak detection procedure which gives best estimates of peak positions and peak intensities along with their uncertainty estimates.

2. Methodology

2.1. *Understanding TOF-MS*

Since the goal here is to develop an algorithm that detects peaks in a TOF-MS spectrum accurately and efficiently, it is important to understand the nature of mass spectrometry.

Mass spectrometry was started by J. J. Thomson, Physics Nobel laureate of 1906, the discoverer of the electron. Since then, mass spectrometry has become one the most useful tools in scientific research. A mass spectrometer differentiates different molecular/atomic ions, which are generated from the sample under investigation, according to their `mass-to-charge ratio` (m/z). It can also give information about the abundance of each species in the sample.

Roughly speaking, a mass spectrometer consists of three important components: ion source, mass analyzer and ion detector. The ion source generates ions from the sample; the mass analyzer separates ions based on their mass-to-charge ratio; the detector records the separated ions.

"`Time-of-Flight`" refers to the way that ions are separated, *i.e.*, the mass analyzer. The concept of a TOF mass analyzer is quite simple. Ions start with the same kinetic energy, *e.g.*, after falling through a fixed electrostatic field Φ, fly through a field-free tube, usually in vacuum, towards an ion detector at the end of the tube. It is easily shown that the time that

ions of charge Ze take to fly through the tube of length D is proportional
to the square root of mass:

$$E_k = Ze\Phi = \frac{1}{2}mv^2; \quad v = \left(\frac{2Ze\Phi}{m}\right)^{\frac{1}{2}}. \tag{1}$$

Using $vt = D$, we find:

$$t = \left(\frac{m}{2Ze\Phi}\right)^{\frac{1}{2}} D. \tag{2}$$

Modern ionization methods like laser desorption ionization (LDI), ESI,
etc., enable ions to be generated efficiently from liquid or solid samples. The
consequences are that increasingly heavier ions like peptides and proteins
can now be generated from a very small amount of sample. For example,
it has been reported that MALDI may achieve a detection limit as low as
zeptomoles $(10^{-21}$ mol)[18]. Together with fast electronics that can work at
nanosecond or sub-nanosecond sample rates to record the mass spectrum,
this has led to rapid developments in instrumentation and applications of
TOF-MS. It is now widely used in chemistry, biochemistry, biology and
biomedical science.

Ideally, ions of a specific m/z would hit the detector after the same time
of flight, resulting in a sharp peak lineshape like a delta function of certain
height. In reality, however, because of the finite time during which the
energy source acts on the sample, sample surface morphology and complex
physical and chemical reactions that occur when energy is deposited onto
the sample, ions of the same m/z are formed at different times and positions
according to some initial time distribution and spatial distribution. They
also come off the sample surface with an initial velocity distribution of finite
width. Though there are ion optics strategies that attempt to correct for
these effects, such as time-lag extraction or reflectrons, ions still enter the
free drift region with velocity and time distributions of finite width, which
results in a finite peak width for ions of a specific m/z. We refer to the sum
of total ions of a given mass peak (integrated intensity) as the intensity of
that peak.

Very often, in a TOF instrument, such as MALDI-MS and secondary ion
mass spectrometry (SIMS), laser/primary ions which are very well focused
can be rastered over the sample surface for a number of irradiations in a
certain pattern. For each irradiation, only a small portion of the scanned

area is irradiated. The sum of the output of each irradiation gives the final spectrum.

The final spectrum can thus be viewed as consisting of measurements repeated many times under nominally identical conditions to gradually build up a portrait of the probability distribution of arrival times for each m/z. Though to derive the exact arrival time distribution is rather complicated, it is clear that, for the sake of reasonable mass resolution, the velocity distribution at the moment that ions enter the drift region should be sharply peaked around some nominal value $v_*(m)$ with certain width $\sigma(m)$. Then from maximum entropy perspective, this would lead to the choice of a Gaussian for the velocity distribution:

$$g\left(v\right) = \frac{1}{\sqrt{2\pi}\sigma} \exp\left(-\frac{\left(v - v_*\right)^2}{2\sigma^2}\right). \tag{3}$$

The choice of the maximum-entropy distribution is founded upon the principle that it maximizes the number of possible outcomes of repeated observations that are consistent with this assignment of the probability[19]. Hence, it is the least biased assignment of the probability that is consistent with our limited knowledge of the initial distribution. Transforming from 3 to the temporal peak shape, *i.e.*, the arrival time distribution, requires solving a Fokker-Planck equation, which defines how the probability density function g evolves along the flying path. The most simple case involves the ions entering the drift region and flying directly to the detector, receiving no extra action. The arrival time distribution would be:

$$p(t_k|v_*, \sigma) = \frac{D}{\sqrt{2\pi}\sigma t^2} \exp\left(-\frac{\left(\frac{D}{t} - v_*\right)^2}{2\sigma^2}\right), \tag{4}$$

where D is the flying distance.

The final spectrum is a summation of many independent, repeated measurements of the sample under identical conditions and each measurement is a sampling from a population characterized by the arrival time distribution $p(t_k|v_*, \sigma)$, which is determined by instrumental function and sample surface. The ion counts between time t_k and $t_k + \Delta t$, s_k, in the final time series $\{s\}$, is then independent of those ion counts that arrive at any other time t_j, even when t_k and t_j are associated with the same ion peak. This independence will be a crucial assumption that underlies the entire analysis we pursue. Any correlations in the signal are assumed to be due to the electronics and should be taken into account as a part of the model used.

2.2. Peak Detection

Having understood the nature of a TOF-MS spectrum, we are ready to set out to detect peaks. We will overview the logic of the peak detection here, for more details, please refer to [20].

But, before we go further to derive formulas for peak detection, let us first introduce some notations that we will use throughout the paper. We are going to use $p(X)$ to denote the probability of some event X; use $p(X|I)$ to denote the conditional probability of X given relevant background information I at hand. We will, when talking about probability, always condition the statements on the background information, as the 'absolute probability' is not well posed. We will use $p(X, Y|I)$ to denote the joint probability of X and Y, conditioned on relevant background information I at hand.

Since a mass spectrum usually consists of a large number of peaks, to identify them, the first step is to put an observation window of carefully chosen width N on the spectrum and thus isolate N data points in the time series. We then compare the hypothesis H_1 that there is a peak in the observation window versus hypothesis H_0 that there is no peak in the window, i.e., just background noise. Once the comparison concludes that there is a peak inside the window, we then estimate its position and intensity via parameter fitting by the `maximum likelihood method`.

It is possible sometimes that there could be more that one peak in an observation window. This can be addressed in several ways. An easy fix is to choose an appropriate observation window width such that the window is wide enough to conclude whether or not there is a peak in the window while it is too narrow for more than one peak to be in the window. This works fine when the instrument is of very high resolving power and peaks are not severely overlapped. If the resolving power of the instrument is not very high and peaks of nearby masses overlap resulting in a broader, fat peak, a test on whether there are multiple peaks in the window will be necessary. The logic of doing such a test would be similar to what we describe below but more computationally involved. Interested readers may refer to [21]. For the moment, let us just consider two possibilities, i.e., there is either a peak, or no peak.

From the previous study of a mass spectrum, it is easy to see that all ions are subjected to the same instrumental function, peaks at different m/z share the same characteristic shape, the peak lineshape at one m/z and another m/z are similar up to a shift and rescaling. Let us assume that we have some peak model, $x = f(t - t_0)$, which maximizes at $t = t_0$, and describes what the peak lineshape, *i.e.*, the arrival time distribution, would be. This function could be obtained either empirically or derived from laws of physics/chemistry, but the bottom line is that it captures most of the characteristics of a typical peak in the spectrum. We are going to use t_0 to label the position of the window.

Thus, for the window at t_0, we have N isolated data points, $s = (s_1, s_2, s_3, \cdots, s_N)$, from the spectrum, and we have an N-component vector that describes the peak lineshape:

$$x = (x_1, \ldots x_N) \equiv (f(t_1 - t_0), \ldots f(t_N - t_0)). \qquad (5)$$

For convenience, let x be normalized to have unit area:

$$\sum_{k=1}^{N} x_k = 1. \qquad (6)$$

This will only introduce a constant correction for the peak intensity computed later.

The first thing we want to determine is whether or not there is a peak in the window. This is a comparison between two hypotheses:

- H_1 = There is a single peak in the window around t_0 with the peak lineshape described by x but of unknown intensity, embedded in noise of assumed type. Deviations from this shape in the data are due to noise. Let us call the associated peak-plus-noise model M_1;
- H_0 = There is no peak in the widow t_0. The data are noise of the assumed type. Let us call the associated pure-noise model M_0;

We want to emphasize that for each model M_0 and M_1, we mean a particular choice of peak lineshape x and noise type. If the noise is additive, for example, the white Gaussian noise, then, hypothesis H_1 is equivalent to assume that the observed signal s within the window is given by:

$$s_k = ax_k + \eta_k, \qquad k = 1, 2, \ldots N, \qquad (7)$$

where a is an unknown intensity and $\eta = (\eta_1, \eta_2 \cdots \eta_N)$ is a random process of the assumed type. Similarly, for hypothesis H_0, we have:

$$s_k = \eta_k \qquad k = 1, 2 \cdots N. \qquad (8)$$

If the noise is Poisson type, then H_1 implies that the local rate r_k is:

$$r_k = ax_k + r_0, \qquad (9)$$

where r_0 characterizes the dark current.

We wish to see that, given the data s, whether H_1 is more favorable or H_0 is. This can be done by computing the **odds**, *i.e.*, taking the ratio of two probabilities $p(H_1|s)$ and $p(H_0|s)$:

$$\frac{p(H_1|s,t_0)}{p(H_0|s,t_0)} = \frac{p(M_1|s,t_0)}{p(M_0|s,t_0)}. \qquad (10)$$

If the odds is large compared to one, we can be confident that there is a peak in the window, while if it is approximately one we interpret that as saying there is only weak evidence of a peak in the window (because $a = 0$ is a possible estimate of the peak intensity, which we interpret as 'no peak'). Therefore, one may set a threshold for peak detection.

In order to compute the odds in 10, let us invoke **Bayes' theorem**:

$$p(X|Y,I) = \frac{p(Y|X,I)p(X|I)}{p(Y|I)}. \qquad (11)$$

Identify Y as data, s, observed in the window, and X as the model M_k:

$$p(M_k|s,t_0) = \frac{p(s|M_k,t_0)p(M_k|t_0)}{p(s|t_0)}. \qquad (12)$$

If there is no reason to prefer M_0 over M_1, then one should assign equal prior probabilities, *i.e.*, $p(M_0|t_0) = p(M_1|t_0) = 1/2$. Then, when take the ratio in 10, the denominator would cancel and we have the simple result that:

$$\frac{p(H_1|s,t_0)}{p(H_0|s,t_0)} = \frac{p(M_1|s,t_0)}{p(M_0|s,t_0)} = \frac{p(s|M_1,t_0)}{p(s|M_0,t_0)}. \qquad (13)$$

Hence, we need to calculate the probability of observing the data s given the model M_k, $p(s|M_k,t_0)$, a quantity called **marginal likelihood**, or **evidence**, and is not conditional on any parameters. It can be computed through marginalization.

Since, M_k implies a particular noise process, we may characterize it by parameter λ (*e.g.*, the variance σ and mean μ for a Gaussian process or the 'dark' current rate r_0 for a Poisson process), and notice that ion counts at different times are independent, then the **likelihood function**, *i.e.*, the probability of observing the particular count sequence $s = (s_1, s_2 \cdots s_N)$ given model M_k and its associated parameters (a, λ) is simply:

$$p(s|a, \lambda, t_0, M_k)$$
$$= p(\{s_1, s_2, \ldots s_N\} | a, \lambda, t_0, M_k) \qquad (14)$$
$$= \prod_{i=1}^{N} p(s_i | a, \lambda, t_0, M_k).$$

$p(s|M_k, t_0)$ can then be computed by marginalizing the likelihood function 14 over the model parameters (a, λ) using an appropriate prior probability $p(a, \lambda | M_k, t_0)$:

$$p(s|M_k, t_0) = \int da d\lambda p(s|a, \lambda, M_k, t_0) p(a, \lambda | M_k, t_0). \qquad (15)$$

For each model class M_k, there will be a prior probability distribution for the parameters. For example, for M_1, *i.e.*, there is a peak present, we choose the prior:

$$p(a, \lambda | t_0, M_1) = p(a | t_0, M_1) p(\lambda | t_0, M_1), \qquad (16)$$

where we have assumed that prior for the intensity and that for the noise are independent. If we know nothing about the values of a and λ, then we choose uniform priors, or some other priors that are very broad in the parameter space on the grounds that when we integrate against 14 only the neighborhood of the maximum likelihood value of (a^*, λ^*) will contribute.

Up to this point, we have set up the concept of doing a model comparison for the data in a window located at t_0, all necessary terms have been computed and the odds is ready to be computed. The window will then slide across the spectrum point by point. When the window is sliding, the window width will get wider accordingly if necessary because of instrumental reasons. For each window, the odds is computed. One can easily imagine that as the window comes across a peak, the odds will increase, and will decrease when the window passes a peak. One can then set a threshold for the confidence we need to have to declare a peak to be detected.

Once we have detected that a peak lies within a certain region of the time axis, we then fix the position and intensity of the peak using the **maximum likelihood method**, *i.e.*, maximizing the likelihood 14 over the parameters (a, λ, t_0). This requires solving the following equations, for a window located at t_0 with isolated data $s = (s_1, s_2 \cdots s_N)$:

$$\frac{\partial L(a, \lambda, t_0)}{\partial a} = 0$$
$$\frac{\partial L(a, \lambda, t_0)}{\partial \lambda} = 0, \qquad (17)$$

where $L(a, \lambda, t_0)$ is the natural logarithm of likelihood function 14:

$$L(a, \lambda, t_0) = \ln(p(s|a, \lambda, M_k, t_0)). \tag{18}$$

Solving equations 17 gives the maximum likelihood estimations of parameters (a^*, λ^*) for the window with a fixed t_0 and data s. If the data is informative, then the likelihood would sharply peak around the point (a^*, λ^*) in the parameter space and die off quickly as we move away from (a^*, λ^*). It is natural to Taylor expand 18 around (a^*, λ^*):

$$\begin{aligned}
&L(a, \lambda, t_0) \\
&\approx L(a^*, \lambda^*, t_0) \\
&\quad + \frac{1}{2}\left[\frac{\partial^2 L}{\partial a^2}\Big|_{a^*,\lambda^*}(a - a^*)^2 + \frac{\partial^2 L}{\partial \lambda^2}\Big|_{a^*,\lambda^*}(\lambda - \lambda^*)^2\right] \\
&\quad + \frac{\partial^2 L}{\partial a \partial \lambda}\Big|_{a^*,\lambda^*}(a - a^*)(\lambda - \lambda^*) \\
&= L(a^*, \lambda^*, t_0) + \frac{1}{2}(X - X^*)'\nabla\nabla L(a^*, \lambda^*, t_0)(X - X^*),
\end{aligned} \tag{19}$$

where $X = \begin{bmatrix} a \\ \lambda \end{bmatrix}$, and:

$$\nabla\nabla L(a^*, \lambda^*, t_0) = \begin{bmatrix} \frac{\partial^2 L}{\partial a^2}\Big|_{a^*,\lambda^*} & \frac{\partial^2 L}{\partial a \partial \lambda}\Big|_{a^*,\lambda^*} \\ \frac{\partial^2 L}{\partial a \partial \lambda}\Big|_{a^*,\lambda^*} & \frac{\partial^2 L}{\partial \lambda^2}\Big|_{a^*,\lambda^*} \end{bmatrix} \tag{20}$$

is the `Hessian matrix` evaluated at (a^*, λ^*).

It follows from 19 that the leading term of the likelihood function in 14 is approximately:

$$\begin{aligned}
&p(s|a, \lambda, M_k, t_0) \\
&= \exp\left[L(a, \lambda, t_0)\right] \\
&\approx \exp\left(L(a^*, \lambda^*, t_0) + \frac{1}{2}(X - X^*)'\nabla\nabla L(a^*, \lambda^*, t_0)(X - X^*)\right) \\
&= e^{L(a^*, \lambda^*, t_0)}e^{\frac{1}{2}(X-X^*)'\nabla\nabla L(a^*, \lambda^*, t_0)(X-X^*)}.
\end{aligned} \tag{21}$$

This implies that the likelihood function looks like a multivariate normal distribution in parameter space, centered at (a^*, λ^*) with the following `uncertainties`, if a and λ are not coupled:

$$\begin{aligned}
\sigma_a &= \left(-\frac{\partial^2 L}{\partial a^2}\Big|_{a^*,\lambda^*}\right)^{-1/2} \\
\sigma_\lambda &= \left(-\frac{\partial^2 L}{\partial \lambda^2}\Big|_{a^*,\lambda^*}\right)^{-1/2}.
\end{aligned} \tag{22}$$

Moreover, the approximation in equation 21 provides a possibly easy way to compute the evidence in equation 15 in the sense that if the prior is independent of (a, λ), for example, a and λ are uniformly distributed in some region (a_{min}, a_{max}) and $(\lambda_{min}, \lambda_{max})$, with substitution of 21 into 15, the integration is readily carried out:

$$p(s|M_k, t_0)$$
$$= \int da d\lambda\, p(s|a, \lambda, M_k, t_0) p(a, \lambda|M_k, t_0)$$
$$= \int_{a_{min}}^{a_{max}} \int_{\lambda_{min}}^{\lambda_{max}} da d\lambda\, e^{L(a^*, \lambda^*, t_0)} e^{\frac{1}{2}(X - X^*)' \nabla\nabla L(a^*, \lambda^*, t_0)(X - X^*)} \frac{1}{a_{max} - a_{min}} \frac{1}{\lambda_{max} - \lambda_{min}}$$
$$= \frac{1}{a_{max} - a_{min}} \frac{1}{\lambda_{max} - \lambda_{min}} e^{L(a^*, \lambda^*, t_0)} \frac{(2\pi)^{m/2}}{\sqrt{|\det[\nabla\nabla L(a^*, \lambda^*, t_0)]|}},$$
$$(23)$$

where m is the dimension of parameter space. In the last step of integration, lower and upper boundaries of integration are extended to infinity. This is valid if the likelihood function is sharply peaked around (a^*, λ^*) and (a_{min}, a_{max}) and $(\lambda_{min}, \lambda_{max})$ are large enough such that contributions from outside these regions are negligible. Otherwise, the integral will result in an error function. Note $|\det[\nabla\nabla L(a^*, \lambda^*, t_0)]|$ is the determinant of the Hessian matrix evaluated at (a^*, λ^*) and $1/\sqrt{|\det[\nabla\nabla L(a^*, \lambda^*, t_0)]|}$ is proportional to the 'volume' within σ_a and σ_λ around (a^*, λ^*) in parameter space, *i.e.*

$$p(s|M_k, t_0) \sim p(s|a^*, \lambda^*, M_k, t_0) \frac{\sigma_a}{a_{max} - a_{min}} \frac{\sigma_\lambda}{\lambda_{max} - \lambda_{min}}. \qquad (24)$$

Notice that solving equation 17 only maximizes the likelihood with respect to (a, λ), the maximizing of likelihood with respect to t_0 is done by computing the likelihood for each window position at (a^*, λ^*), *i.e.*, $p(s|a^*, \lambda^*, M_k, t_0)$ and then find the maximum point of $p(s|a^*, \lambda^*, M_k, t_0)$ with respect to t_0. However, maximizing over t_0 has a different logical character than the other parameters, because we are comparing *different* data sets as we slide the window across the peak. The justification is based upon the physical reasonableness of the approach: the width of the window is large compared to the uncertainty in the position of the peak, hence near the maximum of the likelihood, most of the data being compared comes from overlapping windows. An alternative way of looking at this is that by comparing $p(s|a^*, \lambda^*, M_k, t_0)$ at different t_0 we are actually looking for a window in which the data best support the model M_k.

Before we go any further to give an example, let us summarize the procedure: to detect peaks in a TOF-MS spectrum, we need to put a window of appropriate width on the spectrum that isolates N data points. For these N data points, we want to compare model M_1 versus M_0, in which we need to evaluate the odds 10 and compute the evidence in 15 by marginalizing the likelihood function 14 over the prior distribution $p(a, \lambda | M_k, t_0)$ of parameters (a, λ). If the odds is large compare to one, it strongly suggests that there is a peak in the window; otherwise, it is more likely that there is no peak. Once the odds concludes that a peak is present, parameters may be fit by maximizing the likelihood function 14, via solving equation 17. Equation 23 provides an alternative way of computing the evidence if the likelihood is strongly peaked in parameter space.

3. Example

Here, we give an example of finding peaks in a static TOF-SIMS spectrum. In static TOF-SIMS, many primary ion pulses are used to probe the sample surface and for each pulse only a few secondary ions are generated and detected. The detector usually has sub-nanosecond time resolution and thus counts each secondary ion impact, which implies a Poisson process. The final spectrum is a summation of detected secondary ions from all primary ion pulses. The peak lineshape x is derived using equation 4. The window width N is chosen such that the window covers the region from the left half-max to the right half-max of the peak lineshape x. This is a (rough-and-ready) compromise between the desire to include as much data as possible in the window to improve the sampling statistics and the realization that nearby peaks may overlap and that our peak shape model is probably not very good out on the tails of the peak. An example peak is shown in Fig. 1 (a), overlapped with appropriately scaled peak lineshape (black dots). The natural log of the odds is plotted versus the window position t_0 in Fig. 1(b). It behaves as expected: when the window encounters the peak, it goes up, reaches its maximum when the window is right on top of the peak, and then decreases as the window leaves the peak. This allows a threshold to be set to identify a region where we are confident about peak presence. In Fig. 1(c), log of the maximized likelihood $p(s | a^*, \lambda^*, M_1, t_0)$ for each window position is plotted. The interpretation is the following: when the window is located in a region with only noise, the likelihood remains high. This means it is highly likely that only dark current is observed. As the window encounters the peak, the data in the window begin to climb, the likelihood begins to drop implying data in the window look like neither noise nor a centered peak. As the window eventually overlaps the peak, the likelihood peaks up and forms a spike. When the window leaves the peak, the likelihood decreases again and then recovers as the window totally leaves the peak.

Figure 1(d) is an expansion of Fig. 1(c) such that Fig. 1(a), Fig. 1(b) and Fig. 1(d) have the same y axis coverage. Notice that both Fig. 1(b) and Fig. 1(d) are plotted in log scale while Fig. 1(a) is plotted in linear scale, which means the odds and likelihood are very sharply peaked in the region where there is a peak and the likelihood is even shaper, which implies extreme sensitivity to peak position. Since Fig. 1(d) is plotted in log scale, one can fit the center part of it (inside the rectangle) to a parabola and exponentiate it resulting in a Gaussian-like curve. Then, the center of the parabola would be the center of the Gaussian and is the best estimation of peak position. From the curvature of the parabola one can get the width of the Gaussian that indicates the uncertainty of estimated the peak position.

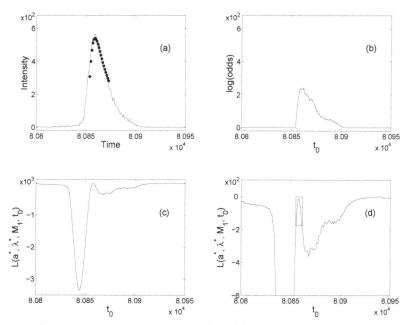

Fig. 1.   Illustration of peak detection procedure: (a) an example peak overlapped with peak lineshape (black dots); (b) log of the odds; (c) log of the maximized likelihood for M_1; (d) expansion of the log of the maximized likelihood.

Having detected peaks using the above method, it is found that there are often shifts in arrival times for the same peak in different spectra, as illustrated in Fig. 2(a), which shows the overlapped, but shifted parent peak of Vasopressin in two different spectra, labeled spectrum 1 and spectrum 2. The multiple peaks seen in Fig. 2(a) are the isotopic pattern. Let p_1 and p_2

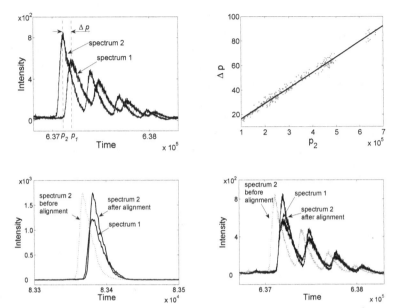

Fig. 2. Illustration of alignment: (a) shift of arrival time for the same peak in two spectra; (b) the linear trend of the shifts with respect to peak arrival time; (c) and (d) after alignment the shift is corrected.

be the estimated peak positions of the first isotopic peak in the two spectra as indicated in Fig. 2(a), then the shift between this peak pair $\Delta p = p_1 - p_2$ is readily computed. Specifically, using the estimated peak positions, the shifts between all paired peaks in the two spectra are easily calculated and are found to increase as peaks arrive at the detector later, as shown in Fig. 2(b), where the shifts are plotted versus peak positions. It is evident from Fig. 2(b) that the shifts, at least to a first order approximation, increase linearly with peak position. A possible cause for this linearly increasing shift may be the difference(s) in surface morphology which affects the kinetic energy that the ejected ions gain during the acceleration stage. There are, of course, many other possible reasons. Nevertheless, the observed linear dependence implies that we can align one spectrum to another by a simple linear operation. An example would be aligning spectrum 2 in Fig. 2(a) to spectrum 1. More specifically, using the least squares method, Δp^i is fit to a linear function of p_2^i as $\Delta p^i = a p_2^i + b$, where the superscript i means the ith peak pair. The resulting a and b give the information about how the time axis of spectrum 2 should be scaled and shifted to match spectrum 1. This simple linear operation is found to effectively enable global alignment of two spectra. The result of this global alignment procedure is illustrated in Fig. 2(c) and Fig. 2(d) for two different mass regions. It is clear that after the linear operation on spectrum 2, peaks in two spectra have been brought into alignment.

It has been shown that this alignment procedure is effective and easy to carry out, as long as two spectra share some known common peaks. After aligning two spectra based on these known common peaks, one may identify if there are other common peaks that are not obvious before alignment. This is performed by comparing the shift in peak positions in all possible peak pairs with the estimated peak position uncertainties. If the shift is large relative to the uncertainties, they will be treated as separate peaks that show in one spectrum but not in the other. Otherwise, they are identified as common peaks in both spectra. After aligning two spectra, this alignment can be extended to multiple spectra in the same fashion.

4. Summary

The peak detection algorithm discussed here is based on a physical understanding of a TOF-MS spectrum and utilizes Bayes' theorem. The peak detection algorithm is automated and can be applied to a variety of TOF-MS spectra, from counting experiments (TOF-SIMS) to instruments like MALDI-TOF which integrate the ion signal rather than counting individual ion. The noise characteristics are different in these devices. The algorithm automatically provides estimates of uncertainties in the peak positions and intensities. This information is used to verify that aligned spectra collected at different spatial positions or at different times are properly aligned.

Acknowledgments

The authors are greatful to Dr. M.W. Trosset for his helpful comments. Financial supports from National Cancer Institute Phase I and II SBIR grant (CA101479) and the Virginia Commonwealth Technology Research Fund (IN2003-04) are also acknowledged. This work was performed in part using computational facilities at the College of William and Mary which were enabled by grants from Sun Microsystems, the National Science Foundation, and Virginia's Commonwealth Technology Research Fund.

References

1. M. Mann, R.C. Hendrickson, and A. Pandey, Analysis of proteins and proteomes by mass spectrometry, *Annu. Rev. Biochem.*, **70** (2001), 437-473.

2. P.L. Ferguson and R.D. Smith, Proteome analysis by mass spectrometry, *Annu. Rev. Biophys. Biomol. Struct.*, **32** (2003), 399-424.
3. B. Adam, A. Vlahou, O.J. Semmes and G.L. Wright, Jr., Proteomic approaches to biomarker discovery in prostate and bladder cancers, *Proteomics*, **1** (2001), 1264-1270.
4. L.H. Cazares, *et al.*, Normal, benign, preneoplastic, and malignant prostate cells have distinct protein expression profiles resolved by surface enhanced laser desorption/ionization mass spectrometry, *Clin. Cancer Res.*, **8** (2002), 2541-2552.
5. B. Adam, *et al.*, Serum protein fingerprinting coupled with a pattern-matching algorithm distinguishes prostate cancer from benign prostate hyperplasia and healthy men, *Cancer Res.*, **62** (2002), 3609-3614.
6. Y. Qu, *et al.*, Boosted decision tree analysis of surface-enhanced laser desorption/ionization mass spectral serum profiles discriminates prostate cancer from noncancer patients, *Clin. Chem.*, **48** (2002), 1835-1843.
7. Y.F. Wong, *et al.*, Protein profiling of cervical cancer by protein-biochips: proteomic scoring to discriminate cervical cancer from normal cervix, *Cancer Lett.*, **211** (2004), 227-234.
8. Y. Hu, *et al.*, SELDI-TOF-MS: the proteomics and bioinformatics approaches in the diagnosis of breast cancer, *The Breast*, **14** (2005), 250-255.
9. J.N. Adkins, *et al.*, Toward a human blood serum proteome, *Mol. Cell. Proteomics*, **1** (2002), 947-955.
10. C. Wrotnowski, The future of plasma proteins, *Genet. Eng. News*, **18** (1998), 14-17.
11. S. Vorderwübecke, S. Cleverley, S.R. Weinberger, and A. Wiesner, Protein quantification by the SELDI-TOF-MS-based ProteinChip system, *Nat. Methods*, **2** (2005), 393-395.
12. W.E. Wallace, A.J. Kearsley, and C.M. Guttman, An operator-independent approach to mass spectral peak identification and integration, *Anal. Chem.*, **76** (2004), 2446-2452.
13. C. M. Guttman, *et al.*, NIST-Sponsored interlaboratory comparison of polystyrene molecular mass distribution obtained by matrix-assisted laser desorption/ionization time-of-flight mass spectrometry: statistical analysis, *Anal. Chem.*, **73** (2001), 1252-1262.
14. Wm.F. Bryant, *et al.*, Data-blocking cross-correlation peak detection in computerized gas chromatography-mass spectrometry, *Anal. Chem.*, **52** (1980), 38-43.
15. R. Gras, *et al.*, Improving protein identification from peptide mass finger-printing through a parameterized multi-level scoring algorithm and an optimized peak detection, *Electrophoresis*, **20** (1999), 3535-3550.
16. K.H. Jarman, D.S. Daly, K.K. Anderson and K.L. Wahl, A new approach to automated peak detection, *Chemo. Intell. Lab. Syst.*, **69** (2003), 61-76.
17. J. S. Morris, *et al.*, Feature extraction and quantification for mass spectrometry in biomedical applications using the mean spectrum, *Bioinformatics*, **21** (2005), 1764-1775.
18. B.O. Keller and L. Li, Detection of 25,000 molecules of substance P by

MALDI-TOF mass spectrometry and investigations into the fundamental limits of detection in MALDI, *J. Am. Soc. Mass Spectrom.*, **12** (2001), 1055-1063.

19. E.T. Jaynes, *Probability Theory*, Cambridge University Press, Cambridge, UK, 2003.

20. H. Chen, *Automated peak identification for time-of-flight mass spectroscopy*, Ph. D. Dissertation, College of William and Mary, Williamsburg, VA, 2005.

21. D.S. Sivia and C.J. Carlile, Molecular spectroscopy and Bayesian spectral analysis–how many lines are there? *J. Chem. Phys.*, **96** (1992), 170-178.

CHAPTER 7

MICROARRAY DATA ANALYSIS IN AFFYMETRIX GENE CHIP

Dung-Tsa Chen[a] and James J. Chen[b]

[a]*Department of Medicine, School of Medicine,*
University of Alabama at Birmingham, Birmingham, AL, USA
[b]*Division of Biometry and Risk Assessment,*
National Center for Toxicological Research, Food and Drug Administration,
Jefferson, AR, USA

Microarray technology has advanced genomic research. Among various platforms, Affymetrix gene chips have been the most widely used to study thousands of genes simultaneously through mRNA expression. Analysis of Affymetrix gene expression data requires multiple steps, including data quality assessment, gene selection, and gene function classification. We describe a 2D image plot approach to assess data quality by examining array comparability. This approach uses a percentile method to group data, and then applies the 2D image plot to display the grouped microarray data with an invariant band to quantify degrees of array comparability. The method provides an efficient way of visually identifying incomparable arrays. Next, we describe a probe rank approach to selecting differentially-expressed genes. The probe rank approach uses rank scores to normalize and analyze probe intensity to control for probe effect, and uses a filter of percentage of probe fold change to account for cross-hybridization and alternative splicing. In the gene function classification, we describe an integrated bioinformatics tool to organize the genomic information of selected genes systematically so that their functional information is readily available for search objectives. The tool integrates a series of major genomic databases, such as Affymetrix's NetAffx Analysis center and Entrez Gene database. The tool classifies genes and generates readable web-based outputs for investigators to easily associate significant genes with biological pathways.

1. Introduction

1.1. *Data Quality*

Microarray is a powerful technology to exploit DNA sequence information[1−5]. Because of the dramatic reduction in labor, time, and costs, this technique has become a popular tool for studying thousands of genes simultaneously. Gene expression profiling through this technology has great promise in biomedicine. For example, the microarray technology can be used in the identification of biomarkers, evaluation of prognoses, classification of disease status, and prediction of clinical outcomes[1,2,6,7]. While this technology has merits of genomic research, assessment of data quality poses a unique challenge because of the enormous volume of data[8,9,10].

There are at least two types of data quality assessment for Affymetrix gene chip: internal and external data quality assessment. Examination of internal data quality focuses on each gene chip, such as inspection of the presence of artifacts, the use of spike-in genes to evaluate sample hybridization efficiency, and the application of actin and GAPDH to detect degradation of RNA and inefficient transcription. Affymetrix software (e.g., GCOS or MAS[11,12]) provides some metrics to evaluate internal data quality, such as scale-factors, percent-present calls, background, and 3'/5' ratios of housekeeping genes. In addition, there are other packages available in R to graphically present these metrics for visual examination of data quality, such as simpleaffy and affyQCReport[13,14].

For external data quality, assessment of array comparability is an important issue because an analysis including incomparable arrays is likely to generate invalid results. Unfortunately, issues of array comparability have not been addressed adequately, either in literature or in practice. For examples, several studies have used the Pearson correlation and/or scatterplot to check degrees of consistency among arrays[15,16,17]. The Pearson correlation is a quantitative measure to describe a linear relationship between two variables[18]. When the correlation is close to 1 (or −1), if one variable increases, then the other variable tends to increase (or decrease). Since data in the gene chips often show a nonlinear pattern, the use of correlation may not be appropriate to examining array comparability. Another approach is scatterplot which is a graphical technique to depict the relationship between two variables with one variable in the x-axis and the other in the y-axis[19,20]. The tool has enjoyed its successful application to graphical exploration. However, its capability to handle large datasets has limitations. A huge dataset could hamper the application of scatterplot by rendering the data both misleading and inefficient. Specifically, its weakness to distinguish the high and low densities for a large dataset could mislead the human eye by overemphasizing the area of a few data points and downplaying the area of high density. Scatterplot also becomes inefficient as data points increase, because the tool often requires a longer time to complete the display especially for data more than million points. The slow display may cause the graphical window to freeze or halt the system when switching from one program window to another window on a PC. Moreover, the resulting huge file (more than 10 MB unit for million points) can cause inconvenience in delivering the information to clients either by email, by a floppy diskette, or by printing.

1.2. Gene-Level Data Analysis

Affymetrix oligonucleotide gene chip has been widely used to study gene expression profiling in the genomic community[21-28]. The Affymetrix array uses a set of probes to interrogate a gene expression, where each array consists of thousands of genes. An experiment routinely collects a huge volume of information; the data structure can be quite complicated. Analyzing such complex data poses a challenge to biostatisticians to develop an approach to summarizing probe-level information that can truly reflect the level of a gene expression adequately, while accounting for probe variation, chip variation, and interaction effects. In addition, due to resource limitations and/or sample availability, many microarray experiments, such as in vitro studies, have only a small number of replicates, statistical inferences such as the p-value significance testing or confidence interval analysis, which work well with a large sample size, often break down and become impractical.

For example, MAS 5 employs the Tukey's Biweight approach to summarizing gene expression intensity from the modified perfect-match (PM) and mismatch (MM) signals[12]. Dchip analyzes probe level intensities using a multiplicative model to decompose each probe signal into a product of gene expression index and probe-sensitivity index[29]. Robust multi-array analysis (RMA) uses a stochastic-model-based approach to improve the preprocessing of array data by taking into account the presence of optical noise, nonspecific binding and probe-specific effects[30]. Specifically, RMA employs a log scale linear additive model to analyze gene expression based on PM intensities which have been background corrected and normalized. The advantage for the use of RMA is the improvement of precision (compared to large variation in MAS 5.0). However, this approach may cause some bias because its global background adjustment does not completely remove nonspecific binding. A modified RMA, GeneChip RMA (GCRMA), has been introduced to improve the accuracy of RMA without much sacrifice in precision[31]. This new approach combines the strengths of stochastic-model algorithms and physical models.

These approaches can be referred to as the gene-level-based approach in which the probe level expression data are summarized into gene level measures, which then are used for a statistical analysis. One advantage of this strategy is that the data dimensions are reduced to a manageable scale. Standard statistical methods can be used to select differentially expressed genes. For example, `Significance Analysis of Microarrays (SAM)` has been widely used as a statistical technique for finding significant genes in a set of microarray experiments[32]. This approach calculates a d-score to each gene which is a ratio of fold-change versus a modified standard deviation (standard deviation plus an exchangeability factor). When genes have higher scores than an adjustable threshold, permutations of the repeated measurements are employed to estimate the false discovery rate (FDR), a measure for multiple comparison.

Since hundreds or thousands of genes are tested simultaneously, simply using the significance level for a p-value cutoff without adjusting for multiple tests will increase the chance of false positives. Traditional multiple testing procedure is to control the family-wise error (FWE) rate[33]. However, the FWE approach tends to screen out all genes except the ones with extreme differential expressions when the number of genes becomes large, as in the case of microarray experiments. The `false discovery rate (FDR)`[32,34] offers a less stringent alternative because it uses the expected proportion of false rejections as an error measure. No matter which criterion is used, determination of the level of significance should depend on the objective of the experiment. For instance, if the objective is to identify a small number of truly differentially expressed genes, then a stringent criterion such as controlling either the family-wise or the false discovery error rate may be appropriate. On the other hand, for prediction purposes in genomic/genetic profiling studies, the omission of informative genes in the development of a predictive classifier generally has a much more serious consequence on predictive accuracy than the inclusion of non-informative genes. In such cases, the stringent control of false-positives may not be essential. In this chapter, we will not consider multiple comparison adjustment.

There are some limitations in using gene-level data for analysis. For example, gene expressions obtained from oligonucleotide arrays often show non-homogeneous probe effects (i.e., different expression intensities among a set of probes). Such non-homogeneous probe effects shown in probe-level expressions may not be reflected in gene-level summary data (see Figure 1). Moreover, expression differences in a two-group comparison could vary among a set of probes. Some probes may have large differential expressions whereas some probes yield similar expressions between the two groups. The dependency of differential expressions on probes indicates an interaction effect between probe and treatment effects. The interaction effect may have potential biological implications, such as alternative splicing[35]. In this case, gene-level data analysis may miss this target gene. Even if the gene is identified, without the information of probe expressions, it is hard to judge the occurrence of alternative splicing. In this chapter, we present a probe rank approach to analyze probe level data.

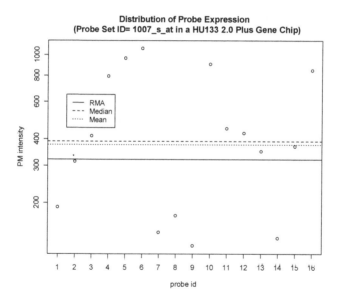

Fig. 1. Heterogeneity of probe effects in a given gene expression. The probe intensity shows large variation, ranging from 100 to 1100 with median 392 (denoted by the dashed line) and geometric mean 376 (denoted by the dotted line). The gene expression using RMA is 321 (denoted by the solid line).

1.3. *Gene Function Classification*

In microarray studies, differentially expressed genes are identified based on descriptive statistics or a test statistics cut-off (e.g., p-value, false discovery rate, or fold change)[36,37,38]. The selected genes indicate their statistical significance of expression change, but researchers would also like to know their biological relevance. Due to recent rapid developments of genomic databases, the gene annotation information is now easily available from the internet. Various tools have been developed to incorporate the information for gene expression profiling. There are many tools available for searching and browsing Gene Ontology (GO)[39], such as AmiGO[40], EPGO[41], GoFish[42], Goblet[43], and CGAP[44]. These are either web-based or java-based tools to search for gene annotations. In addition, numerous tools have been developed to map microarray data onto the GO structure, such as GOstat[45], eGOn[46], DAVID[47], GoMiner[48], and FatiGO[49]. These tools can be used to determine which GO categories are statistically significant for a list of genes, and to suggest the corresponding biological areas to warrant further study. These tools also provide detailed analysis results, such as a hypothesis testing for each GO category, clustering of functionally related genes within a set of genes, interactive graphics, and numerous listings of GO annotations for one or many groups of genes.

Moreover, investigators are interested in gene-gene interaction in particular pathways. Various pathway databases and methods (e.g., KEGG, GENMAPP, REACTOME, CYTOSCAPE, and BIOCARTA) are available on the internet for pathway analysis[50,51,52,53,54,55]. These curated databases are useful resources to study biological processes, such as the pathways of intermediary metabolism, regulatory pathways, and signal transduction. They also help investigators gain insight into the potential functions of new genes. Since the databases contain massive amounts of information, it becomes challenging for researchers to convert the enormous amount of information into useful knowledge. Many approaches have been developed to provide parsimonious models to analyze gene pathways. For example, MAPPFinder and Pathway-Miner are bioinformatics tools to create global gene expression profiles across biological pathways[56,57]. They classify genes by integrating the gene ontology (GO) annotations based on metabolic, cellular and regulatory pathways. Typically, a top list of genes selected by one of these statistical methods is mapped onto pathways with gene product association networks for genes that occur in the pathways. A z-score or the Fisher exact test is then used to test statistical significance of pathways. The pathways can be ranked in accordance with the p-values. Another rigorous approach for gene pathways is the chain reaction model. The chain reaction model has been widely used in the engineering field to simulate chemical reactions that occur in combustion devices such as jet and rocket engines[58,59]. Its application to gene pathways can be done by treating the regulated genes as a set of reacting species and calculating the species changes as the gene expression changes. Since the chain reaction model uses a set of chemical reactions to describe gene-gene interaction in gene pathways, it provides an alternative for pathway level analyses such that parametric studies of various pathways and genes-gene interactions can be performed in an effective manner. Overall, these tools depict biological interaction among genes and provide insights to study associations of the biological pathways with research outcomes (e.g., disease versus non-disease or treatment versus control). In this chapter, we describe a tool for presenting the results in a simple, effective, and self-explanatory format to facilitate the transition from data analysis to biological interpretation.

2. Methods

2.1. *Data Quality Assessment*

This subsection describes a 2D image plot to examine array comparability and to assist verification of differentially expressed genes[60]. The 2D-image plot efficiently sums up the information instead of a scatterplot. Moreover, the 2D image plot can be used as a supplementary tool for gene selection. By using an invariant band as an exploratory criterion, the 2D image plot can be used to help validate whether a gene is differentially expressed.

2.1.1. *2D Image Plot*

The 2D-image plot first reduces the data dimensions by grouping data using percentile cutoffs. The percentiles of intensity in each array are used to form k groups with $x\%$ for the interval length. That is, let $Q_0, Q_x, \ldots, Q_{(k-1) \times x}$, and Q_{100} denote the cutoffs for the k groups, where Q_a represents the ath intensity percentile and $k \times x = 100$. For every two arrays, their percentile cutoffs are used to form $k \times k$ groups. The relative frequency is then calculated to represent density in each subgroup (grid). Thus, the high volume of data is reduced to $k \times k$. The 2D image plot is then applied to the grouped data. The percentile cutoffs of the two array intensities are used as the first two-dimensions in the x-axis and y-axis, respectively. Density in each subgroup is used for the third dimension to display the distribution of two array intensities. When two arrays have comparable intensities, the 2D image plot is likely to show a highly dense thin band along the diagonal percentile curve. We use the invariant band to reflect the degrees of consistency between two arrays' intensities.

2.1.2. Invariant Band

To construct an invariant band, we use $m \times x\%$ deviation to build up a lower boundary curve which is formed by data points (Q_a, Q_b) with $a - b = m \times x$, and an upper boundary curve formed by data points (Q_a, Q_b) with $b - a = m \times x$. Here (A, B) represents data position with A on the x-axis and B on the y-axis. The parameter m is defined as the number of $x\%$ unit to adjust for random variation in the grouped data with $0 < m < k$. For example, when $m = 2$ and $x\% = 5\%$, the $m \times x\%(= 10\%)$ invariant band has a lower boundary curve formed by $(Q_{10}, Q_0), (Q_{15}, Q_5), \ldots, (Q_{95}, Q_{85})$, and (Q_{100}, Q_{90}), and the upper boundary curve formed by $(Q_0, Q_{10}), (Q_5, Q_{15}), \ldots, (Q_{85}, Q_{95})$, and (Q_{90}, Q_{100}). A data point, (Q_a, Q_b), with $|b - a| \leq m \times x$ will be covered by the $m \times x\%$ invariant band. Since the data point is in the tolerable distance away from the diagonal percentile curve, Q_a and Q_b are considered to be comparable. Therefore, if the majority of intensities between two arrays are located within the invariant band, both arrays are likely to have comparable intensity. Thus, given the $m \times x\%$ invariant band, we compute the degrees of array variation by a coverage rate, defined as the number of data points inside the band divided by the total number of data points. A substantial portion of data points outside the band implies a high degree of inconsistency between two arrays. Such incomparability deserves further investigation of data quality before analysis (Figures 2.1-2.2).

2.1.3. A Supplementary Tool for Gene Selection

Microarray data are often normalized prior to data analysis. However, the methods used for **normalization** remain debatable because different normalization procedures often result in selecting different gene lists. Nevertheless, difference in expressions between the two groups can be evaluated in terms of the relative difference in the raw data, where the relative difference in the raw data refers to the degrees of discrepancy of the gene intensity between the control arrays and the experimental arrays. If there is no relative difference in the raw data, but a large absolute difference occurs in

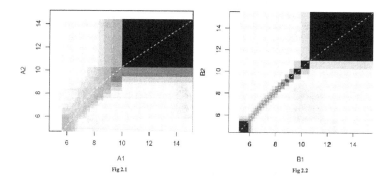

Fig. 2. Figure 2.1 is a 2D image plot for two replicate arrays, A1-A2. The large discrepancy of intensity can be seen by a wide band in the diagonal curve. In contrast, Figure 2.2 shows high degree of consistency between another two replicates (B1-B2).

the normalized data, then it is possible that such difference is caused by over-correction in the normalization procedures. It is useful to verify a set of selected genes in the raw data format (data before normalization) after these genes are selected. The graphical approach described is useful and efficient in displaying the relative difference visually by comparing to the invariant band. We can use the invariant band as an exploratory rule to examine whether a gene has differential expressions from one experiment condition to another.

We illustrate using this approach as a supplementary tool for gene selection by the example of a spike-in gene, CreX_5, in the four arrays E1-E4 (Figures 3.1-3.6). The 2D image plots using the 10% deviation invariant band (i.e., $m = 2, x\% = 5\%$) are displayed to show distribution of probe intensity for the spike-in gene. The pair-wise comparisons of the four arrays show coverage rates of 83% 94%. The high coverage rates suggest these arrays are comparable, and therefore the data are reliable for analysis. Examination of within group variations in Figures 3.1 and 3.6 shows that most probe intensities of CreX_5 are located along the diagonal percentile curve. This observation indicates that probe intensities of CreX_5 are comparable between arrays E1 and E2 and between arrays E3 and E4 (i.e., small replicate variation). On the other hand, examination of between group variation in Figures 3.2-3.5 displays the majority of probe intensities far away from the invariant band. That is, a large discrepancy of CreX_5 intensities occurs

between arrays E1 and E2 versus arrays E3 and E4. The pattern suggests
that the gene CreX_5 has differential expression between the two different
experiment conditions (i.e., arrays E1 and E2 versus arrays E3 and E4).

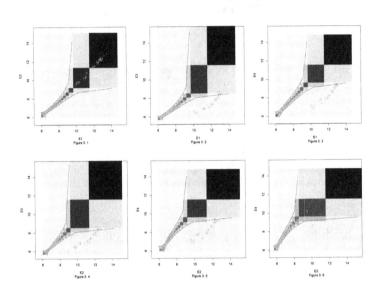

Fig. 3. Verification of differentially expressed genes. Figures 3.1-3.6 are the 6 pair-wise
comparisons between the four arrays, E1-E4. Figures 3.1 and 3.6 show smaller within
group variation. In contrast, large between group variation is graphically observed in
figures 3.2-3.5.

2.2. A Probe Rank Approach for Gene Selection

2.2.1. Rank Normalization for PM Intensity

Rank has been used as a normalization tool in microarray data analysis[61,62],
but its use was limited to the gene level data. We extend its application to
the probe level data in oligonucleotide arrays. Rank avoids assumptions on
distribution of intensity. Rank also provides a better treatment for alleviat-
ing effects of extreme values. Our experiences from various microarray data
analyses have found that probe intensities in the oligonucleotide array data
often show a skewed distribution in extremely high intensities. In this case,
rank is more robust because the ranks of these extreme values are less in-
fluential than their intensity levels. In addition, unlike other measurements

generated by complicated normalization, rank is a simple measure using intensity order.

2.2.2. *The Use of PM*

Affymetrix oligonucleotide gene chips use a set of pairs of probes to interrogate a given gene. Each pair consists of a perfect match probe (PM) and a mismatch probe (MM). PM is used to detect mRNA concentration of a target gene whereas MM is designed to identify background intensity and cross-hybridization. Here we consider only PM probe level data because of potential biases introduced by the use of MM. For example, PM is contaminated with background and cross-hybridization, so PM intensity is supposed to be greater than MM intensity. However, it is common to see a substantial portion of probe pairs with MM>PM (30% $\sim$ 50%) and a high correlation between PM and MM[30]. Such patterns suggest MM also partially measures RNA concentration. Subtraction of MM from PM likely underestimates mRNA concentration. Thus, we consider PM intensity for data analysis. We define PM rank as the rank of PM intensity over all probes in the gene chip. Below we describe a rank approach (un-weighted), and a weighted rank approach[63,64].

2.2.3. *Probe Rank Approach*

Let $Y_{i,j,k}$ be a PM rank for the jth probe in the ith gene on array k. Assume group A has arrays $a_1, a_2, \ldots, a_{n_1}$ and group B has arrays $b_1, b_2, \ldots, b_{n_2}$ (e.g., treatment versus control groups). Consider a difference of two percentiles from the two groups.

$$D_{A,B}^{(i,j)} = (P_a\text{th percentile of } S_a - P_b\text{th percentile of } S_b)/n,$$

where $S_a = \{Y_{(i,j,a_1)}, \ldots, Y_{(i,j,a_{n_1})}\}$, $Sb = \{Y_{(i,j,b_1)}, \ldots, Y_{(i,j,b_{n_2})}\}$, and n represents the total number of probes in an array (e.g., there are 201,807 probes in a HG-u95A gene chip). P_a could be 0 (i.e., the minimum), and P_b could be 100 (i.e., the maximum) when sample size is small (e.g., 2 or 3 in vitro study). $D_{A,B}^{(i,j)}$ is a measure of difference between group A and group B. The measure between group B and group A is defined similarly. Denote the number of probes for gene i as J_i. A gene i is considered to be an altered gene if

$$\frac{1}{J_i} \sum_{j=1}^{J_i} I(D_{A,B}^{(i,j)} > P_{probe,(A,B)}^{(i)}) \geq P_{gene,(A,B)}^{(i)} \text{ or}$$

$$\frac{1}{J_i} \sum_{j=1}^{J_i} I(D_{B,A}^{(i,j)} > P_{probe,(B,A)}^{(i)}) \geq P_{gene,(B,A)}^{(i)},$$

where $P_{probe,E}^{(i)}$ represents a probe level threshold with E as (A, B) or (B, A),

$P^{(i)}_{gene,E}$ represents a gene level threshold, and I is an indicator function. The two thresholds, $P^{(i)}_{probe,E}$ and $P^{(i)}_{gene,E}$, are pre-specified constants. The probe level threshold $P^{(i)}_{probe,E}$ provides a cutoff for probe discrepancy between two groups, and the gene level threshold $P^{(i)}_{gene,E}$ provides a cutoff for determining differential expressions.

2.2.4. Probe Weighted Rank Approach

The probe rank has limitations for detecting expression differences for genes with extremely high intensity (e.g. in the 98th $\sim$ 100th percentile). For genes within this range, their ranks tend to be similar. It becomes difficult to identify altered genes in this range because of a very small rank difference. In practice, this situation is rare and likely occurs in a highly abundant gene. The gene intensity is likely in the range of high percentile at each experimental group (i.e., treatment and control). Though the difference of intensity between the two experimental groups may be substantial (e.g., > 2 fold for treatment versus control), the rank difference remains relatively small. To overcome the problem, we introduce a weighting factor to the rank. By giving the weighting factor, a gene with high intensity is likely to have its rank score amplified substantially because the weighting factor is proportional to the probe intensity. As a result, difference of the weighted rank scores becomes large between treatment and control groups. Mathematically, the weighted rank approach is the same as the rank approach except $Y_{i,j,k}$ multiplied by a weight $w_{i,j,k}$. The weight $w_{i,j,k}$ for the jth probe in the ith gene on array k, is defined as $log_2(PM_{i,j,k})/\sum_{i=1}^{m}\sum_{j=1}^{J_i} log_2(PM_{i,j,k})$ where $PM_{i,j,k}$ is PM intensity for the jth probe in the ith gene of array k, m is the total number of genes in an array, and J_i represents the total number of probes for gene i. The PM weighted rank $Y^{(weighted)}_{i,j,k}$ becomes $Y_{i,j,k} \times w_{i,j,k}$. The probe weighted rank approach uses $Y^{(weighted)}_{i,j,k}$ to compute percentile difference (i.e., $D^{(i,j)}_{A,B}$ and $D^{(i,j)}_{B,A}$) and select differentially expressed genes. By giving a larger weight on high intensity probes, the probe weighted rank approach can increase the power of detecting expression differences for highly abundant genes better than the rank approach does.

2.3. An Integrated Bioinformatics Tool

Analysis of gene selection often yields a long list of genes with detailed information, such as gene expression fold change, p value, and numerous genomic data. Because of the massive quantity of data, investigators may have difficulty sorting through the information. Below, we describe an integrated bioinformatics tool to summarize the long list of genes into a few concise tables which allow researchers to extract relevant biological functions.

2.3.1. *Integration of Genomic Databases*

It is important to have a reliable database in order to yield more accurate results of gene function classification. Our current database collects major gene databases and integrates them into one more comprehensive database for classification. The database includes the Affymetrix gene database[65], NCBI Entrez database[66], GO database[39], and the KEGG pathway database[67]. For example, the database in the Affymetrix's NetAffx Analysis Center contains detailed genomic information for each probe set in Affymetrix gene chips. This information includes probe sequences, gene annotations, and various functional annotations. However, it is not very inclusive, and some important gene variables are not available, such as gene alias (gene synonym, a non-standard name for a gene) and gene RIF (reference into function). For gene alias, it is common to see multiple names published for a particular gene. So, without the gene alias information, it is difficult to recognize a set of different names for the same target gene. For gene RIF, it gives a concise phrase (not a keyword) describing a gene function with a reference to a specific MEDLINE record. The phrase provides a good opportunity to enhance gene classification. Accordingly, inclusion of the gene alias and gene RIF with the Affymetrix's NetAffx database will undoubtedly make the data more valuable. Since the Entrez Gene database includes biological information for genes but with limited probe information for the Affymetrix gene chip, integration of these databases will make gene function classification more accurate.

2.3.2. *Systematic Layout of All Selected Genes*

For a list of significant genes, the integrated bioinformatics tool presents a summary table to list the up- /down- regulated genes. Sorting the selected genes into up- or down- regulation groups is a basic requirement by biomedical researchers because an up-regulated gene has a different biological meaning compared to the same gene having a down-regulation. To get detailed gene information, this summary table is linked to another table where all up- (or down-) regulated genes are listed with their expression data and brief gene description. This table provides testing statistics, such as fold change and p value, for investigators to examine the degrees of expression change. More importantly, the table is readable because it gives only gene names and their description, allowing researchers to quickly obtain biological functions for their interesting genes. This effective layout is different from the standard spreadsheet output, which is hard to read because of the mass of information. In addition, as investigators may want to know detailed information of a particular gene, we provide a table for each gene to give detailed annotations. Boxplots for gene-level data or scatterplots for probe-level data will be displayed to show distribution of expression differences when the data are provided.

2.3.3. *Organization of Selected Genes by GO Annotations*

One research interest in microarray experiments for the biomedical community is to understand the relationship between genes and their biological functions. Because of a large number of selected genes, it is challenging for investigators to identify particular gene functions associated with their genes of interest. One efficient solution is to use GO annotations to sort out the selected genes with similar genomic properties. The GO annotations are structured, controlled vocabularies (ontologies) to describe gene products in terms of their associated biological processes, cellular components and molecular functions. Since the GO terms are concise with consistent descriptions of gene products in different databases, they can be used to facilitate the process of gene function classification. The integrated bioinformatics tool collects all GO annotations of the selected genes and group them by up- and down- regulation. In the application, the tool reports the number of genes at each annotation. This frequency table allows investigators to efficiently explore possible biological functions. A high frequency of genes in an annotation may indicate occurrence of a particular biological functional activity. In addition, this table can be used as prior information to specify relevant keywords for further study. This is especially useful for researchers who are newly involved in genomic research or little background in bioinformatics. Moreover, to further understand the genes in an annotation, a summary table for these genes is given with their expression data, testing statistics, and gene descriptions. This table provides concise and useful information to study the relationship among these genes within the same annotation.

2.3.4. *Classification by Keywords*

Classification based on GO annotations presents useful information to study gene association. However, the lists of annotations may remain large. Investigators would want to narrow down the lists and focus on specific areas of interest. In addition, GO tries to synchronize the description of genes, but there are still wide variations in genomic terminology. Gene alias is an obvious case. For example, the secreted phosphoprotein 1 (SPP1) is a gene associated with ossification. It has various names, such as OP, Bsp, Eta, Ric, Apl-1, and minopontin. These names are quite textually different from the official name. Without the alias information, it would be difficult to relate the various alias names to this gene if they are used. To effectively correlate genes with keywords, we consider various variables, in addition to GO annotations, to search genes associated with the keywords. The current variables included in the search-database are GO annotations, gene alias, gene name, gene description, KEGG pathway, and RIF. Given the keywords, the tool will search the database and identify the genes associated with these keywords. A summarized table of keyword classification will be given. Each keyword classification will include a set of genes associated with the keyword. The generated table will help investigators expedite the process of gene function classification.

2.3.5. *Implementation*

The approach has been written in R software[68] (available on request by email at dtchen@uab.edu). The outputs are a series of html files. Starting with the main.htm file at the root directory, it will guide the user to the whole set of regulated genes, GO classification, or keyword classification.

3. Data Example: A Prolactin Study

3.1. *Background and Study Design*

Prolactin (PRL) is a lactotrophic hormone synthesized and secreted by the pituitary gland[69]. It has been indicated to be associated with regulation of the outgrowth of new capillary blood vessels, a process referred to as angiogenesis[70]. In particular, 23 kDa prolactin (23k PRL) has been shown to be angiogenic while its proteolytic fragment 16 kDa prolactin (16k PRL) has been shown to be antiangiogenic[71]. To address how signaling by 23k and 16k PRL affects endothelial cell function, gene array analysis was performed in the following settings. Recombinant adenovirus expressing the

23-k PRL (Ad-23k PRL) and 16-k PRL (Ad-16k PRL) were generated
to infect human umbilical vein endothelial cells (HUVECs) for 48 hours.
HUVECs infected with Ad-luciferase (Ad-Luc) were used as the control.
Gene expression profiles were analyzed by using HG-u95Av2 gene arrays
(Affymetrix) containing 12,600 genes and ESTs. The numbers of replicates
were 2, 3, and 3, for the 23k PRL sample, the 16k PRL sample, and the
control sample, respectively.

3.2. Assessment of Array Data Quality

Data quality was examined using the 2D image plot for array comparability
between replicate arrays. Results indicated both the 16k PRL group and
the control group had one incomparable array with a coverage rate less than
80% (The results of the 16k PRL group are shown in Figure 4). Thus, data
analysis was performed with the exclusion of these two potential outlier
arrays.

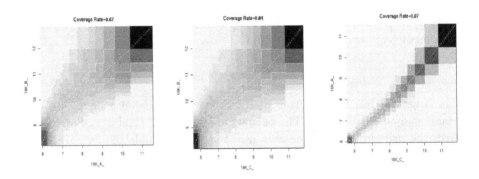

Fig. 4.   Assessment of array data quality. Examination of three arrays in the 16k PRL
group indicated the B array was not comparable to the other two arrays. Data patterns
between the B array versus the A and C arrays were widely spread with 1/3 data points
deviating away from the invariant band (constructed by two yellow curves). In contrast,
the band between the first and third arrays was thinner with coverage rate 97% (coverage
rate is defined the proportion of genes within the yellow upper and lower boundary
curves). This observation indicates the experimental problem in the B array.

3.3. *Gene Selection*

We used the probe rank approach to analyze the prolactin data. Since it was an in vitro study with a small sample size, we use $P_a = 0$ and $P_b = 100$. The probe level threshold was set as 0.05 to calculate the probe percentile difference and the gene level threshold was fixed at 50% to determine differential expression for each gene.

The approach identified 65 regulated genes in the 23k PRL versus the control group. Among them, 55 genes were down-regulated and 10 genes were up-regulated. Similarly, 63 regulated genes (28 down-regulated and 35 up-regulated) were identified in the 16k PRL versus the control group. Here we use the prolactin gene identified from the analysis results to demonstrate the advantage of the probe level data analysis over the gene level data analysis in Figure 5. The probe expressions of this gene showed most probes with differential expressions between the 23k PRL and the control groups. There were 15 probes (probes 1-15) with percentile difference of weighted rank greater than 0.67. This observation indicates a main treatment effect (homogenous differential probe expressions) occurred in the 23k PRL group. In contrast, comparison of the 16k PRL arrays versus the control arrays showed only 10 probes (probes 1-7, 10, 12, and 14) with differential expressions. Specifically, probes 1-7 had a percentile difference of weighted rank greater than 0.9. The result suggests an interaction effect (expression differences depend on probes) occurred in the 16k PRL group. These observations are consistent with the gene structure. The 23k PRL is a wild-type human prolactin in which its mRNA closely matches the probe set of the human prolactin gene in the gene chip. As a result, the expression of the prolactin gene was almost completely differential in the 23k PRL arrays. On the other hand, 16k PRL has a quarter of the PRL molecule truncated (i.e., alternative splicing). Thus, in the gene array analysis, only partial probes showed differential expressions and this explains the occurrence of interaction effect. Clearly, this example highlights the importance of probe level data analysis. If the gene level data analysis is used, we may miss this target gene. Even when we can identify this gene, it only indicates differential gene expression status without knowing probe expression, which may reveal useful biological information.

3.4. *Gene Function Classification*

We used the integrated bioinformatics tool to perform `gene function classification`. The regulated genes were grouped according to similar

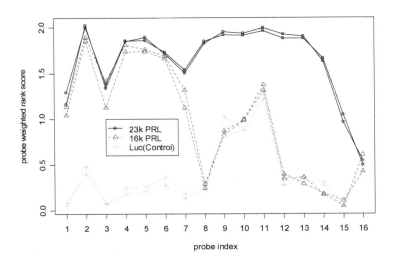

Fig. 5. Prolactin gene profile in probe level expression. The figure is the comparisons of prolactin gene's probe expression among the 23K PRL, 16 PRL, and the control groups. In this figure, a solid curve (-o-) represents probe level expression for the 23K PRL, a dashed curve $(-\Delta-)$ is for the 16 PRL, and a dotted curve (-+-) is for the control group. Most probe expressions were differential in the 23k PRL arrays, but only about half of the probes showed expression changes in the 16k PRL arrays. The results indicate homogenous differential probe expressions occurred in the 23k PRL group, but an interaction effect (expression differences depend on probes) occurred in the 16k PRL group.

biological functions. Here we used the comparison of 16 PRL versus the control groups for illustration. Figure 6.1 is the main output of analysis results. It shows the number of regulated genes (28 down-regulated and 35 up-regulated) in the first table of the figure. The numbers of biological functions related to gene expression change ranged from 8 to 60 in the second table. For example, there were 42 annotations of GO biological process, and 8 pathways involved in the down-regulated genes. A click of the down-regulated cell in the table of total number of selected genes leads to the Figure 6.2, where the 28 down-regulated genes are listed with gene name, fold change, and gene description. The table allows investigators to refine gene selections based on various criteria, such as fold change. Since there may be multiple probe sets listed with the same gene names, the table was sorted by gene name to provide a descriptive assessment of likelihood of true differential expression. If a gene name appears many times, the chance of its being false positive is likely low. For example, the gene chip has two probe sets with the same gene name, ANGPT2. Both of them (i.e., 1951_at and 37461_at) were selected here as down-regulated genes with 1.58 ~ 1.59 fold changes. This information can be used to indicate the likelihood of true differential expression. If investigators want to know more detailed information of the gene (e.g., DKK1), a click of this gene's probe set ID leads to Figure 6.3, which lists most important gene properties, such as alias, locus location, summary, GO annotations, pathway, and reference into function. A scatterplot was given to display data distribution (e.g., gene expressions were well separated for the gene, DKK1). A link to NCBI's Entrez Gene database is given by clicking the Entrez gene ID if investigators want to know most of the detailed information.

To check the results of gene function classification, we can click the cells of the table of "Number of Annotations" in Figure 6.1. For example, Figure 6.4 illustrates the results of pathway classification for the down-regulated and up-regulated genes. A higher frequency may indicate higher likelihood of the corresponding pathway involved in the experiment. A click of a frequency in the cell of the table will generate a table of listed genes. For example, there are 3 selected genes associated with cell cycle in Figure 6.5, which displays gene expression data, gene name, and gene description to check fold change.

3.5. *RT-PCR Validation*

Using the integrated bioinformatics tool, the results of gene function classification led us to identify 6 genes strongly associated with cell proliferation in Table 1. Five of the 6 genes were verified by quantitative RT-PCR. Four of the five genes were confirmed to be differentially expressed in the 23k PRL group. Only one gene, TB1, was misclassified as an up-regulated gene. In the 16k PRL group, only one gene (Asparagine) was a false negative.

4. Discussion

In summary, microarray data analysis is a complicated process. It requires multiple steps in order to yield more comprehensive results. First, we have to check data quality. We describe the 2D image plot to ensure the high quality of microarray array data for analysis. Once we have good quality of data, we perform gene selection to identify differentially expressed genes. We present a probe rank approach to analyze probe level data which has the advantage over the gene level data analysis, such as detection of alternative

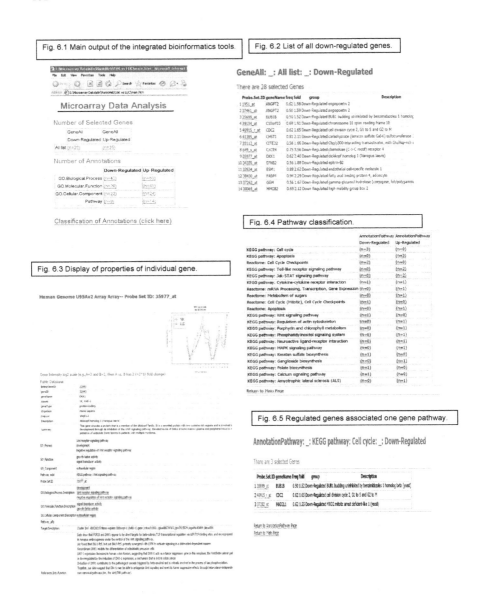

Fig. 6. The Integrated Bioinformatics Tools.

splicing. After we identify a set of regulated genes, we need to classify
and interpret the regulated genes based on biological functions. We use the

Table 1.   Quantitative RT-PCR for the 6 Selected Genes.

Gene Name	Probe Set ID	Gene Description	23k PRL vs. Luc	16k PRL vs. Luc
PRL	878_s_at	Prolactin	—*	—*
IGFBP-5	38650_at	insulin-like growth factor binding protein 5	2.3**	6.5**
CHOP	39420_at	DNA-damage-inducible transcript 3	2.2**	4.5**
Asparagine	36671_at	Asparagines synthetase	5.4**	2.9$^\Delta$
TB1	37178_at	Hypothetical protein BC017169	1.1$^\Delta$	1.14$^\Delta$
DKK1	35977_at	Dickkopf homolog 1 (Xenopus laevis)	0.4**	0.4**

Note.
*: The prolactin gene was not included in quantitative RT-PCR test because it was confirmed in the Kim et al.'s study.[48]
**: Differential expression by microarray.
Δ: Non-differential expression by microarray.

integrated bioinformatics tool to extract the relevant biological information and effectively present the results so investigators can easily convert them into useful knowledge.

4.1. *Quality Control*

The use of 2D image plot is to ensure the high quality of oligonucleotide array data for analysis. The 2D image plot uses percentile methods to group data, and then applies the 2D image plot to display the grouped data. Finally, a coverage rate based on an invariant band is computed to quantify degrees of array comparability. The 2D image plot is limited to pair-wise comparisons. When the number of arrays increases, this pair-wise comparison strategy may become impractical. However, in practice, we found it is not a major issue because, most times, the use of one or two reference arrays is enough for us to screen out incomparable arrays. Alternatively, we can average all arrays as the reference. However, this may introduce a confounding effect between the average and array incomparability, especially when the bias among arrays is nonlinear.

4.2. *Gene Selection*

We use the percentile difference of probe weighted rank to determine the status of probe expression change. When sample size is small, such as the datasets in the data example, the minimum probe rank percentile in one group is compared to the maximum in the other group. This measure is an alternative to mean or median difference, and is potentially useful in basic medical research, especially for in vitro studies where the study is often well-controlled, and the sample sizes are quite small (usually 2-4). For a larger sample size, the difference of probe rank percentile could become median difference. The probe level threshold could be a pre-specified cutoff based on the percentile difference or a p-value (e.g., $p < 0.05$) from the Wilcoxon Mann-Whitney test (a test for median difference between two groups).

In the data analysis of the prolactin study, the use of the probe weighted rank approach leads us to identify a subset of genes strongly associated with cell proliferation. Quantitative RT-PCR confirmed most genes. Moreover, an alternative splicing form of the prolactin gene was identified. By taking these observations together, the probe weighted rank approach provides an alternative for analyzing oligonucleotide gene array data.

4.3. *Integrated Bioinformatics Tool*

The integrated bioinformatics tool can be used to extract relevant biological functions associated with gene expression changes efficiently, and generate a simplified web-based output for investigators to expedite their research. The tool has the following unique features: (1) Integration of genomic database. The database is sufficient for researchers to study the association of regulated genes with biological functions and pathways. Classification based on GO annotations and KEGG pathway in the database lists all biological processes, cellular components, molecular functions, and pathways involved in the regulated genes. Utilizing the corresponding frequency tables to indicate the likelihood of particular biological functional activities, investigators can easily identify pathways associated with regulated-genes. In addition, the integrated database includes useful variables, such as gene alias, gene name, gene description, KEGG pathway, and RIF, to identify genes associated with keywords of interest; (2) Effective presentation of analysis results. The results of data analysis are presented in an easily readable format. The outputs are self-tutorial and easy to operate with very basic knowledge of using internet web browsers. Starting with a simple main HTML file, users can easily browse the results from the whole set of regulated-genes to a single differentially expressed gene. For all regulated-genes, the tool will group them into subgroups based on their differential expressions, GO annotations, pathways, or special keywords. For each sub-group, the tool summarizes genes in the group with valuable biological information to study relationships among these genes. For a single regulated gene, the tool details the gene information such that researchers can have a better understanding of this gene. A link is provided in the HTML file to connect to NCBI database for further examination. To visualize gene expression change, various graphical outputs are given, such as scatterplots for probe level data and boxplots for gene level data.

Acknowledgments

This work was supported by grants from the National Institute of Health (5P30 CA-13148, 1P50 CA89019, P30 AI 27767, N01-DC-5-0008, and 1U54 CA100949). We thank Laura Gallitz for secretarial assistance.

References

1. C. Sotiriou, et al., *Proc Natl Acad Sci* **100**, 10393 (2003).
2. J. R. Nevins, et al., *Hum Mol Genet.* **12** , R153 (2003).
3. A. Seth, et al., *Anticancer Res.* **23** , 2043 (2003).
4. S. Swami, et al., *Breast Cancer Res Treat* **80**, 49 (2003).
5. T.J. Yeatman, *The American Surgeon* **69**, 41 (2003).
6. L. Benimetskaya, et al., *Clin Cancer Res.* **10**, 3678 (2004).
7. K.L. Schaefer, et al., *Cancer Res.* **64** ,3395 (2004).
8. J.J. Going, et al., *Eur J Cancer* **37**, S5 (2001).
9. Y. Luo, et al., *Stem Cells* **21**, 575 (2003).
10. S. Bilke, T. Breslin, and M. Sigvardsson, *BMC Bioinformatics* **4**, 40 (2003).
11. Affymetrix, *Affymetrix GeneChip Operating Software with AutoLoader*, Version 1.4, Affymetrix, Santa Clara (2005)
12. Affymetrix, *Affymetrix Microarray Suite User Guide*, Affymetrix, Santa Clara, (2002).
13. C.L. Wilson and C.J. Miller , *Bioinformatics* **21**, 3683 (2005).
14. AffyQCReport: *http://bioconductor.org/packages/1.8/bioc/html/affyQCReport.html.*
15. A. Bhattacharjee, et al., *PNAS* **98**, 13790 (2001).
16. J.H. Kim, et al., *Experimental And Molecular Medicine* **34**, 224 (2002).
17. T. Beissbarth, et al., *Bioinformatics* **16**, 1014 (2000).
18. R. Rosner R. *Fundamentals of Biostatistics (5th ed.)*, Duxbury, Pacific Grove, California, (2000).
19. J.M. Chambers, et al., *Graphical Methods for Data Analysis*, Wadsworth, Belmont, California (1983).
20. W.S. Cleveland, *The Elements of Graphing Data*, Wadsworth, Monterey, California (1985).
21. D. Singh, et al., *Cancer Cell* **1**, 203 (2002).

22. N.N. Hansel, et al., *J. Lab Clin Med* **145**, 263 (2005).
23. C. Holmen, P. Stjarne, and S. Sumitran-Holgersson, *Am. J. Respir. Cell Mol. Biol.* **32**, 18 (2005).
24. D.R. Shaffer, et al., *PNAS* **102**, 210 (2005).
25. P.A. Horwitz, et al., *Circulation* **110**,3815 (2004).
26. J. Lunec, E. Halligan, N. Mistry, and K. Karakoula, *Ann N Y Acad Sci* **1031**, 169 (2004).
27. I. Rioja, et al., *Arthritis Res Ther* **7**, R101 (2005).
28. G.A. Toruner, et al., *Cancer Genet Cytogenet* **154** ,27 (2004).
29. C. Li, and W.H. Wong, *Proc. Natl. Acad. Sci. U S A* **98**, 31 (2001).
30. R.A. Irizarry, et al., *Nucleic Acids Research* **31**, e15 (2003).
31. Z. Wu and R.A. Irizarry, *J Comput Biol.* **12**,882 (2005).
32. V. Tusher, et al, *PNAS* **98**, 5116 (2001).
33. S. Dudoit,S., et al., *Statistica Sinica* **12**, 111 (2002).
34. Y. Benjamini and Y. Hochberg, *Journal of the Royal Statistical Society B* **57**, 289 (1995).
35. B. Modrek, and C. Lee, *Nature Genetics* **30**, 13 (2002).
36. M.C. Thompson, et al., *J Clin Oncol* **24**, 1924 (2006).
37. J.N. McClintick, et al., *J Nutr Biochem* (2005).
38. S.E. Hannema, et al., *Horm Res* **65**, 200 (2006).
39. Gene Ontology: *http://www.geneontology.org.*
40. AmiGO: *http://godatabase.org.*
41. EP: *GO http://ep.ebi.ac.uk/EP/GO.*
42. G.F. Berriz, J.V. White, O.D. King, and F.P. Roth, *Bioinformatics* **19**, 788 (2003).
43. D. Groth, H. Lehrach, and S. Hennig, *Nucleic Acids Res* **32**, W313 (2004).
44. Cancer Genome Anatomy Project: *http://cgap.nci.nih.gov/Genes/GOBrowser.*
45. T. Beissbarth, T.P. Speed. *Bioinformatics* **20**, 1464 (2004).
46. http://www.genetools.no.
47. G.J. Dennis, et al. *Genome Biol* **4**,P3 (2003).
48. W. Feng, et al. *AMIA Annu Symp Proc* **839**, (2003).
49. F. Al-Shahrour, R. Diaz-Uriarte, J. Dopazo. *Bioinformatics* **20**, 578 (2004).
50. M. Kanehisa, et al. *Nucleic Acids Res* **32**, D277 (2004).
51. M. Kanehisa, et al. *Nucleic Acids Res* **34**, D354 (2006).
52. K.D. Dahlquist, et al. *Nat Genet* **31**, 19 (2002).
53. G. Joshi-Tope, et al. *Nucleic Acids Res* **33**, D428 (2005).
54. P. Shannon, et al. *Genome Res* **13**, 2498 (2003).
55. biocarta: *http://www.biocarta.com.*
56. S.W. Doniger SW, et al. *Genome Biol.* **4**, R7 (2003).
57. R. Pandey, et al. *Bioinformatics* **20**, 2156 (2004).
58. G.C. Cheng, et al. *6th AIAA/ASME Joint Thermophysics and Heat Transfer Conference*, 2026 (1994).
59. G.C. Cheng, et al. *33rd AIAA/ASME/SAE/ASEE Joint Propulsion Conference and Exhibit*, 3228 (1997).
60. D.T. Chen, *Journal of Biopharmaceutical Statistics* **14**, 591 (2004).

61. T.C. Kroll, and S. Wolfl, *Nucleic Acids Research* **30**, e50 (2002).
62. D.C. Hoyle, M. Rattray, R. Jupp, and A. Brass, *Bioinformatics* **18**, 576 (2002).
63. D.T. Chen, S.H. Lin, and S.-J. Soong, *Bioinformatics* **20**, 854 (2004).
64. D.T. Chen, J. Chen, and S.-J. Soong, *Bioinformatics* **21**, 2861 (2005).
65. Netaffx Analysis Center: *http://www.affymetrix.com/analysis/index.affx.*
66. Entrez: *The Life Sciences Search Engine www.ncbi.nlm.nih.gov/Entrez.*
67. KEGG: *http://www.genome.jp/kegg.*
68. R: *http://www.r-project.org.*
69. C. Bole-Feysot, et al., *Endocr. Rev.* **19**, 225 (1998).
70. A. Ochoa, et al., *Investigative ophthalmology & visual science* **42**, 1639 (2001).
71. J. Kim, et al., *Cancer Research* **63**, 386 (2003).

CHAPTER 8

WAVELETS AND PROJECTING SPECTRUM BINNING FOR PROTEOMIC DATA PROCESSING

Don Hong[a], Huiming Li[b], Ming Li[c], and Yu Shyr[c,d]

[a] *Department of Mathematical Sciences, Middle Tennessee State University, Murfreesboro, Tennessee, USA*
E-mail: dhong@mtsu.edu
[b] *ITS, Peabody College, Vanderbilt University, Nashville, Tennessee, USA*
[c] *Department of Biostatistics, Vanderbilt University, Nashville, Tennessee, USA*
[d] *Department of Statistics, National Cheng Kung University, Taiwan, ROC*

High throughput mass spectrometry (MS) has been motivated greatly from recent developments in both chemistry and biology. Its technology has been extended to proteomics as a tool in rapid protein identification and is emerging as a leading technology in the proteomics revolution. However, key challenges still remain in the processing of proteomic MS data. It is substantial to develop a comprehensive set of mathematical and computational tools for proteomic MS data analysis. The processing goal is to effectively and correctly obtain the true information from the raw MS data for further statistical analysis. To provide a final peak list for future statistical analysis, the whole processing procedure usually takes the following steps: data registration (calibration), denoising (smoothing), baseline correction, normalization, peak detection, and peak alignment (binning). In this chapter, a wavelet-based approach for data denoising is discussed and a so-called projecting spectrum binning (PSB) method for proteomic MS cross samples peaks alignment is introduced. Applications to real MS datasets for different cancer research projects in Vanderbilt Ingram Cancer Center show that the approach is efficient and satisfactory.

1. Introduction

Proteomics is the study of the function of all expressed proteins. Mass Spectrometry (MS) technology makes it possible to study various biological samples at their protein level. High-throughput Mass Spectrometry, including Matrix-Assisted Laser Desorption/Ionization, Time-of-Flight (MALDI-TOF) and Surface-Enhanced Laser Desorption/Ionization Time-of-Flight

(SELDI-TOF) mass spectroscopy, is becoming a leading technology in finding disease-related proteomic patterns in tissue, blood, or other biological samples. The data generated by this technology holds invaluable information leading to the disease diagnosis and treatment[1,22,26]. However the raw mass spectrometric data reflects not only the protein information but also noise information. The data processing goal then is to effectively and correctly obtain the useful information from the MS data for bimarkers discovery. Biomarkers are biological features such as molecules that are indicators of physiologic state and also of change during a disease process. At the protein level, distinct changes occur during the transformation of a healthy cell into a neoplastic cell, including altered expression, differential protein modification, changes in specific activity, and aberrant localization, all of which may affect cellular function. Identifying and understanding these changes is the underlying theme in cancer proteomics[28].

Mass spectrometers are ion optical devices that produce a beam of gas-phase ions from samples. They sort the resulting mixture of ions according to their mass-to-charge (m/z) ratios or a derived property, and provide analog or digital output signals (peaks) from which the mass-to-charge ratio and intensity (abundance) of each detected ionic species may be determined. Masses are not measured directly. Mass spectrometers are m/z analyzers. The mass-to-charge ratio of an ion is obtained by dividing the mass of the ion (m), by the number of charges (z) that were acquired during the process of ionization. The mass of a particle is the sum of the atomic masses (in Dalton) of all the atoms of the elements of which it is composed.

Mass spectrometers attempt to answer the basic questions of *what* and *how much* is present by determining ionic masses and intensities. MALDI-TOF MS is emerging as a leading technology in the proteomics revolution. Indeed, the year 2002 Nobel Prize in chemistry recognized MALDI's ability to analyze intact biological macromolecules. Though MALDI-TOF MS allows direct measurement of the protein "signature" of tissue, blood, or other biological samples, and holds tremendous potential for disease diagnosis and treatment, key challenges still remain in the processing of MALDI MS data. As shown in Figure 1, MALDI MS data sets from the same sample have obvious intensity noises, baseline artifacts, and m/z location variations.

Mass spectrometry based proteomics experiments usually comprise a data generation phase, a data preprocessing phase, and a data analysis phase. In early applications of MALDI-TOF analyzers, the mass resolution was poor and the mass accuracy was limited. A mathematical model of

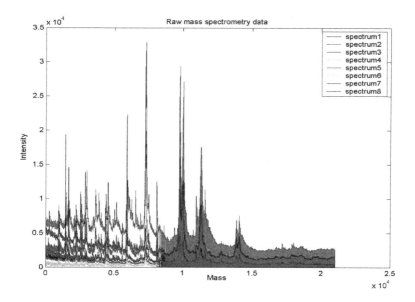

Fig. 1. Raw Data Sets of MALDI-TOF MS.

systems employing uniform electric fields is presented in [29], which allows "exact" calculations of flight times as functions of mass-to-charge ratio, initial velocity and position, applied voltages, and instrument geometry.

The whole mathematical processing procedure of MS signals can be roughly divided into two steps. First, in the "preprocessing" step, we attempt to recover from the time of arrival data, as accurately as possible, the "true" signal reflecting the mass/charge distribution of the ions originating from the sample. The preprocessing step includes registration, denoising, baseline correction, and deconvolution. In the preprocessing step, these operations are performed independently of any biological information one seeks to extract from the data. The second type of processing attempts to represent the data in a form that facilitates the extraction of biological information. This step involves operations such as dimension reduction, feature selection, clustering, and pattern recognition for classification. Recently, many efforts have been put into preprocessing of proteomic MS data using mathematical tools[2,15,25], statistical techniques[3,7,31,32], as well as computing skills and machine learning methods[4,10,30].

In the following, we focus on the preprocessing phase using mathematical tools such as wavelets and a new developed peak alignment method, namely the projecting spectrum binning (PSB).

The paper is organized as follows: mass spectrometric data preprocessing procedures, GG procedure – Gaussian smoothing and Genetic algorithm for final peak binning, WW procedure – Wavelet denoising and Window-based peak alignment, as well as the WG procedure – Wavelet denoising and Genetic algorithm for peak binning, will be briefly reviewed in the next section. In section 3, the projecting spectrum binning (PSB) method will be introduced and a new MS data preprocessing procedures using wavelet denoising and PSB, named as WPSB procedure is proposed. Comparison results are shown in Section 4. Final remarks and questions for future study are discussed in the final section.

2. Review of MS Data Processing Procedures

2.1. *The GG procedure*

The GG procedure was based on Gaussian smoothing and Genetic algorithm for final peak binning, which was adopted by Vanderbilt Medical Center and can be described as follows.

Step 1, Raw data smoothing and calibration: Use a Gaussian smoothing function provided by the Data Explorer software (Applied Biosystems, Foster City, CA). After smoothing, each spectrum was internally calibrated to minimize the inevitable mass shifts with a single sample as well as between different samples. The spectra were calibrated using four fixed m/z values.

Step 2, Baseline correction: A piecewise linear function interpolates the lowest intensity within a series mass windows. The baseline corrected spectrum is generated by subtracting the area under the fit.

Step 3, Normalization: Compare each spectrum to one pre-specified reference spectrum. For each comparison, the common peaks between two spectra are identified. Calculate the "intensity ratio" for each peak in common. Fit a linear equation to these ratios. Remove those ratios bigger that two standard deviations from the fit. Then fit the remaining intensity ratios again. Rescale the intensity for each spectrum by multiplying the correspondence value of the fitted equation.

Step 4, Peak selection: Based on a pre-specified S/N ratio, decide the number of peaks for each spectrum[27].

Step 5, Peak alignment (binning): Genetic Algorithm (GA) is customized to search the best bins for combining the peaks represent the same protein. A search started to find the optimal window width and location if it can maximize $\sum n^2$, n is the number of peaks within that window, while the maximum width of a window is constrained by $3 + 0.001 \times$ Mass in Dalton[18].

After alignment (binning), the GG procedure provides a $p \times n$ matrix (p rows of mass/charge (m/z values for n samples) for further statistical analysis. Each row of the final matrix stands for intensities at a certain m/z value for n samples. The m/z value actually represents the median value of a binning range involved in GG procedure.

2.2. The WW procedure

The WW procedure applied wavelet denoising with window-based peak alignments, which was adopted by MD Anderson Cancer Center. The word "wavelets" means "small waves" (the sinusoids used in Fourier analysis are "big" waves), and in short, wavelet is an oscillation that decays quickly. Mathematically, wavelets usually are basis functions of an L^2 space that satisfy so-called multiresolution analysis requirements[6,9,16]. In recent years, wavelets have been applied to a large variety of signal processing and image compression[19]. Also, there is a growing interest in using wavelets in analysis of biomedical signals and functional genomics data[14]. The major steps of WW procedure can be summarized in the following.

Step 1, Raw data calibration: The calibration was made based on the three known proteins[8] as well as applying linear interpolation method. Thus, the raw MS data have the common mass for all different spectra at the very beginning of the processing.

Step 2, Wavelet denoising (Smoothing): To implement the undecimated discrete wavelet transform (UDWT), and choose a Daubechies wavelet of certain degree.

Step 3, Baseline correction: Estimate the baseline by fitting a monotone local minimum curve to the denoised spectra.

Step 4, Normalization: Normalize each spectrum by dividing the total ion current (summing the observed intensities) in a certain mass/charge region and then multiplying by the arbitrary constant of 10000. It is motivated by the idea that the total ion current is a surrogate for the total amount of protein being measured in the sample.

Step 5, Peak detection: Peak detection has two stages, first, identify and quantify peaks by simply identifying the local maxima in a processed spectrum and recording their heights and locations; second, refine the list of potential peaks found from the first stage by considering the signal-to-noise ratio S/N greater than a pre-specified value.

Step 6, Peak alignment (binning): To match (align) peaks across spectra takes two rounds: the first round only considers the set of peaks with S/N greater than a pre-specified value m_1, pool the list of detected peaks and combine peaks that differ in location by no more than 7 clock ticks or in relative mass by 0.003, thus the peaks classified within one range corresponds to the same protein. The second round is going back to add the peaks greater than another pre-specified value m_2 ($m_2 \leq S/N \leq m_1$) to above list only if they fall within the same range limits (7 clock ticks or 0.003 relative mass) of above peaks just identified.

2.3. *The WG procedure*

The WG procedure is a relatively new method by using wavelets for denoising and genetic algorithm (or PSB) for final peak alignment. The WG procedure combines different portion of WW and GG procedures and the rationale for proposing it are explained below.

First of all, denoising (smoothing) is an especially important step for detecting true peaks. The GG procedure used Gaussian smoothing, a default machine software for smoothing and it may have problems, for example, closely overlapping peaks may not be distinguished[27]. On the other hand, the WW procedure applied wavelet smoothing, a very flexible and powerful method for the signal process like MS data. `Wavelet denoising` normally starts by transforming from the time domain to the wavelet domain and then estimating the variability of the coefficient. Then it sets up a threshold parameter and applies either soft or hard thresholding, and finally, transforms back to the time domain. More descriptions on advantages of wavelets methods for MS data processing and medical data analysis can be found in [5, 8, 14, 15].

For the whole MS data processing procedure, the final peak alignment is an inevitable step due to the drift in the locations of spectral peaks from on experiment to another even though they represent the same biochemical substance across different spectra. Nevertheless, the quality of alignment method directly affects the final $p \times n$ matrix for further statistical analysis. The alignment (binning) idea of WW method (combining the peaks that differ by no more than a certain clock tick or a certain relative mass) sounds reasonable, but in practice, it might be problematic. For example, consider 20 consecutive peaks found by peak selection. If any two adjacent peaks meet the above criteria for combining peaks, we might end up combining all 20 peaks together. In applications (see section 4), it actually shows the implementation algorithm by the WW procedure having trouble distinguishing distinctive peaks for certain spectral data. As a result, it may combine some different peaks together in a wide bin range. While the alignment (binning) algorithm of the GG procedure, or the projecting spectrum binning (PSB) method, can effectively identify these distinct peaks. The basic idea of PSB is to projects all MS peaks, from the view of the top of MS spectra, to a plane, in which one MS spectrum is one row and a MS peak is one dot on the row. These dots represent the peak distribution in spectra. The peak distribution has been used to determine bin location and bin width. The results show that PSB bins peaks both effectively and efficiently (see next section for details).

If we adapt the strengths of WW and GG procedure, then we have a sketch of the WG procedure:

Step 1 to 5: adopt the WW procedure for (1) raw data calibration, (2) wavelet denoising, (3) baseline correction, (4) normalization, and (5) peak detections.

Step 6: adopt the GG procedure for final peaks alignment (binning).

In the next section, we intruduce the `projecting spectrum binning` (PSB) method. PSB is an equivalent yet more efficient method for peak final alignment than that of the GA binning method. It gaves similar results with less computation time.

3. Projecting Spectrum Binning Method

Now, let us discuss the cross sample alignment of MS data. For data samples from patients, as it is mentioned above, the data first has to be preprocessed with the proper background subtracted, normalized, and the different fractions combined to obtain one integrated spectrum for each patient. The integrated spectrum is then binned or aligned so that the data for all patients in the sample is formatted in a matrix with one index representing the patients and the other index the peaks (discrete m/z's corresponding to the mean of the m/z of each bin).

The spectral data sets that result from MS experiments consist of the sequentially recorded numbers of ions arriving at the detector (intensity) corresponding to the mass-to-charge ratio (m/z) values. Although variation occurs in MS data, the following two assumptions are commonly used in MS data processing and analysis: (i) The peaks from a protein in the spectra should be positioned in an extremely tight mass range; (ii) the peaks, located in an extremely tight mass range in the spectra, should be generated by a protein. According to these two assumptions and after the peak selection process, for a given appropriate binning location and binning window, the bin could contain all peaks of a protein in spectra. These peaks in the bin can be assigned a mass ID of the same protein.

As a powerful searching method, Genetic Algorithm (GA) has been implemented in many search problems (see [11] for instance). Genetic algorithms are randomized optimization methods that need minimal information on the problem to guide the search. They use a population of multiple structures, each one encoding a tentative solution, to perform a search from many zones of the problem space at the same time[12]. GA was customized to search bins for mass spectra in [6]. Although it performs very well, GA Binning (GAB) is a computation-intensive method and theoretically obtains only a local optimum solution in binning search because the search space in GAB is incompact[18]. In [20], though it tried to avoid binning the peaks in the data processing, the binning idea actually is presented by using a mean spectrum. The bin locations are determined by the peaks in the mean spectrum. One of its drawbacks is that the mean spectrum usually cannot represent the peak distribution of spectra in an acurate manner. It is desired to find a simple binning method, by which bin locations are determined by two criteria: (1) the peaks selected in one bin should meet the requirement for a certain signal to noise (S/N) ratio, and (2) one bin combines only the peaks that differ by no more than a certain clock tick or a certain relative mass. This binning method actually uses a constant initial bin width. Some clustering techniques are applied in [5] to determine a so-called center spectrum for a binning procedure. In the following, we present a new binning method, named the projecting spectrum binning (PSB). This method mainly consists of two major steps: spectrum projection and bin determination. Comparing PSB with GAB, the results show that PSB bins peaks both effectively and efficiently. Binning approach reduces the dimension of data significantly.

Given a mass window with window location and window width, the peak frequency in the mass window for a given set of spectra is easy to be calculated. Moving the mass window with a certain shifting unit from lower mass to higher mass, we obtain a set of mass-frequency pairs (x, n), where the mass x, can be the middle value of the mass window and the frequency n, is the peak frequency of the spectra in the mass window. In other words, if $w(x)$ is the window width associated with the mass value x, then the peak frequency f of the spectra can be expressed as $f(x) = f(x, w(x))$. According to the assumptions mentioned above, it is obvious that a protein would generate a peak in the mass-frequency spectrum and a peak in the mass-frequency spectrum may represent a protein. If the peak distribution of the spectra in a small neighborhood is about symmetric, then $f(x)$ will have a bell shaped graph in the neighborhood with a peak at x.

Since $f(x)$ projects a stack of mass spectra, which can be viewed as a 3D image, into a 2D mass-frequency graph, we call the peak frequency function $f(x)$ the projecting spectrum. Following the notation in [5], we define maximum bin width function to determine the window width as $w(x) = a + b \times x$, where a and b are parameters and x is the current mass value. The window width can be a function other than the linear format. To generate a projecting spectrum in real application as the mass window moving along the whole mass range, we need to discretize the mass range by defining a so-called shifting unit $s(x)$, which is usually a function of x. In practice, the parameters a and b, along with the shifting unit function are determined by empirical experiences. They can be defined using more sophisticated statistical estimating models. In the shifting process, we use the middle mass value x of the window to represent the window location. Associating with each window, the peak frequency is calculated as the number of peaks in the window across all spectra. Thus, each window has a pair of mass value and peak frequency. In this way, we obtain a discrete data set, the projecting spectrum of the given spectra.

Figure 2 shows an example of a segment of projecting spectrum with mass range from about 5,000 Da to 6,000 Da. The entire spectrum has about 19,087 mass-frequency pairs generated using our empirical parameters with mass ranging from 2,000 Da to 25,000 Da. From the projecting spectrum, we can see the peak locations clearly. Afterwards, a binning procedure can be carried out.

In a mass-frequency spectrum, peaks can be quite close to each other. To prevent two bins from being too close, we add a restriction that if the distance of the two peaks is less than certain shifting units, they will be combined as a one-bin. The peak location of the projecting spectrum is considered as the middle point of each bin. Following this, the bin range is then extended to certain shifting units from the binning center. The binning width should be controlled by an upper bound, which is usually called the maximum window width function, $w(x)$. If overlapping occurs between two bins, the dip point between the two peaks is the splitting point of two bins.

In the projecting spectrum, there are many small peaks representing a small percentage of peaks that appeared in the spectra at those points. In most cases, those small peaks of projecting spectrum represent the "noisy" peaks in the spectra. Therefore, we need to set up a percentage cut-off level

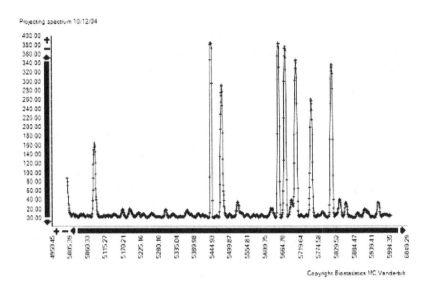

Fig. 2.   Part of the mass-frequency spectrum. The mass range is from 4950Da to 5994Da.

to remove the "noisy" bins. Again, the cut-off level can be an empirical value or it can be determined by statistical estimation. In our procedure, we use the cut-off level of 5%. That is, if the number of samples is 100, then the bins with 5 peaks or less will be considered as invalid bins.

Experimental results show that PSB reaches about the same goal as GAB does. In GAB, the initial step and crossover operations contain random factors. Therefore, the result can not be exactly reproduced. Compared with GAB, PSB has at least the following two advantages: First, PSB consistently generates the same bins on a given dataset, while GAB creates slightly different bins in each run. Second, PSB is more efficient than GAB. In particular, when the size of spectra increases, time for PSB consumes has little change, while time for GAB increases vastly. Figure 3 shows the bins, generated by PSB, with the mass peak distribution of the spectra. We plot the peaks as dots in the graph and each row as a representative of a spectrum. The x-axis is mass value and y-axis is the labeled spectrum number.

The proposed PSB method gives a fast and accurate binning process for high-throughput mass spectrometry data. It organizes and expresses MS peak data in an innovative way, which makes binning process simpler and easier. It performs well with profiles from different research projects

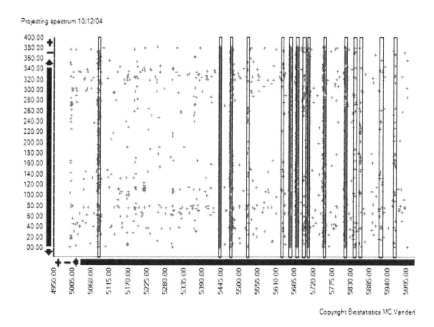

Fig. 3. Part of mass peak distribution with bins generated by PSB. The total number of spectra is 382.

and is insensitive to various parameters in preprocessing steps. In the PSB process, there is no precondition of bin location or bin width. The bins are generated completely from the distribution of peaks in spectra. The method introduces the window width function and the shifting unit. They are the tools to characterize the spectrum data. The parameters used in the functions of window width as well as the shifting are experimental. The method only involves the presence of peaks, not the intensities of peaks and the peak determination. Also, the PSB results are not affected much by small variation in the data registration.

Remark 1. PSB can be used to generate a more reasonable mean spectrum compared to the one derived in [20]. The direct comparisons between the projecting spectra between normal tissues and cancer tissues should be very helpful in biomarkers discovery as well.

Remark 2. Similar to many other computer algorithms, one concern of PSB is the stability of its performance when the size of the spectra is exceeding to certain number, say 700. In this case, we suggest adding in some statistical sub-sampling techniques when one applys PSB.

The PSB software package is available for downloading on the website: http://www.vicc.org/biostatistics/. Combined with the wavelet denoising for MS proteomic data, the preprocessing procedure using PSB is called the WPSB procedure for MS data preprocessing.

4. Applications

4.1. Data

The MS data sets for this application are obtained from the mass spectrometry laboratory at the Vanderbilt Medical Center. The 20 replicate spectra are from two mice with 10 spectrum each. These two mice can be treated as identical, both having caecal tumor but no liver metastasis. The mass/charge range we studied is from 4000 Da to 25000 Da. Figure 1 showed these raw spectral data before any preprocessing procedure.

4.2. Results

We applied the GG, WW and WG procedure to this spectral data respectively. The results are summarized in the following plots and tables.

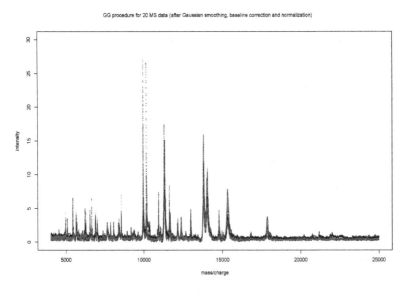

Fig. 4.   Results of GG procedure for 20 MS data sets after denoising, baseline correction, and normalization.

Figure 4 shows the Gaussian smoothed, baseline corrected and normalized data by the GG procedure for the mass/charge range from 4000 Da to 25000 Da. Figure 5 displays the wavelet smoothed, baseline corrected and normalized data by WW and WPSB methods within the mass/charge range 4000 Da to 25000 Da. The results for WW and WPSB method are the same until this step.

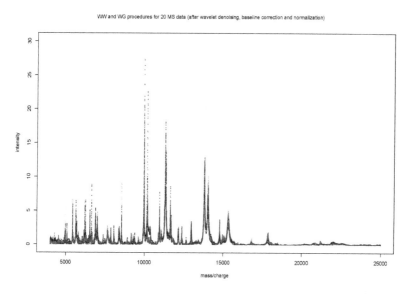

Fig. 5.   Results of WW or WG procedure for 20 MS data sets after denoising, baseline correction, and normalization.

From these two plots, we may agree that the wavelet method did a better job in terms of denoising since it filtered out more noise than that of the Gaussian smoothing method. It clearly demonstrated that the wavelet is much more powerful in removing the noise components.

This application, at this stage, showed that WPSB (WW) procedure is better than the GG procedure.

Figure 6, 7, and 8 show the final bin range of the selected peaks for the mass/charge range from 4000 Da to 25000 Da by the GG, WW and WPSB procedures respectively. In these plots, we use a pair of parentheses to represent a bin and a "⋆" to stand for the peaks detected. The peaks within a ( ) will be treated to represent the identical biological substance.

We use the median value of this range to stand for the mass/charge for all the peaks all in this range. Thus, we are able to provide a $p \times n$ matrix.

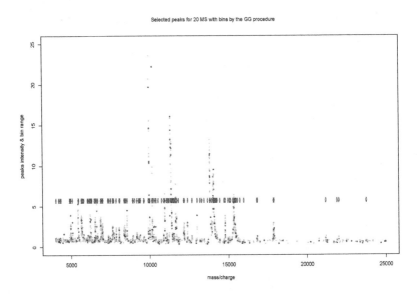

Selected peaks for 20 MS with bins by the GG procedure

Fig. 6.   Peaks and the bin ranges of 20 MS data sets after GG binning.

In Table 1, we made some summary statistics for these methods. For these 20 spectra, the alignment method by the GG procedure provides 258 bins, which means it identified 258 peaks. Equivalently, the alignment method by the WW procedure identified 60 peaks, and that of WPSB procedure identified 674 peaks. Obviously, it showed that the window-based alignment by the WW procedure generated relatively wide bin range compare to the PSB alignment method.

Figure 9 gives comparisons on the alignment results for the WW and WPSB procedures. To take a closer look at this, we only plotted the mass/charge range between 10000 Da and 12000 Da in the figure. We can see that the bins from WW procedure (with ( ) in red color) could not able to separate some distinctive peaks, while the bins from WPSB procedure (with ( ) in blue color) look very reasonable.

This application shows that the WPSB procedure has advantages among these procedures.

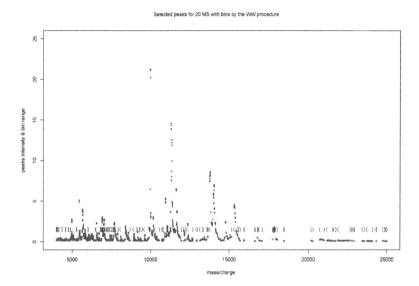

Fig. 7.   Peaks and the bin ranges of 20 MS data sets after WW binning.

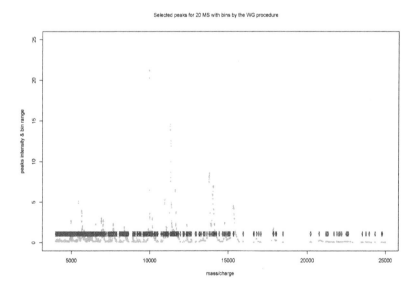

Fig. 8.   Peaks and the bin ranges of 20 MS data sets after WG or WPSB binning.

Table 1. Results of GG, WW and WPSB

Summary	Three procedures		
	GG	WW	$WPSB$
Number of peaks class	258	60	474
Number peaks in one class			
(minimum)	2	1	2
(1st Quintile)	2	15	4
(Median)	5	20	6
(Mean)	7.63	17	7
(3rd Quintile)	12	20	10
(Maximum)	20	20	20
Range of the bin			
(minimun)	3.6	0	1.89
(1st Quintile)	9.53	37.75	6.89
(Median)	12.85	122.5	9.51
(Mean)	13.87	200	11.34
(3rd Quintile)	17.37	257	14.35
(Maximum)	30.89	1382	32.33

5. Discussion and Future Study

The new procedure, WPSB, provides a potential framework for the feature extraction method in general. Within this framework, every step has some room to improve. For example, in the future, different types of wavelets may be adopted for different types of MS data; more flexible semi-parametric functions may be considered to fit the baseline; and normalization part requires more understanding on the biological knowledge to come up a better schema for spectra comparisons.

It is important to ascertain whether or not the peaks being found by the algorithm correspond to real phenomena in the spectra. So for searching a criteria for evaluating a procedure, we need to relay on the biological knowledge. Statistical results alone may not be adequate to demonstrate it as a reasonable method or not. Therefore, the idea of evaluating the methods itself is still an open research topic.

The new generation of mass spectrometers produces an astonishing amount of high-quality data in a brief period of time, leading to inevitable data analysis bottlenecks. Automated data analysis algorithms are required for rapid and repeatable processing of proteomic MS data. Toward this end a mathematical algorithm is presented in [17] that automatically lo-

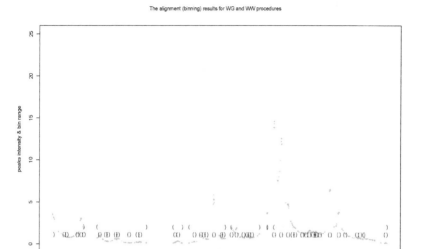

Fig. 9. Comparison binning results of WW (upper-row) and WPSB (lower-row) procedures.

cates and calculates the area beneath peaks. As mentioned in [21], a broad range of mass spectrometers are used in MS based proteomics research. Each type of instrument processes a unique design, data system and performance specifications, resulting in strengths and weaknesses for different types of experiments. However, the original raw data formats produced by each type of mass spectrometer also differ. A so-called *mzXML* format was introduced, using instrument-specific converters, as an open, genetic XML (extensible markup language) representation of MS data[21]. To find a common mathematical representation of MS data signals, we assume, in a very recent discussion[13], the ion cloud as $\sum_k \alpha_k \delta_{\beta_k}$ and model the output MS data f after the TOF instrument I as

$$I(\sum_k \alpha_k \delta_{\beta_k}) = \sum_k \alpha_k \psi_k(\cdot - \beta_k).$$

We hope to separate the output signal into two parts:

$$\sum_{|\alpha_k| \geq \epsilon} \alpha_k \psi_k(\cdot - \beta_k) + \sum_{\alpha_k < \epsilon} \alpha_k \psi_k(\cdot - \beta_k)$$

and expect the second term to be used to remove both baseline and noise. If the peak locations are determined, say by the mean spectrum method[20], then in such a model, the most challenge part will be the selection of the "bump" functions ψ_k and to determine the the parameters α_k and β_k. Though some basic ideas and tools are mentioned in [15], many challenges remain in the area of research along this direction.

Acknowledgments

The authors would like to thank Jonathan Xu at the Mass Spectrometry Research Center and Cancer Biology, Vanderbilt University for evaluating the performance of PSB and providing many useful suggestions. This research was supported in part by Lung Cancer SPORE (Special Program of Research Excellence) (P50 CA90949), Breast Cancer SPORE (1P50 CA98131-01), GI (5P50 CA95103-02), and Cancer Center Support Grant (CCSG) (P30 CA68485) for Y. Shyr, by GI SPORE (5P50CA95103-05) for M. Li, and by NSF IGMS (#0408086 and #0552377) and by MTSU REP for D. Hong.

References

1. P. J. Adam, et al., Comprehensive proteomic analysis of breast cancer cell membranes reveals unique proteins with potential roles in clinical cancer, *Journal of Biological Chemistry*, **278** (2003), 6482-6489.

2. K.A. Baggerly, et al., A comprehensive approach to the analysis of matrix-assisted laser desorption/ionization-time of flight proteomics spectra from serum sample, *Proteomics*, **3** (2003), 1667-1672.

3. S.A. Beausoleil, J. Villèn, S.A. Gerber, J. Rush, and S.P. Gygi, A probability-based approach for high-throughput protein phosphorylation analysis and site localization, *Nature Biotechnology*, **24** (2006), 1285-1292.

4. H. Chen, E.R. Tracy, W.E. Cooke, O.J. Semmes, M. Sasinowski, and D.M. Manos, Automated peak identification in a TOF-MS spectrum, in: *Quantitative Medical Data Analysis Using Math Tools and Statistical Techniques* (this volume), World Scientific Publication, LLC, Singapore, 2007.

5. S. Chen, D. Hong, and Y. Shyr, Wavelet-Based Procedures for Proteomic MS Data Processing, *Computational Statistics and Data Analysis*, in press (doi:10.1016/j.csda.2007.02.022).

6. C.K. Chui, An Introduction to Wavelets, Academic Press, New York, NY, 1992.

7. M.A. Clyde, L.L. House, and R.L. Wolpert, Nonparametric models for proteomic peak identification and quantification, In: *Bayesian Inference for Gene Expression and Proteomics*, (K.A Do, P. Mller, and M. Vannucci Eds.), Cambridge University Press, pp. 293-308, 2006.

8. K.R. Coombes, et al., Improved peak detection and quantification of mass spectrometry data acquired from surface-enhanced laser desorption and ion-

ization by denoising spectra with the undecimated discrete wavelet transform, *Proteomics*, **5** (2005), 4107-4117.

9. I. Daubechies, Ten Lectures on Wavelets, Society for Industrial and Applied Mathematics, Philadelphia, Pennsylvania, 1992.

10. J.E. Elias, F.D. Gibbons, O.D. King, F.P. Roth, and S.P. Gygi, Intensity-based protein identification by machine learning from a library of tandem mass spectra, *Nature Biotechnology*, **22** (2004), 214-219.

11. L. Franconi and C. Jennison, Comparison of a genetic algorithm and simulated annealing in an application to statistical image reconstruction, *Statistics and Computing*, 7 (1997), 193-207.

12. D.E. Goldberg, Genetic Algorithm in Search, Optimization and Machine Learning, Addison-Wesley, Reading, MA, 1989.

13. D. Hardin, D. Hong, and Q. Sun, private communications, 2006.

14. D. Hong and Y. Shyr, Wavelet applications in cancer study, *J. Concrete and Applicable Mathematics*, **4** (2006), 505-521.

15. D. Hong and Y. Shyr, Mathematical Framework and Wavelets Applications in Proteomics for Cancer Study, In: *Handbook of Cancer Models With Applications to Cancer Screening, Cancer Treatment and Risk Assessment*, (Wai-Yuan Tan and Leonid Hannin Eds.), World Scientific Publication, Singapore, 2007 (to appear).

16. D. Hong, J.Z. Wang, and R. Gardner, Real Analysis with an Introduction to Wavelets and Applications, Academic Press, New York, 2005.

17. A.J. Kearsley, W.E. Wallace, J. Bernal, and C.M. Guttman, A numerical method for mass spectral data analysis, *Applied Math Letters*, **18** (2005), 1412-1417.

18. H. Li, B. White, and J. Moore, Binning of high-throughput mass spectrometry data with genetic algorithm, *manuscript*, 2004.

19. S. Mallat, A Wavelet Tour of Signal Processing, Academic Press, New York, 1999.

20. S.J. Morris, et al., Feature extraction and quantification for mass spectrometry in biomedical applications using the mean spectrum, *Bioinformatics*, **21** (2005), 1764-1775.

21. P.G.A. Pedrioli, et al., A common open representation of mass spectrometry data and its application to proteomics research, *Nature Biotechnology*, **22** (2004), 1459-1466.

22. C.P. Paweletz, et al., Rapid protein display profiling of cancer progression directly from human tissue using a protein biochip. *Drug Development Research*, **49** (2000), 34-42.

23. Y. Qu, et al., Data reduction using a discrete wavelet transform in discriminant analysis of very high dimensionality data, *Biometrics*, **59** (2003), 143-151.

24. J. Ramasay and B.W. Silberman, *Functional Data Analysis*, Springer, New York, 1997.

25. T.W. Randolph and Y. Yasui, Multiscale processing of mass spectrometry data, *Biometrics*, **62** (2006), 589-597.

26. S. Schaub, et al., Urine protein profiling with surface-enhanced laser-

desorption/ionization time-of-flight mass spectrometry, *Kidney International*, **65** (2004), 323-332.

27. A.S. Schwartz, et al., Proteomic-Based Prognosis of Brain Tumor Patients Using Direct-Tissue Matrix-Assisted Laser Desorption Ionization Mass Spectrometry, *Cancer Research*, **65** (2005), 7674-7681.

28. P.R. Srinivas, et al., Proteomics for cancer biomarker discovery, *Clinical Chemistry*, **48** (2002), 1160-1169.

29. M. Vestal and P. Juhasz, Resolution and mass accuracy in matrix-assisted laser desorption ionization time-of-flight, *J. Am. Soc. Mass. Spectrom.*, **9** (1998), 892-911.

30. Z.R. Yang and K.-C. Chou, Bio-support vector machines for computational proteomics, *Bioinformatics*, **20** (2004), 735-41.

31. W. Yu, B. Wu, T. Huang, X. Li, K. Williams, and H. Zhao, Statistical methods in proteomics, In: *Handbook of Engineering Statistics*, Springer, pp. 623-638, 2005.

32. W. Yu, B. Wu, N. Lin, K. Stone, K. Williams, and H. Zhao, Detecting and aligning peaks in mass spectrometry data with applications to MALDI, *Computational Biology and Chemistry*, **30** (2006), 27-38.

UNIT III

SURVIVAL MODELING
AND ANALYSIS

CHAPTER 9

APPLICATION OF THE NON-PROPORTIONAL RATES MODEL TO RECURRENT EVENT DATA: ANALYSIS OF RISK FACTORS FOR PRE-SCHOOL ASTHMA

Jianwen Cai

Department of Biostatistics,
University of North Carolina at Chapel Hill,
Chapel Hill, NC, 27599-7420, USA

Douglas E. Schaubel

Department of Biostatistics,
University of Michigan,
Ann Arbor, MI, 48109-2029, USA

Asthma remains one of the most common chronic childhood illnesses and a leading cause of hospital admissions. Our clinical objective was to assess the effect of gender, birth characteristics and neonatal respiratory disorders on pre-school asthma rates of (i) hospitalization and (ii) days hospitalized. The proportional rates (PR) model is a flexible adaptation to recurrent event data of the well-known Cox proportional hazards model. The PR model is related to Poisson regression, but relaxes the often untenable assumption that the events within a subject are independent. Despite having been originally proposed over a decade ago, examples of the use of the proportional rates model in the medical literature are quite rare. Moreover, little attention has been devoted to the extension of the PR model to accommodate covariate effects which vary over time. We evaluate the non-proportional rates model through simulation. We then apply the non-PR model to asthma data from a retrospective birth cohort study.

1. Introduction

Asthma remains one of the most common chronic childhood illnesses, and a leading cause of hospital admissions[19,22]. Rates of hospitalization for asthma have increased in several countries during the last two decades including Canada[11,27] and the United States[26]. Childhood `asthma` usually begins in infancy or early childhood[18]; most children that suffer the disease have their first asthmatic episode before their third birthday[9]. Pre-school children hospitalized for asthma reportedly account for a disproportionately large fraction of total acute pediatric asthma admissions and tend to present the most difficult long-term disease management problems[9].

Several previous studies have examined the relationship between neonatal conditions and asthma. For example, Schaubel *et. al.*[21] conducted a retrospective cohort study that examined the effect of a wide variety of suspected risk factors for pre-school asthma incidence using a large health administrative database. Of current interest are risk factors for asthma-attributable hospitalizations and days hospitalized, since both quantities reflect disease severity as well as health care costs. Since the correlation among within-subject hospitalizations was not of direct interest, a marginal model was chosen for our analysis.

Lawless and Nadeau[13] proposed a general class of marginal means models for recurrent event data. The class can accommodate `time-dependent` `effects`. However, to the best of our knowledge, the appropriateness of asymptotic results in finite samples in the presence of time-dependent effects has not been evaluated.

In this investigation, we examine the finite-sample properties of the `non-proportional rates model` through simulation. We then assess the effect of birth characteristics on hospitalizations and days hospitalized for pre-school asthma using semi-parametric marginal rates models with time-dependent covariates. The remainder of this article is organized as follows. In Section 2, we describe the data sets used in this study. In Section 3, the marginal rates model is described, with comparisons made to alternative approaches. A simulation study to evaluate the non-proportional rates model is presented in Section 4. An analysis of the asthma data set is presented in Section 5. The article concludes with a discussion in Section 6.

2. Data Sources

Data were obtained from Manitoba Health, a provincial health administration organization in Canada. Health care in Canada is publicly funded and hence is, in theory, universal. For example, residents do not pay when they go to the hospital. Manitoba was among the first provinces in Canada to assign a unique identifier to residents at birth; the identifier is known as the Personal Health Identification Number (PHIN). Through the PHIN, it is possible to track utilization of various health services (e.g., physician office visits; hospital admissions) longitudinally.

Two Manitoba Health files were utilized: hospital admission/discharge records and a birth information file. From the birth file, data were obtained on variables which were suspected of being associated with an increased risk of childhood asthma, such as low birth weight, prematurity and neonatal respiratory conditions (e.g., respiratory distress syndrome (RDS), transient tachypnea of the newborn (TTN)). The birth and hospital files were linked using the PHIN, assigned to each child at birth. Children in the (fiscal) 1984 birth cohort (i.e., born between April 1, 1984 and March 31, 1985) were followed retrospectively until March 31, 1989 for hospitalizations resulting from asthma (ICD-9: rubric 493). All newborns had at least 4 years of observation, each being censored some time between ages 4 and 5. Further details pertaining to data collection and record linkage are available in Johansen et. al.[11]. We now discuss the statistical model of interest.

3. Model and Methods

We begin by defining the requisite notation. Let $N_i^*(t)$ be the total number of events for subject i $(i = 1, \ldots, n)$ as of time t. The censoring time for subject i is given by C_i and we define $\tau = \max\{C_1, \ldots, C_n\}$. The covariate vector, which may contain time-dependent elements, is denoted by $\mathbf{Z}_i(t)$.

The observed number of events is denoted $N_i(t) = N_i^*(t \wedge C_i)$, where $a \wedge b = \min\{a, b\}$. Event times for subject i are denoted $T_{i1}, \ldots, T_{iN_i}$, where $N_i = N_i(C_i)$. Expressed in terms of stochastic integrals, $N_i^*(t) = \int_0^t dN_i^*(s)$, where $dN_i^*(s) = N_i^*(s) - N_i^*(s-)$ and $s-$ is the time instant immediately preceding s. We assume that $N_i^*(t)$ is a `counting process` (e.g., Chiang[3]), such that $N_i^*(t_2) \geq N_i^*(t_1)$ for $t_2 > t_1$, $dN_i^*(t) = 0$ or 1, and $dN_i^*(t)dN_j^*(t) = 0$ for $i \neq j$. The $dN_i^*(s)$ quantities are referred to as the counting process increments.

The proportional means model[13,16] is given by:

$$\mu_i(t) \equiv E[N_i^*(t)|\mathbf{Z}_i] = \mu_0(t)\exp\{\boldsymbol{\beta}_0^T\mathbf{Z}_i\}, \qquad (1)$$

where $\mu_0(t)$ is an unspecified baseline mean function and $\boldsymbol{\beta}_0$ is the parameter of interest. In the case of time-dependent covariates, the `proportional rates model` is given by:

$$d\mu_i(t) \equiv E[dN_i^*(t)|\mathbf{Z}_i(t)] = d\mu_0(t)\exp\{\boldsymbol{\beta}_0^T\mathbf{Z}_i(t)\}, \qquad (2)$$

where $d\mu_0(t)$ is the `baseline rate` function (the rate being interpreted as the derivative of the mean). Model (1) is more restrictive in that it applies to covariates that do not vary over time, $\mathbf{Z}_i(t) = \mathbf{Z}_i$ for all t. Since it can accommodate time-dependent covariates (which play a key role in our application), we focus on model (2).

The proportional means/rates models, (1) and (2), can be considered recurrent event analogs of the Cox[5] `proportional hazards model`, for application to recurrent event data. Model (2) also has a close connection to the Andersen-Gill[2] model, which can be written as:

$$d\Lambda_i(t) \equiv E[dN_i^*(t)|\mathcal{F}_i(t-)] = d\Lambda_0(t) \exp\{\boldsymbol{\theta}_0^T \mathbf{Z}_i(t)\}, \tag{3}$$

where $\mathcal{F}_i(t)$ can be thought of as the event history for subject i at time t. One could refer to (3) and (2) as conditional and marginal models, respectively. Practitioners may prefer the latter for at least two reasons. First, it is often difficult to capture $\mathcal{F}_i(t-)$ through the covariate vector; e.g., by including $N_i^*(t-)$ or various other related functions of $\mathcal{F}_i(t)$ as elements in $\mathbf{Z}_i(t)$. Second, consider a study with one covariate, $\mathbf{Z}_i(t) = Z_i$, which takes the value 1 for 'treated' subjects and 0 for those receiving placebo. Compare two models, a marginal model,

$$E[dN_i^*(t)|Z_i] = d\mu_0(t) \exp\{\beta_0 Z_i\}, \tag{4}$$

and a conditional model,

$$E[dN_i^*(t)|Z_i, N_i^*(t-)] = d\Lambda_0(t) \exp\{\theta_0 Z_i + \theta_N N_i^*(t-)\}. \tag{5}$$

The quantity $\exp\{\beta_0\}$ from (4) can be interpreted as the ratio of the event rate, treated versus placebo (reference) subjects; that is,

$$\frac{E[dN_i^*(t)|Z_i = 1]}{E[dN_i^*(t)|Z_i = 0]} = \exp\{\beta_0\}.$$

The quantity $\exp\{\theta_0\}$ from model (5) would be making the same comparison, but restricting attention to subjects with the same number of previous events; i.e.,

$$\frac{E[dN_i^*(t)|Z_i = 1, N_i^*(t-) = m]}{E[dN_i^*(t)|Z_i = 0, N_i^*(t-) = m]} = \exp\{\theta_0\}.$$

If Z_i affects the event rate, $E[dN_i^*(t)]$, then it will also affect the $N_i^*(t-)$ and, provided events within-subject are positively correlated, conditioning on the previous number of events will attenuate the estimated marginal effect of Z_i; i.e., $|\theta_0| < |\beta_0|$.

The estimate of the parameter of interest in the proportional rates model, β_0, is the solution to the estimating equation,

$$\sum_{i=1}^{n} \int_0^\tau \{\mathbf{Z}_i(t) - \overline{\mathbf{Z}}(t; \boldsymbol{\beta})\} dN_i(t) = \mathbf{0}, \tag{6}$$

where $\mathbf{0}$ is a vector of 0's and the risk-weighted covariate mean is given by:

$$\overline{\mathbf{Z}}(t;\boldsymbol{\beta}) = \frac{\sum_{i=1}^{n} I(C_i > t)\mathbf{Z}_i(t)\exp\{\boldsymbol{\beta}^T\mathbf{Z}_i(t)\}}{\sum_{i=1}^{n} I(C_i > t)\exp\{\boldsymbol{\beta}^T\mathbf{Z}_i(t)\}}.$$

We can re-express the left side of (6) in a perhaps more familiar form as

$$\sum_{i=1}^{n}\sum_{j=1}^{N_i}\{\mathbf{Z}_i(T_{ij}) - \overline{\mathbf{Z}}(T_{ij};\boldsymbol{\beta})\}, \tag{7}$$

without the stochastic integral. In the univariate survival setting, where time until a single event is studied and subjects cannot experience multiple events (i.e., $N_i \leq 1$), the left side of (7) reduces to the partial likelihood[6] score equation,

$$\sum_{i=1}^{n}\Delta_i\{\mathbf{Z}_i(T_{ij}) - \overline{\mathbf{Z}}(T_{ij};\boldsymbol{\beta})\},$$

where $\Delta_i = I(T_i < C_i)$. The correspondence between the Cox score equation and (7) makes sense in light of the close connection between the proportional hazards and proportional rates models. As such, standard software (e.g., PROC PHREG in SAS; coxph in R) can be used to fit the proportional rates model, as described in Allison[1] and Therneau and Hamilton[23].

The model of current interest is given by:

$$E[dN_i^*(t)|\mathbf{Z}_i] = d\mu_0(t)\exp\{\boldsymbol{\beta}(t)\mathbf{Z}_i\}, \tag{8}$$

the **non-proportional rates model**, which allows the covariate effects to depend on time. Since the software cannot tell the difference between $\boldsymbol{\beta}(t)\mathbf{Z}_i$ and $\boldsymbol{\beta}\mathbf{Z}_i(t)$, we can estimate $\boldsymbol{\beta}(t)$ in (8) by fitting (2) and adding time-dependent elements to $\mathbf{Z}_i$ which reflect the nature of the hypothesized time-dependence of the effects suspected of being non-proportional. For example, returning to (4), a time-dependent treatment effect could be specified by the model,

$$E[dN_i^*(t)|Z_i] = d\mu_0(t)\exp\{(\beta_0 + \phi t)Z_i\}, \tag{9}$$

where estimators $\widehat{\beta}$ and $\widehat{\phi}$ could be computed by fitting the model,

$$E[dN_i^*(t)|Z_i] = d\mu_0(t)\exp\{\beta_0 Z_i + \phi Z_i \times t\}. \tag{10}$$

Model (9) allows the effect of Z_i on the event rate to change exponentially with time. Naturally, other functional forms are possible. Depending on the application, it may be desirable to shift the time-dependent term. For example, a model equivalent to model (10) is:

$$E[dN_i^*(t)|Z_i] = d\mu_0(t) \exp\{\beta_0 Z_i + \phi Z_i \times (t - t_0)\}, \tag{11}$$

where t_0 would be chosen to be some readily intuited time; e.g., mean, median, mid-point of follow-up distribution. Due to the non-proportionality, the rate ratio ($Z_i = 1$ vs. $Z_i = 0$) varies with t in model (10) and equals $\exp\{\beta_0\}$ at $t = t_0$ in model (11).

4. Simulation Study

To assess the performance of the non-proportional rates model in finite samples, we conducted a simulation study. A wide range of scenarios were examined. The number of subjects was set to $n = 30$, 50, 100 and 200. Censoring times, C_i, were generated from a Uniform(0,2.5) distribution. The simulated non-proportional rates model was given by:

$$d\mu_0(t) = Q_i d\mu_0 \exp\{\beta_0 Z_i + \phi_0 Z_i \times (t - 1.25)\}, \tag{12}$$

with $d\mu_0 = 0.5$, $\beta_0 = \log(2)$, $\phi_0 = 0.5$, and Q_i followed a Gamma distribution with mean 1 and variance, σ^2. The covariate was set to $Z_i = \text{mod}(i, 2)$, where mod is the remainder operator.

The frailty variate, Q_i, was included in order to accommodate positive intra-subject event time correlations. Frailty variances employed included $\sigma^2 = 0$, 0.5, 1.0, and 2.0. For $\sigma^2 = 0$, within-subject event times are independent. Setting σ^2 to 0.5 and 1.0 results in positive correlation among event times for each subject, with $\sigma^2 = 2.0$ resulting in extremely strong event time correlations. In the analysis of **recurrent events**, at least among human subjects in biomedical studies, it would be rare to observe $\sigma^2 = 0$ or $\sigma^2 > 2$.

For each subject, $N_i^* = 25$ events were generated from a non-homogeneous Poisson process (Chiang[3]), with the j'th event time generated as:

$$T_{i,j} = T_{i,j-1} - \frac{1}{\phi_0} \log\left\{1 - \frac{\phi_0 \log(U_i)}{Q_i d\mu_0 \exp\{Z_i(\beta_0 - 1.25\phi_0)\}}\right\}, \tag{13}$$

for $j = 1, \ldots, 25$, where the U_{ij} are Uniform(0,1) variates and $T_{i,0} \equiv 0$. Events with ($T_{i,j} > C_i$) were treated as unobserved.

Due to the non-proportionality ($\phi_0 \neq 0$), the effect of Z_i on the event process is not constant over time. The shift in the $Z_i \times t$ term allows that β_0 represents the log rate ratio at $t = 1.25$, the mid-point of the observation period or, equivalently, the mean observation time, since $E[C_i] = 1.25$.

The parameter ϕ_0 reflects the degree of non-proportionality. In our set-up, the effect of Z_i increases with increasing follow-up time, ranging from $\beta_0 - 0.5 \times 1.25 = 0.068$ at $t = 0$ to 1.318 at $t = 2.5$. The mean number of observed events was 0.625 for the $Z_i = 0$ subjects and 1.06 for subjects with $Z_i = 1$. The number of observed events ranged from 0 to 25.

A total of 5,000 replications per data configuration were generated. Bias was estimated by comparing the mean parameter estimate (across the 5,000 replicates) with its true value. The accuracy of the asymptotic robust standard error estimators were assessed by comparing their average values (denoted ASE) with the empirical standard deviation (ESD) and through comparing the empirical coverage probability (ECP) with its nominal value of 0.95.

Simulation results are presented in Table 1. For all data configurations, $\widehat{\beta}$ and $\widehat{\phi}$ were approximately unbiased, even for $n=30$. Generally, the accuracy of asymptotic standard errors increased as the intra-subject event time correlation decreased. Coverage probabilities for the asymptotic confidence intervals for β_0 and ϕ_0 were approximately equal across all parameter combinations, and increased as intra-subject event time correlation decreased. For uncorrelated intra-subject event times, $n=50$ was required to obtain ECP of at least 0.92; for moderate to high event time correlations ($\sigma^2=0.5$, 1.0), $n=100$ was required. A sample size of $n=100$ failed to yield ECP> 0.92 in the case of extremely high event-time correlation ($\sigma^2=2.0$), although this was achieved with $n=200$.

5. Analysis of Preschool Asthma Data

We fitted separate rate models for asthma-attributable hospitalizations and days hospitalized. Time, t, was measured in days; since $t = 0$ corresponded to the child's date of birth, the times axis was also the age axis. The selected set of covariates included binary indicators of low birth weight (LBW), respiratory distress syndrome (RDS), transient tachypnea of the newborn (TTN), birth asphyxia, and gender, with each coded as 1 for 'present' and 0 for 'absent'. Gender was coded as 0 for females and 1 for males. Initially, rate models were fitted, with the degree of departure from proportionality examined separately for each covariate by sequentially fitting models with $Z_{ij} \times t$ interactions, and examining the corresponding Wald statistic (using a robust SE estimate) and degree of improvement in fit as depicted by plots of the residual, $N_i - \widehat{\mu}_i(C_i; \widehat{\beta})$, suggested by Lawless[12]. The final model is

Table 1
Simulation Results: Non-proportional Rates Model

		$\widehat{\beta}$				$\widehat{\phi}$			
n	σ^2	BIAS	ASE	ESD	ECP	BIAS	ASE	ESD	ECP
30	0	0.017	0.429	0.345	0.903	0.001	0.610	0.504	0.913
50		0.012	0.294	0.265	0.927	0.004	0.422	0.384	0.934
100		0.007	0.197	0.187	0.936	0.009	0.286	0.269	0.937
200		0.004	0.135	0.132	0.946	0.007	0.191	0.189	0.945
30	0.5	0.010	0.609	0.460	0.888	-0.002	0.718	0.549	0.887
50		0.010	0.420	0.361	0.904	0.009	0.481	0.416	0.913
100		-0.008	0.279	0.259	0.930	-0.005	0.315	0.294	0.932
200		0.002	0.190	0.185	0.946	0.000	0.215	0.207	0.945
30	1.0	0.010	0.790	0.544	0.868	0.004	0.827	0.587	0.881
50		0.015	0.513	0.428	0.896	0.001	0.529	0.442	0.905
100		0.005	0.335	0.312	0.927	0.000	0.346	0.316	0.928
200		-0.004	0.236	0.223	0.938	-0.004	0.234	0.224	0.940
30	2.0	-0.006	1.331	0.668	0.846	-0.004	1.204	0.653	0.862
50		0.015	0.677	0.522	0.880	0.004	0.627	0.489	0.883
100		0.001	0.436	0.384	0.913	-0.009	0.402	0.350	0.910
200		-0.001	0.292	0.280	0.937	-0.001	0.270	0.253	0.931

given by:

$$d\mu_i(t) = d\mu_0(t)\exp\{\beta_1 LBW_i + \beta_2 RDS_i + \beta_3 TTN_i + \beta_4 ASPH.mod_i$$
$$+ \beta_5 ASPH.sev_i + \beta_6 MALE_i + \beta_7 MALE_i(t - 2.5\text{yrs})\}. \quad (14)$$

Having selecting the final model, fitted means and their corresponding point-wise 95% confidence intervals were computed for selected covariate patterns.

A risk factor profile of the study population is presented in Table 2, with respect to all covariates retained in the final model. Each of the birth conditions studied was relatively rare. A summary of the event history of the

Table 2
Risk factor profile of 1984/85 Manitoba birth cohort (n=16,207)

Characteristic	Variable	n	%
Low birth weight (< 2500 g)	LBW	703	4.3
Respiratory distress syndrome	RDS	247	1.5
Transient tachypnea of newborn	TTN	326	2.0
Birth asphyxia mild-to-moderate	ASPH.mod	918	5.7
severe	ASPH.sev	307	1.9
Male gender	MALE	8,357	51.6

birth cohort is provided in Tables 3 and 4. A total of 376 hospitalizations and 1,377 hospital days were experienced by the 207 children hospitalized for asthma during age 0 to 4. Among those hospitalized, 65% were hospitalized only once. The mode of the length-of-stay distribution was 2 days (28%); almost 5% of hospitalizations were for 10 days or more.

Results of the non-proportional rates models are listed in Tables 5 and 6 for asthma-attributable hospitalizations and days hospitalized, respectively. Significant increases in hospitalization rates were associated with low birth weight (Rate Ratio(RR)=2.03), respiratory distress syndrome (RR=3.65), severe birth asphyxia (RR=3.41) and male gender (RR=1.89, at t =2.5 years), while an important but not statistically significant increase was associated with mild-to-moderate birth asphyxia. As indicated in Table 6, all covariates having a significant effect on mean number of hospitalizations were also associated with significant increases in mean days hospitalized. For each parameter estimate, there was great disparity between the naive and robust standard error estimates indicating strong intra-subject event correlations, particularly for the days-hospitalized model (Table 6).

As indicated in both Tables 5 and 6, significant departure from proportionality was detected for the gender effect. The trend in the mean

Table 3
Distribution of number of hospitalizations: 1984/85 Manitoba birth cohort

Hospitalizations	n	%
1	134	64.7
2	37	17.9
3	18	8.7
4	6	2.9
≥ 5	12	5.8
Total	207	100.0

Table 4
Distribution of number of days hospitalized per hospitalization: 1984/85 Manitoba birth cohort

Days hospitalized per hospitalization	n	%*
0	7	1.9
1	73	19.4
2	105	27.9
3	54	14.4
4	34	9.0
5	35	9.3
6	21	5.6
7	11	2.9
8	7	1.9
9	11	2.9
≥ 10	18	4.8
Total	376	100.0

*percentage among children hospitalized at least once.

ratio by age is displayed in Figure 1 for the hospitalization model. The smooth line represents the RR for the gender covariate estimated by a model that contained a MALE$\times(t - 2.5$ yrs) interaction term, which assumes an exponential trend in the RR across the 0-4 age interval. The step function pertains to a model which contained MALE$\times I(0 \leq t \leq 1$ year), ..., MALE$\times I(4$ years $< t \leq 5$ years), assuming a constant RR within each one-year age interval. As Figure 1 indicates, the decrease in the RR for MALE is consistent with an exponential decrease; hence, the continuous form of the time interaction was retained for the remainder of the analysis in the interests of parsimony and efficiency. As implied by Tables 5 and 6, the interaction term was centered at the mid-point of the observation period (i.e., 2.5 years). Hence, the rate ratio parameter for MALE (main effect) refers to the RR for male gender at age 2.5 years.

Table 5
Risk factors for pre-school asthma: Hospitalizations

k	Covariate	$\widehat{\beta}_k$	naive $\widehat{SE}(\widehat{\beta}_k)$	robust $\widehat{SE}(\widehat{\beta}_k)$	$\exp\{\widehat{\beta}_k\}$	(95% CI)
1	LBW	0.708	0.192	0.257	2.03	(1.23, 3.36)
2	RDS	1.295	0.226	0.313	3.65	(1.98, 6.75)
3	TTN	0.469	0.269	0.339	1.60	(0.82, 3.10)
4	ASPH.mod	0.517	0.181	0.319	1.68	(0.90, 3.14)
5	ASPH.sev	1.227	0.201	0.471	3.41	(1.36, 8.58)
6	MALE ($t = 2.5$ yrs)	0.598	0.110	0.202	1.89	(1.22, 2.70)
7	MALE$\times t$	-0.001	0.0003	0.0004	0.9989	(0.9981, 0.9998)

The lack of proportionality with respect to the gender effect was also suggested by the gender-specific residual plots in Figure 2, where the residuals were computed as $\sum_{i=1}^{n} MALE_i\{N_i - \widehat{\mu}_i(C_i; \widehat{\beta})\}$ and $\sum_{i=1}^{n}(1 -$

Table 6
Risk factors for pre-school asthma: Days hospitalized

k	Covariate	$\widehat{\beta}_k$	naive $\widehat{SE}(\widehat{\beta}_k)$	robust $\widehat{SE}(\widehat{\beta}_k)$	$\exp\{\widehat{\beta}_k\}$	(95% CI)
1	LBW	0.863	0.095	0.353	2.37	(1.19, 4.74)
2	RDS	1.233	0.112	0.411	3.43	(1.53, 7.68)
3	TTN	0.400	0.139	0.460	1.49	(0.60, 3.68)
4	ASPH.mod	0.212	0.110	0.324	1.24	(0.65, 2.34)
5	ASPH.sev	1.745	0.085	0.590	5.73	(1.80, 18.21)
6	MALE $(t = 2.5$ yrs)	0.604	0.059	0.279	1.83	(1.06, 3.16)
7	MALE$\times t$	-0.002	0.0002	0.0005	0.9981	(0.9972, 0.9991)

$MALE_i)\{N_i - \widehat{\mu}_i(C_i; \widehat{\boldsymbol{\beta}})\}$ for males and females, respectively. Residuals for the proportional rates model (denoted by 'o') are of far greater magnitude than those for the time-dependent model ('t'). While residuals from the proportional rates model display a distinct pattern (i.e., bow-shaped), residuals for the time-dependent model display much little trend and appear to oscillate about 0. Careful examination of the 't's reveals that some pattern in the residuals persists even for the non-proportional rates model; it is possible that a more flexible specification of the time-dependence (e.g., including a $(t - 2.5$ yrs$)^2$ term) may be warranted.

The baseline asthma rate per 1,000 children per day, is plotted against age in Figure 3 for hospitalizations (top panel) and days hospitalized (bot-

Results were quite similar for the days hospitalized model (data not shown). Such plots were examined for several covariate combinations. Other checks of proportionality included examining the Wald statistics of various interaction terms with time. Evidence of non-proportionality was not found for any covariate besides gender.

Rate Ratio: M/F, Asthma hospitalizations

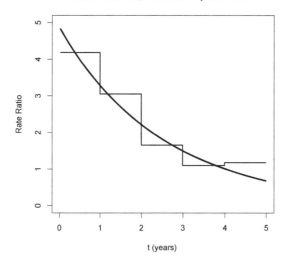

Fig. 1. Mean ratio ($\exp\{\widehat{\beta}_k\}$), male:female, for asthma hospitalizations. The curve equals $\exp\{\widehat{\beta}_6 + \widehat{\beta}_7(t - 2.5\text{yrs})\}$ from model (14), while the step function corresponds to a model with separate year-specific MALE coefficients.

tom). The baseline rates were smoothed using local regression via the *loess*($\cdot$) function in R. For both hospitalizations and days hospitalized, the baseline rate tends to increase with age.

Estimated **cumulative mean numbers** of asthma-attributable hospitalizations and days hospitalized are depicted in Figure 4. For children with no neonatal risk factors (i.e., $LBW_i + RDS_i + \ldots + ASPH.sev_i = 0$), the model predicts a mean (and 95% CI) of 13.9 (8.7, 19.0) hospitalizations per 1,000 females (top left panel) and 24.9 (18.7, 31.1) per 1,000 males (top right panel) during the first 5 years of life. For days hospitalized, the corresponding model predicted means (95% CIs) are 43.8 (24.4, 63.1) per 1,000 females (bottom left panel) and 89.5 (54.2, 124.8) per 1,000 males (bottom right panel) during the same period.

As a check of the adequacy of the final models, the fitted cumulative mean number of asthma events is plotted against time, and compared with the observed counts in Figure 5. These two quantities are the components of the residuals discussed previously. Several covariate patterns were examined; two are presented for illustration, and labelled 'unexposed' (LBW+RDS+... +ASPH.sev=0) and exposed (LBW+RDS+...

Residuals: Females

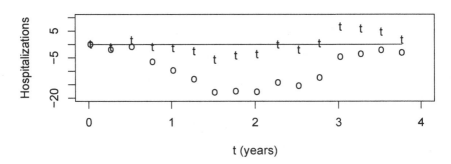

t (years)

Residuals: Males

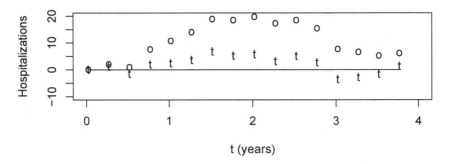

t (years)

Fig. 2. Residuals: for females (left panel) and males (right panel) for asthma hospitalizations. Comparing models which did (t) and did not (o) include the MALE$\times(t-2.5$ yrs) term, respectively.

+ASPH.sev>0), referring to presence or absence of adverse birth conditions within the same gender, respectively. Fitted means approximated observed event counts very closely within both groups for each model, as was observed across most covariate patterns.

6. Discussion

Through simulation, we found that the finite-sample performance of the semi-parametric `non-proportional rates model` is generally comparable to that of its proportional rates counterpart; results are not shown for the

Baseline rate: hospitalizations per 1,000 children per day

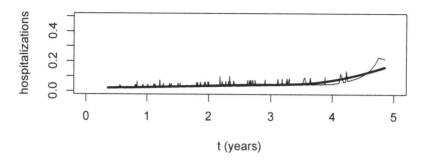

Baseline rate: hospital days per 1,000 children per day

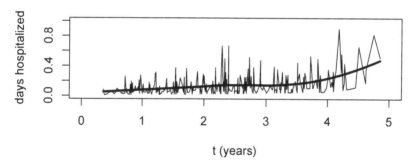

Fig. 3.   Baseline rate of hospitalization (top panel) and days hospitalized (bottom panel) for asthma per 1,000 children per day during age 0-5.

proportional rates case since pertinent simulation results were already reported by Lin *et. al.*[16]. Slightly greater sample size is required for approximate unbiasedness of the time-dependent (non-proportionality) parameter; the same holds for its asymptotic variance. For example, in the proportional means case, even $n=30$ subjects was sufficient for coverage probabilities to approximate their nominal values, while $n=50$ was required in the non-proportional setting. Hence, for very small data sets, investigators would be prudent to **bootstrap**[8] SEs and/or CIs since the normal approximation may lead to false conclusions, particularly when the proportional means assumption fails to hold or when intra-subject correlations are high. Although

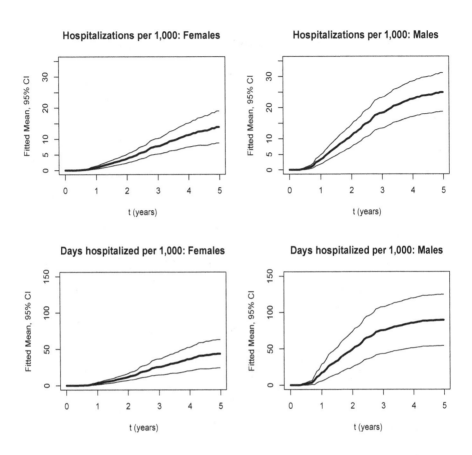

Fig. 4. Mean number of asthma-attributable hospitalizations (per 1,000 children) and days hospitalized with 95% confidence intervals for female (left panels) and male (right panels) children free of other birth risk factors listed in Table 1, for $t \in (0, 5]$ yrs.

the literature on the bootstrap is quite sparse regarding recurrent events, general bootstrap methods for the censored data, described by Efron[7], could probably be extended to the multiple failure time setting.

We assessed the effect of gender, birth weight and adverse neonatal respiratory conditions on the mean number of hospitalizations (event count increment=0 or 1) and mean days hospitalized (increments of size ≥ 0) for pre-school asthma using the non-proportional means model. Male gender, birth weight <2.5 kg, respiratory distress syndrome and severe birth asphyxia were all independently associated with an increase in mean number

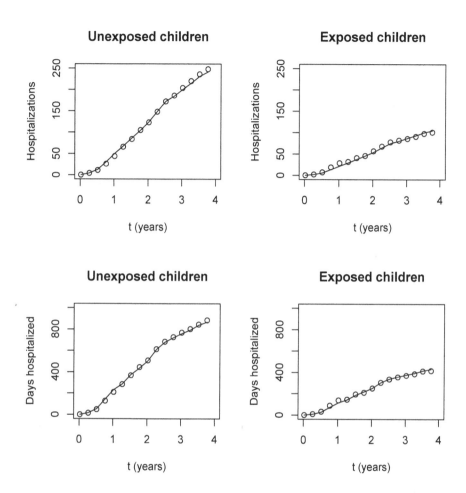

Fig. 5.   Fitted (solid lines) versus observed (dots) number of asthma-attributable hospitalizations (top two panels) and days hospitalized (bottom panels) among "unexposed" (i.e., $LBW_i + \ldots + TTN_i = 0$) (left panels) and "exposed" (i.e., $LBW_i + \ldots + TTN_i > 0$) children (right panels) for $t \in (0, 5]$ yrs.

of hospitalizations and mean days hospitalized. The increase associated with male gender was found to decrease steadily and monotonically during the 0 to 4 age interval.

We then fitted semi-parametric marginal rates models with time-dependent covariates to data from a retrospective birth cohort study. Among all simulation trials, the last of line of Table 1 is most relevant in terms of evaluating the appropriateness of asymptotic results in the current investigation, due to parallels with respect to expected number of events and intra-subject event time correlations. For this data configuration, no evidence of inappropriateness is revealed for the large sample approximations employed.

A previous analysis of this birth cohort[21] treated hospitalization for asthma during age 0-4 as a binary variable and employed logistic regression. Under the assumption that most children who experience asthma very early in life tend to suffer it the rest of their lives, not incorporating information on the number of episodes per child or their timing was deemed appropriate at the time given the goals of the study. Our objective in the current investigation was to assess the effect of birth characteristics on the number of asthma-attributable hospitalizations and days hospitalized. It is reasonable to assume that both quantities reflect disease severity as well as health care costs. Hence, while the original study served strictly an etiologic purpose, the objectives of the current analysis were also pertinent from a public health perspective.

Often in biomedical studies when patients are followed either prospectively or retrospectively over time, multiple occurrences of the event of interest are possible. Patients may leave the study before its conclusion, or may complete the study without experiencing the event of interest. Methods are well-established to analyze the potentially censored time until first event by survival analysis. A more informative analysis would incorporate all event times, requiring a multivariate survival analysis, for which methods are now fairly well known (Prentice et. al.[20]; Andersen and Gill[2]; Wei et. al.[25]; Lin et. al.[15]). Most multivariate failure time methods involve modelling the hazard function. However, in the context of recurrent event data, the mean or rate is often of direct interest, and is a more interpretable quantity. Compared to the marginal hazards model, an advantage of the marginal means/rates model is that estimates of the mean number of events are directly obtainable from model parameters. Both models could be used to generally assess the effect of covariates on the event process of interest; both have appeal from an etiologic perspective. However, among clinicians, public policy officials and health administrators, direct interest often lies in the mean number of events and, in such cases, the marginal means/rates model would be preferred. A natural area of application for the marginal means/rates model is health economics. For example, if cost data are available for the event of interest, the mean increase in costs associated with various attributes could be estimated and compared with the costs of primary prevention (e.g., through education or intervention programs) to project the net savings of such programs to the health organization of concern. From a public health perspective, parameters from the marginal means/rates model have a direct, intuitive and functional interpretation.

Despite its utility, the marginal means/rates model is inappropriate in certain settings due to its underlying assumptions. The requirement that censoring time be independent of the event process may be clearly untenable, particularly for biomedical studies. As an obvious example, suppose that hospitalizations are the event of interest. Subjects can be censored for a variety of reasons, including death, and increasing numbers of hospitalizations may well be associated with increased mortality rates. Many interesting approaches exist for modelling **recurrent events** in the presence of a terminating event (e.g., Cook and Lawless[4]; Li and Lagakos[14]; Ghosh and Lin[10]) and this remains an active area of research (e.g., Liu, Wolfe and Huang[17]; Wang, Qin, and Chiang[24]). The issue of informative censoring is not prominent in our study, as children seldom die from asthma attacks.

Acknowledgments

This research was supported in part by National Institutes of Health grants R01 HL-57444 (JC) and R01 DK-70869 (DES).

References

1. P.D. Allison, *Survival Analysis using the SAS System: A Practical Guide*, SAS Institute Inc., Cary, 1995.
2. P.K. Andersen and R.D. Gill, Cox's Regression Model for Counting Processes: A Large Sample Study, *The Annals of Statistics* **10** (1982), 1100-1120.
3. C.L. Chiang, *An Introduction to Stochastic Processes and their Applications*, Kreiger, New York, 1980.
4. R.J. Cook and J.F. Lawless, Marginal analysis of recurrent events and a terminating event, *Statistics in Medicine*, **16** (1997), 911-924.
5. D.R. Cox, Regression models and life-tables (with discussion), *Journal of the Royal Statistical Society, Series B* **34** (1972), 187-220.
6. D.R. Cox, Partial likelihood, *Biometrika* **62** (1975), 262-276.
7. B. Efron, Censored data and the bootstrap, *Journal of the American Statistical Association*, **76** (1981), 312-319.
8. B. Efron, *The Jackknife, the Bootstrap and Other Resampling Plans*, SIAM, Philadelphia, 1982.
9. P. Gergen and K. Weiss, Changing patterns of asthma hospitalization among children: 1979 to 1987, *Journal of the American Medical Association*, **264** (1990), 1688-1692.

10. D. Ghosh and D.Y. Lin, Marginal regression models for recurrent and terminal events, *Statistica Sinica*, **12** (2002), 663-688.

11. H. Johansen, M. Dutta, Y. Mao, K. Chagani, and I. Sladece, An investigation of the increase in pre-school age asthma in Manitoba, Canada, *Health Reports*, **4** (1992), 379-402.

12. J.F. Lawless, The analysis of recurrent events for multiple subjects, *Applied Statistics*, **44** (1995), 487-498.

13. J.F. Lawless and C. Nadeau, Some simple robust methods for the analysis of recurrent events, *Technometrics*, **37** (1995), 158-168.

14. Q.H. Li and S.W. Lagakos, Use of the Wei-Lin-Weissfeld method for the analysis of a recurring and a terminating event, *Statistics in Medicine*, **16** (1997), 925-940.

15. D.Y. Lin, Cox regression analysis of multivariate failure time data: The marginal approach, *Statistics in Medicine*, **13** (1994), 2233-2247.

16. D.Y. Lin, L.J. Wei, I. Yang, and Z. Ying, Semiparametric regression for the mean and rate functions of recurrent events, *Journal of the Royal Statistical Society, Series B* **62** (2000), 711-730.

17. L. Liu, R.A. Wolfe, and X. Huang, Shared frailty model for recurrent events and a terminal event, *Biometrics*, **60** (2004), 747-756.

18. B.G. Loftus and J.F. Price, Clinical and immunological characteristics of pre-school asthma, *Clinical Allergy*, **16** (1986), 251-257.

19. W.J. Miller and G.B. Hill, Childhood asthma, *Health Reports*, **10** (1998), 9-21.

20. R.L. Prentice, B.J. Williams, and A.V. Peterson, On the regression analysis of multivariate failure time data, *Biometrika*, **68** (1981), 373-389.

21. D. Schaubel, H. Johansen, M. Dutta, M. Desmeules, A. Becker, and Y. Mao, Neonatal characteristics as risk factors for preschool asthma, *Journal of Asthma*, **33** (1996), 255-264.

22. E. Skobelhoff, W. Spivey, S. St. Clair, and J. Schoffstall, The influence of age and sex on asthma admissions, *Journal of the American Medical Association*, **268** (1992), 3437-3440.

23. T.M. Therneau and S.A. Hamilton, rhDNase as an example of recurrent event analysis, *Statistics in Medicine*, **16** (1997), 2029-2047.

24. M.C. Wang, J. Qin, and C.T. Chiang, Analyzing recurrent event data with informative censoring, *Journal of the American Statistical Association*, **96** (2001), 1057-1065.

25. L.J. Wei, D.Y. Lin, and L. Weissfeld, Regression analysis of multivariate incomplete failure time data by modelling marginal distributions, *Journal of the American Statistical Association*, **84** (1989), 1065-1073.

26. K. Weiss and D. Wagener, Asthma surveillance in the United States: a review of current trends and knowledge gaps, *Chest*, **98** (1990), 179S-184S.

27. K. Wilkins and Y. Mao, Trends in rates of admission to hospital and death from asthma among children and young adults in Canada during the 1980's, *Canadian Medical Association Journal*, **148** (1993), 185-190.

CHAPTER 10

SURVIVAL MODEL AND ESTIMATION FOR LUNG CANCER PATIENTS

Xingchen Yuan[a], Don Hong[b], and Yu Shyr[c,d]

[a] Fermilab, Batavia, IL 60510, USA
[b] Department of Mathematical Sciences, Middle Tennessee State University,
P.O. Box 34, Murfreesboro, Tennessee 37132, USA
E-mail: dhong@mtsu.edu
[c] Department of Biostatistics, Vanderbilt University, Nashville, TN 37232, USA
[d] Department of Statistics, National Cheng Kung University, Taiwan, ROC

Lung cancer is the most frequently occuring fatal cancer in the United States. By assuming a form for the hazard function for a group of lung cancer patients for survival study, the covariates in the hazard function are estimated by the maximum likelihood estimation following the proportional hazards regression analysis. Although the proportional hazards model does not give an explicit baseline hazard function, the function can be estimated by fitting the data with non-linear least square technique. The survival model is then examined by a neural network simulation. The neural network learns the survival pattern from available hospital data and gives survival prediction for random covariate combinations. The simulation results support the covariate estimation in the survival model.

1. Introduction

Cancer develops when cells in a part of the body begin to grow out of control. It is the second most significant reason for US mortality. In 2001, cancer caused 553,768 deaths in the United States, accounting for 22.9% of all deaths in that year [13]. In the past fifty years, efforts have been made to reduce death rates for different diseases, but the death rate for cancer remains almost unchanged ([14], [15]). Among the various types of cancers, lung cancer is the most frequently occuring fatal cancer, for both men and women, in the United States. Each year there are about 170, 000 new cases of lung cancer in the U.S.A. and 150,000 deaths attributable to this disease. Men are affected somewhat more frequently (100,000 cases/year) than women (70,000 cases/year). Worldwide, there are 1 million new cases per year. Over the past 5 decades the number of yearly cases has increased, and the worldwide incidence may double to 2 million per year in the coming decade. The average patient is 60 years old, and only 1% of cases are under 40 years old. About 90% of patients have historically died from their disease.

Recently, there has been a great deal of interest in modeling survival data of cancer patients (see [2], [8], [12] for example). Survival analysis is concerned with studying the time between entry to a study and a subsequent event, such as death. In practice, after a lung cancer patient is hospitalized, a set of medical data regarding the patients' condition is recorded. This data set may include information such as the patient's survival time, the tumor's stage, the health grade, the disease free time, etc. With the data set, we wish to study how the patient's conditions might be associated with the survival pattern and also a lung cancer patient's survival chance, or a group of patients' survival distribution over time.

The goal of this study is to develop a survival model for relating the hospital data profile to censored survival data such as time to cancer death or recurrence. Censored survival times occur if the event of interest, i.e., the death, does not occur for a patient during the study period. Traditionally, there are two approaches to model the unknown survival distribution. One is to assume a classical parametric model such as normal, lognormal, gamma, Weibull, Pareto or beta, then use a histogram, kernel or other nonparametric estimate of the unknown density function. This method is straightforward but cannot reflect the contribution of patients' hospital conditions to the survival distribution. Another is the proportional hazards model, which was first proposed by D.R. Cox [1] in 1972 to investigate the effects of covariates on survival patterns, also known as Cox regression model [7]. The model permits having the patients' hospital conditions as a vector of covariates in the hazard function and can estimate the unknown parameters for the covariates by partial likelihood without putting a structure of baseline hazard. In this study, however, we propose a structure of the baseline hazard function, and estimate the parameters by the available censored survival data so that the explicit survival function is determined. This estimation is achieved by a least square fit for the cum hazard value computed by SPSS.

In a survey study, the design parameters for the survey are sometimes related to the hazard function but do not fit in the model. On some other occasions, the independence assumption of the covariates may be violated.

Sometimes correlations exist within each level of nesting. These could cause biases and affect variances of parameter estimation [10, 11]. Therefore, tests need to be done to evaluate the goodness of the estimated survival function. There are two popular ways to test the model. One is to use $1/2$ or $2/3$ of the time scale in the survival data to determine the parameters, and then use the whole data set to examine the model; another is to use the whole data set to set up the model, then using resample methods to check the model. Neural networks are increasingly being seen as an addition to the statistics toolkit which should be considered alongside both classical and modern statistical methods. It has been pointed out in [16] many different ways that classification networks have been used for survival data. In this study, due to the lack of patient data, we propose a neural network model to simulate the patients' survival pattern and use the neural network to generate a long list of "virtual data" to test the survival model.

The remainder of the paper is organized as follows: In Section 2, we give a description for the survival model. We first introduce the conception of hazard function and survival function as well as their relationship. We then outline the method of proportional hazard model and propose and justify the exponential form for baseline hazard function. In Section 3, we discuss the parameter estimation by statistical methods including maximum likelihood estimation (MLE) and non-linear least square estimation (LSE). We also introduce the idea and conception of the neural network and set up the proper neural network by MATLAB programs for testing. In Section 4, we present the computational result with actual patient data. Discussions and conclusions are given in Section 5.

2. Description of Model

2.1. *Survival Function and Hazard Function*

Following the notations in Actuarial Mathematics [4], we let T be a nonnegative random variable representing the failure time of an individual in the population. Assume T is distributed with the probability density function (pdf) $f(t)$, then the cumulative distribution function (cdf) is

$$F(t) = Pr[T \leq t] = \int_0^t f(z)dz \tag{2.1}$$

giving the probability that the event has duration t. The **survival function**, $S(t)$, is defined as the complement of the c.d.f., that is

$$S(t) = Pr[T < t] = 1 - F(t) = \int_t^\infty f(z)dz. \tag{2.2}$$

The survival function gives the probability of being alive at duration t. Naturally, when $t = 0$, $S(t) = 1$ and $t \to \infty$, $S(t) \to 0$.

An alternative characterization of the distribution of T is given by the **hazard function**. Sometimes it is also called the **force of mortality**, the mortality intensity function, or the failure rate. The hazard function is the probability that an individual will experience an event (for example, death) within a small time interval, given that the individual has survived up to the beginning of the interval. It can therefore be interpreted as the instantaneous risk of occurrence of dying at time t. The hazard function $h(t)$ can be estimated using the following equation:

$$h(t) = \lim_{\Delta t \to 0} \frac{Pr[t < T \leq t + \Delta t | T > t]}{\Delta t}. \tag{2.3}$$

The numerator of this expression is the conditional probability that the event will occur in the interval $(t, t + \Delta t)$ given that it has not occurred before, and the denominator is the width of the interval. We obtain a rate of event occurrence per unit of time. Taking the limit as the width of the interval decreases to zero, we obtain an instantaneous rate of occurrence.

The conditional probability in the numerator may be written as the ratio of the joint probability that T is in the interval $(t, t + \Delta t)$ and $T > t$ (which is, of course, the same as the probability that t is in the interval), to the probability of the condition $T > t$. The former may be written as $f(t)\Delta t$ for small Δt, while the latter is $S(t)$ by definition. Dividing by dt and passing to the limit gives the useful result

$$h(t) = \frac{f(t)}{S(t)} = \frac{F'(t)}{S(t)} = \frac{(1 - S(t))'}{S(t)} = -\frac{S'(t)}{S(t)}. \tag{2.4}$$

This equation suggests the relationship between the survival function and the hazard function. That is, the rate of occurrence of the event at duration t equals the density of events at t divided by the probability of surviving to that duration without experiencing the event. Furthermore, equation (2.4) suggests that

$$h(t) = -\frac{d}{dt} \log S(t), \tag{2.5}$$

then

$$\log S(t) = -\int_0^t h(z)\, dz + C. \tag{2.6}$$

Considering the boundary condition $S(0) = 1$ as we mentioned before, we have $C = 0$, and thus

$$S(t) = \exp\{-\int_0^t h(z)\,dz\}. \tag{2.7}$$

Combining (2.7) with (2.4), we obtain

$$f(t) = h(t)S(t) = h(t)\exp\{-\int_0^t h(z)\,dz\}. \tag{2.8}$$

A recent survey on dynamic mortality modeling in actuarial mathematics is given in [17].

2.2. *Cox Regression*

A Cox model is a well-recognized statistical technique for exploring the relationship between the survival of patient and a set of explanatory variables (see [1], [16] for example). We call these explanatory variables covariates.

Suppose that we have collected n patients with lung cancer. For the ith patients, let $(t_i; \delta_i)$ be the observed phenotype, where t_i is the failure time (in other words, when death occurs) when $\delta_i = 1$, and is the censoring time (e.g., last time known of a patient being cancer-free) when $\delta_i = 0$. Let $x_i = (x_{i1}, \cdots, x_{ip})$ be the vector of p covariates for the ith sample taken from the ith patient. We assume that a general Cox model with the hazard function for the ith patient is modeled as

$$h(t|x_i) = h_0(t)\exp(f(x_i)), \tag{2.9}$$

where $h_0(t)$ is called the baseline hazard function. Although $f(x_i)$ may assume many formats, the most popular and also the simplest model for $f(x)$ is

$$f(x_i) = x_i \cdot \beta = x_{i_1}\beta_1 + \cdots + x_{i_p}\beta_p, \tag{2.10}$$

where β is a column vector of coefficients. In this equation, it is assumed that the effects of the different covariates on survival are constant over time and are addictive in a particular scale. The Cox model makes no assumptions about the form of $h_0(t)$, but assumes the parametric form for the effect of the covariates (predictors) on the hazard. In this sense, the Cox model is a semi-parametric model.

The vector β of parameters can be estimated by the partial likelihood method. Let the observed follow up time of the ith individual be t_i with corresponding covariates x_i, $i = 1, .., n$. The conditional probability for the

ith individual failing at t_i given that the individual is from the risk set $R(t_i)$ (i.e., $R(t_i) = \{j \,|t_j \geq t_i\}$) is [10]:

$$\frac{h_0(t) \exp(x_i\beta)}{\sum_{\ell \in R(t_i)} h_0(t_i) \exp(x_\ell\beta)}. \tag{2.11}$$

Assuming that there are K failures. The partial likelihood function is then:

$$\prod_{i=1}^{K} \frac{\exp(x_i\beta)}{\sum_{\ell \in R(t_i)} h_0(t_i) \exp(x_\ell\beta)}. \tag{2.12}$$

Recalling the definition of δ_i at the beginning of this section, the partial likelihood function can be expressed as:

$$L(\beta) = \prod_{i=1}^{n} \left[\frac{\exp(x_i\beta)}{\sum_{j=1}^{n} y_j(t) \exp(x_j\beta)} \right]^{\delta_i}, \tag{2.13}$$

where $y_j(t) = 0$ when $t \leq t_j$, otherwise $y_j(t) = 1$. Equation (2.13) can be written in another way to remove the expression of δ_i:

$$L(\beta) = \prod_{i \ uncensored} \left[\frac{\exp(x_i\beta)}{\sum_{j=1}^{n} y_j(t) \exp(x_j\beta)} \right]. \tag{2.14}$$

For a sample of size n, the log partial likelihood for expression (2.14) is

$$l(\beta) = \log L(\beta) = \prod_{i \ uncensored} \left\{ x_i\beta - \log \left[\sum_{j=1}^{n} y_j(t) \exp(x_j\beta) \right] \right\}. \tag{2.15}$$

The maximum partial likelihood estimation of β can be obtained as a solution to the equation

$$\frac{\partial l(\beta)}{\partial \beta} = 0,$$

and thus,

$$\sum_{i \ uncensored} x_i - \frac{\sum_{j=1}^{n} y_j(t) x_j \exp(x_j\beta)}{\sum_{j=1}^{n} y_j(t) \exp(x_j\beta)} = 0. \tag{2.16}$$

Cox and others have shown that this partial log-likelihood can be treated as an ordinary log-likelihood to derive valid (partial) MLE of β. Therefore, we can estimate hazard ratios and confidence intervals using maximum likelihood techniques whose principal will be discussed in the next section. To avoid the baseline hazard, estimates are based on the partial as opposed to the full likelihood.

Usually, the Cox proportional hazard regression model is a very useful tool to estimate the coefficients in a linear combination of covariates in survival analysis since both SAS PHREG procedure and SPSS Survival Package perform regression analysis of the survival data based on the proportional hazards model. However, because of the nature of proportional hazard regression, neither software packages give an explicit function expression for the baseline hazard function $h_0(t)$. In the next section, we will justify an explicit function of the baseline hazard function $h_0(t)$ and also estimate the parameters in $h_0(t)$ using non-linear least square technique based on the result obtained from the Cox regression for the survival function fitting the data set of lung cancer patients.

2.3. *Baseline Hazard for Lung Cancer Patients*

Like any cancer, the exact reason why one particular person is diagnosed lung cancer and another does not remains unknown. However, certain factors are strongly correlated with an increase in lung cancer, when groups of patients are studied. By rank, these factors are listed below [13]:

(i) Tobacco Smoking or exposure to smoke

(ii) Carcinogen Exposures

(iii) Radiation Exposure

(iv) Miscellaneous Risks Factors, including old scars in the lungs.

The first three factors involve an interaction between the individual and the environment. Presumably an individual is continuously exposed to and absorbs certain levels of smoke, radiation, or some kind of toxic material (like carcinogen) which then lead to lung cancer. Though a portion of the absorbed toxic materials is discharged from the body, the cumulative effect of retained toxins contributes to the individual's death [6].

For every given τ in $[0, t]$ and the infinitesimal time element $[\tau, \tau + d\tau]$, let the sum $\delta d\tau + o(d\tau)$ be the probability that a unit of toxic material is absorbed during $[\tau, \tau + d\tau]$ and the sum $\nu d\tau + o(d\tau)$ be the probability that a unit of toxic material in the body is discharged during $[\tau, \tau + d\tau]$. Assuming that δ and ν are independent of time, then the probability that an individual will absorb a unit of toxic material during $[\tau, \tau + d\tau]$ and will retain it in his/her body up to time t is given by [6]

$$\delta d\tau \, \exp\{-(t - \tau)\nu\}. \tag{2.17}$$

Integrating (2.17) over all possible value of τ yields

$$\int_0^t \delta \exp\{-(t - \tau)\nu\} d\tau = \frac{\delta}{\nu}[1 - \exp\{-\nu t\}]. \tag{2.18}$$

The quantity in (2.18) is the expected amount of toxic material absorbed during the interval $[0, t]$ and present in the body at time t, which leads to a possible suggestion of a function format for the hazard for cancers caused through exposure to factors. Suppose the baseline hazard for lung cancer patients is proportional to the quantity in the following equation:

$$h_0(t) = \frac{a}{b}(1 - \exp(-bt)). \tag{2.19}$$

Defining the cumulative baseline hazard function, $H_0(t)$, by integrating $h_0(t)$ and applying boundary condition that $h_0(0) = 0$ yield:

$$H_0(t) = \int_0^t h_0(x)dx = \frac{a}{b}[x - \frac{1}{b}(1 - \exp(-bt))]. \tag{2.20}$$

3. Statistics Methods and Neural Network

3.1. *Maximum Likelihood Estimation*

Maximum likelihood estimation begins with writing a mathematical expression known as the likelihood function of the sample data. Roughly speaking, the likelihood of a set of data is the probability of obtaining that particular set of data, given the chosen probability distribution model. This expression contains the model's unknown parameters. The values of these parameters that maximize the sample likelihood are known as the Maximum Likelihood Estimates, or MLE. Maximum likelihood estimation is a totally analytic maximization procedure. It applies to every form of censored or multi-censored data, and is even able to be used across several stress cells and estimate acceleration model parameters at the same time as life distribution parameters. Moreover, MLE and likelihood functions generally have very desirable large sample properties because they: (a) become unbiased minimum variance estimators as the sample size increases, (b) have approximate normal distributions and approximate sample variances that can be calculated and used to generate confidence bounds, and (c) likelihood functions can be used to test hypotheses about models and parameters. Although it has many good attributes, MLE has an important drawback, that is, with a small number of failures (say, less than 30, and oftentimes, less than 50), MLE may be heavily biased and the large sample optimality properties do not apply.

If X is a continuous random variable with *pdf*

$$f(x, \beta_1, \beta_2, \cdots, \beta_p), \tag{3.1}$$

where $\beta_1, \cdots, \beta_p$ are p unknown constant parameters which need to be estimated. Denote $\beta^\tau = (\beta_1, \cdots, \beta_p)$. Conduct an experiment and obtain N independent observations, $x_1, \cdots, x_N$, which correspond in the case of life data analysis to failure times. The likelihood function is given by

$$L = L(x_1, \cdots, x_N | \beta_1, \cdots, \beta_p) = \Pi_{i=1}^N f(x_i | \beta_1, \cdots, \beta_p). \quad (3.2)$$

The Logarithmic function is

$$l = \log L = \sum_{i=1}^N \log f(x_i | \beta_1, \cdots, \beta_p). \quad (3.3)$$

For the survival analysis, we assume (2.9) and (2.10). Then the *pdf* becomes

$$f(t_i | x_i) = h(t_i | x_i) S(t_i | x_i) = h_0(t_i) \exp\{x_i \beta - \int_0^{t_i} h_0(z) \exp(x_i \beta) \, dz\}. \quad (3.4)$$

The log-likelihood function $l(\beta)$ has the expression

$$l = \sum_{i=1}^N \log f(t_i | x_i) = \sum_i [\log h_0(t_i) + (x_i \beta - \int_0^{t_i} h_0(z) \exp(x_i \beta) \, dz)]$$

$$= N \log h_0(t_i) + h_0(t_i) + \sum_i x_i \beta - \sum_i \int_0^{t_i} h_0(z) \exp(x_i \beta) \, dz. \quad (3.5)$$

When taking partial derivatives with respect to β to maximize $l(\beta)$, the computation often becomes very difficult due to the presentation of $h_0(z)$ in the integration term. That is why a proportional hazard model is used in the Cox models so that the term $h_0(z)$ can be canceled out in MLE calculation.

Recall (2.15), the MLE for $\hat\beta$ is $s(\hat\beta) = 0$, where the score function is

$$s(\beta) = \begin{pmatrix} \frac{\partial l(\beta)}{\partial \beta_1} \\ \cdots \\ \frac{\partial l(\beta)}{\partial \beta_p} \end{pmatrix}. \quad (3.6)$$

One of many nonlinear algorithms to compute this maximization is the Newton-Raphson iteration. The Newton-Raphson algorithm for computing $\hat\beta$ starts with an initial guess $\hat\beta^{(0)}$ and then iteratively determines $\hat\beta^{(m)}$ from the formula

$$\hat\beta^{(m)} = U^{-1}(\hat\beta^{(m-1)}) s(\hat\beta^{(m-1)}), \quad (3.7)$$

where

$$U(\beta) = -N \cdot Hessian(\beta) = N \cdot \begin{pmatrix} \frac{\partial^2 l(\beta)}{\partial^2 \beta} & \frac{\partial^2 l(\beta)}{\partial \beta_1 \partial \beta_2} & \cdots & \frac{\partial^2 l(\beta)}{\partial \beta_1 \partial \beta_p} \\ \frac{\partial^2 l(\beta)}{\partial \beta_2 \partial \beta_1} & \frac{\partial^2 l(\beta)}{\partial^2 \beta_2} & \cdots & \frac{\partial^2 l(\beta)}{\partial \beta_2 \partial \beta_p} \\ \cdots & \cdots & \cdots & \cdots \\ \frac{\partial^2 l(\beta)}{\partial \beta_p \partial \beta_1} & \frac{\partial^2 l(\beta)}{\partial \beta_p \partial \beta_2} & \cdots & \frac{\partial^2 l(\beta)}{\partial^2 \beta_p} \end{pmatrix}. \tag{3.8}$$

The Hessian matrix is positive definite, so it is strictly concave on β. However, the computation is obviously more complex. In practice, we use software to carry out this process for the MLE.

3.2. Non-Linear Least Square Fit

Least square regression (LSE) is a very popular and useful tool used in statistics and other fields. Suppose we want to find a relationship between a dependent (response) variable Y and an independent (predictor) variable X, in which a statistical relation is

$$Y = g(X|\theta) + \epsilon, \tag{3.9}$$

where ϵ is the error, and θ is a vector of parameters to be estimated in function g. If g assumes a non-linear format in terms of X, we are facing a non-linear regression. Suppose $X = (x_1, \cdots, x_m)^\tau$, $Y = (y_1, \cdots, y_m)^\tau$. We define

$$f_i(\theta) = y_i - \hat{y}_i = y_i - g(x_i|\theta) \tag{3.10}$$

The non-linear least square regression is to find $\hat{\theta}$ which minimizes $F(\hat{\theta})$, where $F(\theta)$ is defined as

$$F(\theta) = \frac{1}{2} \sum_{i=1}^m (f_i(\theta))^2 = \frac{1}{2} \|f(\theta)\|^2 = \frac{1}{2} f(\theta)^\tau f(\theta). \tag{3.11}$$

There are many non-linear algorithms for finding $\hat{\theta}$. These well-developed algorithms include the Gauss-Newton method, the Levenberg-Marquardt method, and Powell's Dog Leg method (see [7] for example). In this study, we use the Gauss-Newton method. It is based on the implementation of first derivatives of the components of the vector function. In special cases, it can give quadratic convergence as the Newton-method does for general optimization [8]. The Gauss-Newton method is based on a linear approximation to the components of f (a linear model of f) in the neighborhood of θ: For small $\|h\|$, we see from the Taylor expansion that

$$f(\theta + h) \approx \ell(\theta) := f(\theta)J(\theta)h, \tag{3.12}$$

where J is the Jacob matrix. Inserting this to the definition for F, we obtain

$$F(\theta + h) \approx L(\theta) := \frac{1}{2}\ell(h)^t\ell(h) = \frac{1}{2}f^t f + h^t J^t f + \frac{1}{2}h^t J^t J h$$

$$= F(\theta) + h^t J^t f + \frac{1}{2}h^t J^t J h. \tag{3.13}$$

The Gauss-Newton step $\hat{h}$ minimizes $L(h)$. In practice, the Gauss-Newton least square fitting the baseline hazard function can be achieved by using MATLAB software.

3.3. *Neural Network Testing*

In the Cox model, the main interest is usually about the parameter vector β. However, when one is interested in making predictions about the failure time for a given set of covariates, or when one assumes a parametric family for the baseline hazard function, just as what we have performed, then testing that h_0 is equal to a specified hazard rate function or evaluating how stable h_0 is for varying data source becomes important [12]. In the field survival analysis, there are two popular methods in order to test a model. One is to use $1/2$ or $2/3$ of the time scale in the survival data to determine the parameters and then use the whole data set to examine the model. In our study, however, to the short length of data (total of 66 rows, in which approximately two-thirds are censored) and the high data demand from MLE (refer to section 3.1), this solution is not feasible. Another way is to use the whole data set to set up the model and then use a resample method to check the model. This solution also has a problem on the principle by which we resample the original data. As we have known, MLE relies heavily on the given data set especially when the length of data is not exceptionally long. If we randomly resample the original data, the selected data for testing may be far from the "pattern" of the whole data set, e.g., having quite different mean and standard deviation.

In this study, we propose an artificial neural network testing model. First, we let the neural network "learn" the patients' survival pattern from the given hospital data. We then use the neural network to generate a long list of "virtual data" and "simulate" the survival pattern to test our covariate estimation and baseline hazard estimation. By this process, we also show that the neural network has great potential as a research tool in survival analysis.

The conception of neural network came up as early as the middle of this century. A **Neural Network** (NN) is an information processing paradigm that is inspired by the way biological nervous systems, such as the brain, process information. Simply speaking, it is software that is "trained" by having its examples of input and the corresponding desired output presented to it.

Neural networks, with their remarkable ability to derive meaning from complicated or imprecise data, can be used to extract patterns and detect trends that are too complex to be noticed by either humans or other computer techniques. A trained neural network can be thought of as an "expert" in the category of information it has been required to analyze.

The typical structure of neural network consists of a layer of d (the dimension of the futures) input units, a layer of output units, and a variable number of hidden layers of units, as shown in Figure 1. Generally more layers result in higher accuracy, but also are more time-consuming on computation.

The construction of the NN for this study and test results will be shown in the next section.

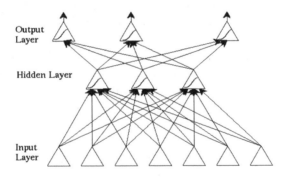

Fig. 1.   Typical Structure of Neural Network.

4. Application to Lung Cancer Data

4.1. *Data Structure*

A data set records the survival times (S_INT, in months) of the patients seen at Vanderbilt University School of Medicine Hospital. The data set also records patients' hospital condition including

PT: patient term, ranges from $T1$ to $T4$

PN: occurrence of lymph notes, a symptom of cancer invasion, ranges from *N*0 to *N*2

STAGE: pathological diagnosis of cancer and it is ordinal, ranges from 1*A* to *IV*

DF_INT: disease free time, in months

GRADE: the fitness condition when patient in hospital, ranges from well to poor

STATUS: indicating if the patient is still alive (A) or deceased (D). If the *STATUS* of a patient is "A" (alive), this row of data is censored.

In our study, we take *PT, PN, STAGE, DF_INT*, and *GRADE* six variables as covariates to be estimated. The original hospital data set records information for 66 patients and is listed in Appendix 1.

4.2. *Estimation for Covariates*

The proportional hazard regression to estimate β is performed by SPSS. The results are shown in Appendix 2:

The Cox regression gives the mean and standard deviation for each covariate in given data. The β is estimated at a certain significance level. For "patient term" and "grade," β is positive, which means a higher value for these two variables will result in higher hazard or risk of death. For "disease free time," β assumes a negative value. This means that the longer the patient is disease free, the less likely that he or she will die shortly, which is reasonable. The β values for *PN* and *STAGE* are both near zero, which indicates that these two variables do not associated much with the hazard rate.

The Cox regression gives baseline cumulative hazard and overall cumulative hazard vs. survival time, at mean value of covariates. To estimate the hazard function, we fix the covariates at their mean values, then use least square regression to estimate the parameters a and b in (2.20), by fitting two columns of data in the survival table in Appendix 2.

4.3. *Estimation for Baseline Hazard Function*

Starting from the results of the Cox regression, let

$$X^\tau = \text{SurvivalTime} = [1\ 2\ 3\ 4\ 5\ 6\ 8\ 9\ 11\ 16\ 17\ 18\ 33],$$
$$H^\tau = \text{CumBaselineHazard}$$
$$= [.006\ .010\ .022\ .029\ .037\ .054\ .065\ .089\ .129\ .163\ .303\ .377\ .991].$$

Following the Gauss-Newton least square estimation discussed by section 3.2, we find estimations for a and b. The MATLAB computation results are summarized below.

```
FITTEDMODEL =
General model:
FITTEDMODEL(x) = a/b*(x-1/b*(1-exp(-b*x)))
Coefficients (with 95% confidence bounds):
a = 0.002185 (0.001524, 0.002845)
b = 0.01727 (-0.01574, 0.05029)
GOODNESS =
sse: 0.0129
rsquare: 0.9854
dfe: 11
adjrsquare: 0.9840
rmse: 0.0342
OUTPUT =
numobs: 13
numparam: 2
residuals: [13x1 double]
Jacobian: [13x2 double]
exitflag: 1
iterations: 7
funcCount: 22
firstorderopt: 1.4601e-004
algorithm: 'Gauss-Newton'
```

The estimated baseline hazard function is

$$h_0(t) = 0.1265(1 - \exp(-0.01727t)). \tag{4.1}$$

Figure 2 shows the fit for the cumulative baseline hazard. Figure 3 plots the baseline hazard as a function of time.

4.4. Survival Model Testing

With the help of MATLAB command newff, a feed-forward backpropagation network is constructed to simulate the survival model. This network has a total of three layers: an input layer of dimension 6, a hidden layer of dimension 3, and an output layer of dimension 1. The unit of output layer may assume a value of "0" or "1", representing "alive" and "dead" respectively. More hidden levels are proven not to improve NN performance. Since

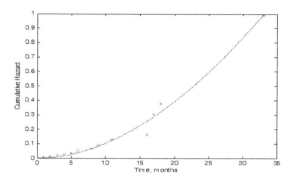

Fig. 2. Fit for Cumulative Hazard.

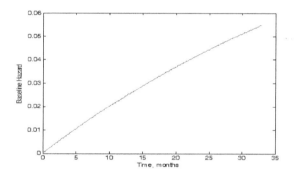

Fig. 3. Baseline Hazard as a Function of Time.

the output values assume only two possible values, we use `logsig` as the nonlinear transfer function between layers.

When having `traingda/learngdm` as the training/learning function, the NN reaches best performance, and the error rate for training set is 9%. The error rate is defined as the rate of false "alive-dead" judgment for all 66 training cases. The network performance is shown in Figure 4.

After the NN is set up, we generate a 1000×6 matrix to simulate 1000 patients' record. Each column of the matrix corresponds to a covariate, and each row stores a patient's information on $PT, PN, STAGE, S\_INT, D\_INT$, and $GRADE$. Then we use the trained NN to judge the $STATUS$ of the patient, as we "believe" the NN

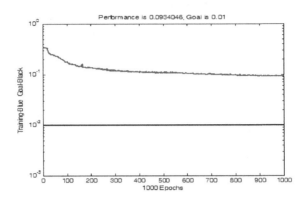

Fig. 4.   Network Performance over Epochs.

has learned the "right" survival pattern of lung cancer patients.

At first, we generate the data for each column randomly and uniformly distributed in the domain. For example, the domain for *PN* column is the closed interval $[1, 4]$. All numbers are rounded to integers. After a Cox regression analysis, the computation cannot be converged. This result shows that randomly generated data is not acceptable. The covariates for lung cancer patients must be distributed with a certain pattern.

Recall the Cox regression results for original hospital data. The mean and standard deviation for each covariate are calculated. Respecting this result, another 1000×6 matrix is generated. For each column, the generated data assume normal distribution with a corresponding mean and standard deviation that are rounded to integers (disregarding that the rounding may shift the mean and deviations for each column).

After a Cox regression and a least square fit for the cumulative baseline hazard as we did before, the baseline hazard for the NN generated data is plotted as a function of time. It is compared to the baseline hazard function we found before for the original hospital data, as shown in Figure 5.

Further more, define the score function

$$s(x, \beta) = x^\tau \cdot \beta. \tag{4.2}$$

Then the hazard function changes to be

$$h(t|x_i) = h_0 \exp(s). \tag{4.3}$$

The score function determines the risk of death. The higher score, the more likely a patient will die (or will die sooner).

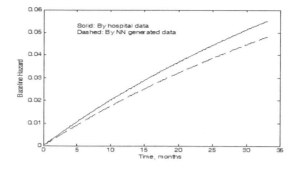

Fig. 5.   Estimated Baseline Functions.

A scatter plot for "score vs. survival time" is shown in Figure 6. Notice that time assumes a negative value if it is censored (patient is still alive.)

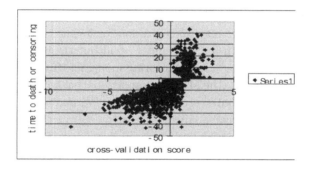

Fig. 6.   Scores vs. Time to Death or Censoring.

Figure 6 shows that when a patient scores negative or very small value, he or she tends to survive; the lower the score is, the longer he or she will live. On the other hand, a high positive score means death. This proves that proportional hazard regression is a beneficial way to estimate β coefficients.

Final Remarks: 1. In this study, we set up a survival model for lung cancer patients. This was achieved by three steps: using proportional hazard regression to estimate the coefficients for five covariates, using non-linear least square fit to estimate the exponential baseline hazard function, and using a neural network to exam the survival model. The analysis tools used in this research were SPSS, EXCEL and MATLAB.

2. MLE is a powerful statistical tool but it has its own limitation. When the data length is short, MLE might be heavily biased. In this study, there were data for 66 patients, but two thirds were censored and only one third is used in MLE. The shortage of data resulted in a unideal significance level of the estimation.

3. Neural network simulation is a new idea for testing the model, especially when the original data set is short. Neural network application in survival analysis has promising prospects.

4. Although we assume a linear combination format in the score function, the five covariates are believed to be correlated with each other. A randomly generated covariate matrix may not result in a convergent Cox regression.

5. When the NN generated data assume the same mean and SD with the original data, they tend to have similar baseline hazard functions by LSE. This supports our assumption on the format of baseline function.

6. The score function provides a good indication for the risk of death. This supports the Cox regression for β estimation.

7. In future work, we may do regression for longer hospital data for a more stable β estimation and attempt to find out the correlation among the parameters, assuming a more accurate model for $f(x|\beta)$ in the hazard function and re-formulate the MLE in proportional hazards regression. This is quite complex work but truly worth to do. We may also explore more NN applications in survival analysis.

8. In survival analysis with long-term survivors, handling situations consisting of a proportion of subjects under study that may never experience the event of interest, one proposes to formulate the model as a mixture of long-term survivors (subjects that will never "fail") and susceptibles (subjects that will "fail" eventually). In [18], comparing (4.3), the hazard rate function is modeled as $h(t|x_i) = h_0(t)\exp(s)$ with $h_0(t) = \frac{pf_0(t)}{1-pF_0(t)}$ and $0 < p \le 1$, here, $f(t)$ and $F(t)$ are defined in (2.1). Partial likelihood and full likelihood are then used to obtain the estimators of the coefficients of covariates and the proportion of long-term survivors.

Acknowledgments

The authors would like to thank William Wu, Department of Biostatistics, Vanderbilt University for providing data sets for this study. This research was supported in part by Lung Cancer SPORE (P50 CA90949), Breast

Cancer SPORE (1P50 CA98131-01), GI (5P50 CA95103-02), and Cancer Center Support Grant (CCSG) (P30 CA68485) for Y. Shyr, and by NSF IGMS (#0408086 and #0552377) and MTSU REP for D. Hong.

References

1. D.R. Cox, Regression models and life tables, *Journal of the Royal Statistical Society*, Series B, **34** (1972), 187-220.
2. N.L. Bowers et al, Actuarial Mathematics, Second Edition, Society of Actuaries, 1997.
3. S.J Walters, What Is a Cox Model, Hayward Medical Communications, volume 1, number 10, May 2001.
4. Hsi-Wen Liao, A simulation study of estimation in stratified proportional hazards model, In: NESUG 1998 Proceedings, pp. 118-125, Pittsburgh, PA, 1998.
5. Lung Cancer Transcripts, www.canceranswers.com.
6. C.L. Chiang and P.M. Conforti, A survival model and estimation of time to tumor, *Mathematical Biosciences*, **94** (1989), 1-29.
7. K. Madsen, H.B. Nielsen, and O. Tingleff, Methods for Non-Linear Least Squares Problems, 2nd Edition, Informatics and Mathematical Modeling, Technical University of Denmark, April 2004.
8. P.E. Frandsen, K. Jonasson, H.B. Nielsen, and O. Tingleff, Unconstrained Optimization, 3rd Edition, IMM, DTU, 2004.
9. P.K. Andersen and R.D. Gill, Cox's regression model for counting processes: a large sample study, *The Annals of Statistics*, **10** (1982), 1100-1120.
10. D.Y. Lin and L.J. Wei, The Robust inference for the Cox proportional hazards model, *Journal of American Statistician Association*, **84** (1989), 1074-1078.
11. D.A. Binder, Fitting Cox's proportional hazards models from survey data, *Biometrika*, **79** (1992), 139-147.
12. E.A. Pena, Smooth goodness-of-fit tests for the baseline hazard in Cox's proportional hazards model, *Journal of American Statistical Association*, **93** (1998), 673-692.
13. US Mortality Public Use Data Tape 2001, National Center for Health Statistics, Centers for Disease Control and Prevention, 2003.
14. 1950 Mortality Data CDC/NCHS, NVSS, Mortality Revised.
15. 2001 Mortality Data – NVSR, Death Final Data 2001, Vol. 52, No. 3.
16. B.D. Ripley and R.M. Ripley, Neural networks as statistical methods in survival analysis, In: Artificial Neural Networks: Prospects for Medicine, (R. Dybowski and V. Grant Eds.), pp. 237-255, Cambridge University Press, 2001.
17. E. Pitacco, Survival models in a dynamic context: a survey, *Insurance: Mathematics and Economics*, **35** (2004), 279–298.
18. X. Zhao and X. Zhou, Proportional hazard models for survival data with long-term survivals, *Statistics and Probability Letters*, **76** (2006), 1685-1693.

Appendix 1: Patients Data

#	PT	PN	STAGE	STAT	S_INT	DF_INT	GRADE
1	T1	N2	IIIA	D	11	5	mod
2	T4	N2	IIIB	D	11	9	poor
3	T1	N1	IV	D	17	0	poor
4	T2	N0	IB	A	24	24	well-mod
5	T2	N0	IV	D	9	0	mod-poor
6	T2	N2	IIIA	A	21	7	well-mod
7	T4	N0	IV	D	1	1	poor
8	T1	N0	IA	A	21	13	well-mod
9	T3	N0	IIB	D	2	0	mod-poor
10	T2	N0	IB	A	20	20	mod
11	T1	N0	IA	D	3	3	mod
12	T2	N0	IB	A	23	23	poor
13	T1	N0	IA	D	8	8	mod-poor
14	T2	N1	IIB	A	21	21	mod
15	T2	N0	IB	A	20	20	mod
16	T2	N0	IB	D	33	30	mod-poor
17	T2	N0	IB	A	18	18	mod-poor
18	T2	N2	IIIA	D	6	0	poor
19	T2	N2	IIIA	D	3	3	mod-poor
20	T1	N1	IIA	D	5	0	poor
21	T2	N2	IIIA	A	21	17	poor
22	T2	N0	IB	A	23	10	mod-poor
23	T2	N0	IB	A	26	26	well-mod
24	T2	N0	IB	A	26	26	mod
25	T1	N2	IIIA	D	18	0	poor
26	T2	N1	IIB	A	17	17	mod-poor
27	T2	N0	IIB	A	33	9	mod
28	T2	N0	IB	D	17	17	mod
29	T2	N0	IIB	A	42	42	mod-poor
30	T2	N0	IIB	D	16	5	poor
31	T1	N1	IIA	D	1	0	poor
32	T2	N0	IB	D	17	15	poor
33	T2	N2	IIIA	D	9	0	poor
34	T2	N2	IIIA	D	4	0	mod-poor

Appendix 1: Patients Data (Cont.)

#	PT	PN	STAGE	STAT	S_INT	DF_INT	GRADE
35	T2	N0	IB	A	2	1	poor
36	T2	N0	IB	A	5	1	well-mod
37	T2	N2	IIIA	A	6	6	mod
38	T1	N0	IA	A	1	1	well
39	T1	N0	IA	A	1	1	mod
40	T1	N0	IA	A	3	3	mod-poor
41	T1	N0	IA	A	1	1	mod-poor
42	T1	N0	IA	A	1	1	well-mod
43	T3	N0	IIB	A	1	1	well
44	T1	N0	IA	A	1	1	poor
45	T2	N0	IB	A	2	2	poor
46	T2	N0	IB	A	1	1	well-mod
47	T2	N0	IB	A	1	1	mod
48	T1	N0	IA	A	12	0	mod-poor
49	T1	N2	IIIA	A	6	4	mod-poor
50	T2	N0	IB	A	1	1	mod
51	T2	N0	IB	A	3	3	poor
52	T3	N0	IIB	A	10	4	poor
53	T3	N1	IIIA	D	6	6	poor
54	T2	N0	IB	A	1	0	mod
55	T4	N1	IIIB	A	2	0	mod-poor
56	T2	N0	IB	A	1	1	mod
57	T2	N0	IB	A	1	1	mod-poor
58	T2	N0	IB	A	5	4	poor
59	T1	N2	IIIA	A	1	1	poor
60	T1	N0	IA	A	1	1	mod
61	T1	N0	IA	A	7	7	poor
62	T2	N0	IB	A	2	2	mod
63	T2	N1	IIB	A	1	1	mod
64	T2	N2	IIIA	A	11	4	poor
65	T1	N0	IA	A	10	3	poor
66	T1	N0	IA	A	1	1	poor

Appendix 2: Cox Regression Results

Covariate Means

	Mean
PT	1.833
PN	.515
STAGE	3.000
D_FREE	6.879
GRADE	2.788

Survival Table

			At mean of covariates	
Time	Baseline Cum Hazard	Survival	SE	Cum Hazard
1.00	.006	.983	.012	.017
2.00	.010	.971	.018	.029
3.00	.022	.939	.030	.062
4.00	.029	.922	.036	.082
5.00	.037	.903	.042	.102
6.00	.054	.860	.053	.151
8.00	.065	.835	.061	.181
9.00	.089	.780	.073	.248
11.00	.129	.698	.091	.359
16.00	.163	.635	.105	.455
17.00	.303	.431	.123	.842
18.00	.377	.350	.121	1.050
33.00	.991	.064	.115	2.755

CHAPTER 11

NONPARAMETRIC REGRESSION TECHNIQUES IN SURVIVAL ANALYSIS

Chin-Shang Li

Department of Biostatistics, St. Jude Children's Research Hospital,
332 N. Lauderdale St., Memphis, TN, USA
E-mail: chinshang.li@stjude.org

Some nonparametric regression techniques for estimating hazard or log-hazard functions and functional forms of covariate effects in Cox's proportional hazard model are introduced. Some nonparametric and semi-parametric regression models for a conditional hazard function are discussed as alternatives to the proportional hazard model.

1. Introduction

In biomedical follow-up or industrial life-testing studies, the time to occurrence of a certain event of interest (generically called a failure) is the primary endpoint, e.g., time to hypothyroidism after treatment for pediatric Hodgkin lymphoma. The interval of interest, called failure time, survival time, or event time, is often subject to right censoring, that is, the value of the event time is not known but only that it is greater than or equal to the censoring time. Other censoring forms include left censoring and interval censoring . In left censoring, some observed times are greater than or equal to the actual failure times. Interval censoring means that some failures have occurred only within some time interval. We will confine this discussion to right-censored data.

Of particular interest are the survival and hazard functions in summarizing failure time data. Let T be a nonnegative, continuous random variable representing the failure time of an individual in a homogeneous population (i.e., no explanatory variables). The **survival function** is the probability that the individual survives until time t, i.e., $S(t) = \Pr(T \geq t)$. The **hazard function** is the risk or hazard of failure at time t given that failure has not occurred before time t and is expressed as

$$h(t) = \lim_{\Delta t \to 0^+} \frac{\Pr(t \leq T < t + \Delta t | t \leq T)}{\Delta t} = \frac{f(t)}{S(t)}, \qquad (1)$$

where $f(t) = \lim_{\Delta t \to 0^+} \Pr(t \leq T < t + \Delta t)/\Delta t = -dS(t)/dt$ is the probability density function of T. The hazard function is also called the hazard rate, the age-specified death rate, the conditional failure rate, the instantaneous death rate, the intensity rate, the mortality intensity, or the force of mortality. It follows from (1) that the survival function may be written as $S(t) = \exp(-H(t))$, where $H(t) = \int_0^t h(u)du$ is referred to as an integrated or cumulative hazard function. Therefore, the probability density and survival functions can be completely characterized by the hazard function. For a homogeneous population, parametric models for failure time include the exponential, Weibull, extreme value, gamma, log-normal, log-logistic, and generalized gamma distributions, among others. The exponential, Weibull, and gamma distributions are special cases of the generalized gamma distribution. For nonparametric methods, the Kaplan-Meier(product-limit) (K-M) estimator[80] is the most commonly used nonparametric maximum likelihood (ML) estimator of the survival function; the Nelson-Aalen (N-A) estimator [103,1], also called Altshuler's estimator[7], estimates the cumulative hazard function, which is an alternative nonparametric ML estimator of the survival function. In the absence of censoring, the K-M estimator is an empirical survival function. The asymptotic properties of the K-M estimator have been studied by Breslow and Crowley[24], Földes and Rejtö[52], and Wellner[151], among others. Padgett and McNichols[109] reviewed nonparametric density estimation from censored data.

The failure times of individuals usually depend on characteristics that are also referred to as explanatory variables, covariates, regressors, or predictor variables. The explanatory variables may include demographic variables such as age, sex, and race; physiological variables such as weight, height, and blood pressure; and behavioral factors such as smoking history and dietary habits. One can use parametric regression models such as the exponential, Weibull, and log-normal models to include explanatory variables. See [79] and [90] for detailed discussions of parametric failure time models.

Let $\mathbf{X} = (X_1, \ldots, X_p)$ be a p-vector of covariates assumed to be time independent for simplicity of discussion throughout this chapter. To explore the possible relationship between the censored failure time and covariates, it is often convenient to work with the conditional hazard function of T given $\mathbf{X} = \mathbf{x}$, $h(t|\mathbf{x})$. The Cox or proportional hazards (PH) model[34] is the most commonly used conditional hazard model. The PH model assumes that the covariates act multiplicatively on the conditional hazard function and is expressed as follows:

$$h(t|\mathbf{x}) = h(t)\exp(\mathbf{x}\boldsymbol{\beta}), \tag{2}$$

where $h(t)$ is the conditional hazard function of T given $\mathbf{X} = \mathbf{0}$, which is called the baseline hazard function, and $\boldsymbol{\beta} = (\beta_1, \ldots, \beta_p)^{\mathrm{T}}$ is a p-vector of parameters with T denoting transposition. Because no particular functional form of $h(t)$ is assumed, the PH model (2) is referred as a semiparametric regression model. The parameter vector $\boldsymbol{\beta}$ can be estimated by maximizing the partial likelihood[34,35,153]. Kalbfleisch and Prentice[79] derived an exact expression for the partial likelihood to accommodate tied observations. A number of approximation methods have been proposed by Peto[112], Breslow[23], and Efron[42], among others. The asymptotic properties of the maximum partial likelihood estimator has been studied by Tsiatis[144] and Andersen and Gill[9].

The PH model does not propose a direct relationship between failure time and covariates. In contrast, the accelerated failure time (AFT) model[79,97,36] has an intuitive physical interpretation in which the effect of covariate $\mathbf{x}$ is assumed to act multiplicatively on the failure time T or additively on the log failure time, $\log T$, expressed as $\log T = \mathbf{x}\boldsymbol{\beta} + \epsilon$ with error density $f_\epsilon(e)$. The AFT model with unspecified error distribution is called a semiparametric accelerated failure time model semiparametric accelerated failure time model and can be considered a semiparametric alternative to the PH model. Let $h(u)$ be the hazard function of $T^* = \exp(\epsilon)$. The conditional hazard function can be written in terms of this baseline hazard function as

$$h(t|\mathbf{x}) = \exp(-\mathbf{x}\boldsymbol{\beta})h(t\exp(-\mathbf{x}\boldsymbol{\beta})), \tag{3}$$

where $\exp(\mathbf{x}\boldsymbol{\beta})$ is referred to as the accelerated factor. In this model, the role of covariates is to accelerate or decelerate the time to failure. The Weibull, log-logistic, the log-normal, gamma, and inverse Gaussian distributions have the AFT property. Among them, the Weibull distribution is the only one that has both the PH property and the AFT property. See [114, 118, 145, 150, 87, 88, 159, 55, 78] and [77] for semiparametric inference procedures for the AFT model.

Hazard functions play a fundamental role in understanding and modeling failure time data. See [36] and [21] for a detailed discussion of the role of the hazard function. In addition, Aalen and Gjessing[2] considered the shape of the hazard function from a process point of view. In Sec. 2, we will discuss some nonparametric regression techniques used to estimate hazard or log-hazard functions. In Sec. 3, we will review nonparametric modeling of covariate effects in the PH model when the linear effects of the covariates are not appropriate and some semiparametric and nonparametric regression models for the conditional hazard model (i.e., hazard function with covariates) as alternatives to the PH model. A discussion is given in Sec. 4.

2. Smooth Estimation of Hazard Function

One can estimate a hazard function in at least two ways. The first is to estimate the density and cumulative distribution functions and then use their estimates to yield an estimate of the hazard function[148,4]. However, the shape of the estimate of the hazard function can exhibit serious departures from the functional form of the hazard function. More specifically, when the estimate of the density function is smooth and unimodal and when the hazard function has a smooth monotone increasing form, as it does with a gamma distribution, the estimate of the hazard function can still have a major peak and major valley in the middle of the distribution[20].

The second way is to estimate the hazard function directly. Once the hazard function is estimated, one can obtain the estimates of the density and cumulative distribution functions. The primary advantage of estimating the hazard function directly is that it can simplify the process when constraints are placed on the form of the estimate. Therefore, we will review some nonparametric regression techniques used to directly estimate the hazard or log-hazard functions in this section. A review of estimation of the hazard function with nonparametric methods was given by Singpurwalla and Wong[128] and Padgett and McNichols[109]. Wu[154] discussed issues of smoothing empirical hazard functions.

2.1. *Kernel-based Estimation*

Let $Y = \min(T, C)$, where T denotes the failure time, C denotes the corresponding censoring time, and T and C are assumed to be independent. Let $\Delta = I(T \leq C)$ be a censoring indicator for $I(\cdot)$ being the indicator function. Let (Y_i, Δ_i), $i = 1, \ldots, n$, be a sample of independent and identically distributed (i.i.d.) random variables, each having the same distribution as (Y, Δ). Let (y_i, δ_i) denote the observed data, where $\delta_i = 1$ if $y_i = \min(t_i, c_i) = t_i$; 0, otherwise.

Ramlau-Hansen[116], Tanner and Wong[136], and Yandell[157] investigated the asymptotic properties of the following **kernel estimator** of the hazard function $h(t)$ with different techniques:

$$\hat{h}_{\vartheta}(t) = \sum_{j=1}^{n} \frac{\Delta_{(j)}}{n-j+1} \mathsf{K}_{\vartheta}\left(t - Y_{(j)}\right) = \sum_{i=1}^{n} \frac{\Delta_i}{n - R_i + 1} \mathsf{K}_{\vartheta}\left(t - Y_i\right). \quad (4)$$

Here $Y_{(1)}, \ldots, Y_{(n)}$ are the ordered Y_i's; $\Delta_{(1)}, \ldots, \Delta_{(n)}$ are the corresponding censoring indicators; R_i is the rank of Y_i; and ϑ is either a positive valued bandwidth (smoothing parameter) or bandwidth vector. For the kernel estimator of $h(t)$, $\vartheta = \mathsf{b}$ and $\mathsf{K}_{\vartheta}(u) = \mathsf{b}^{-1}\mathcal{K}(u/\mathsf{b})$ for $\mathcal{K}(\cdot)$, which is a symmetric nonnegative kernel with integral $\int \mathcal{K}(u)du = 1$. The kernel estimator $\hat{h}_{\vartheta}(t) = \hat{h}_{\mathsf{b}}(t)$ is referred to as a 1-parameter estimator and can be regarded as a convolution smoothing of the formal derivative of the empirical cumulative hazard function $\hat{H}(t) = \sum_{Y_i \leq t} \Delta_i/(n - R_i + 1)$ that is an N-A estimator of the cumulative hazard function $H(t)$. The kernel estimator $\hat{h}_{\mathsf{b}}(t)$ is a generalized version of the kernel estimator of Watson and Leadbetter[149] for the uncensored case.

Tanner and Wong[137] proposed a 3-parameter estimator $\hat{h}_{\vartheta}(t)$ (4) with $\vartheta = (\mathsf{b}_1, \mathsf{b}_2, \mathsf{k})$, and $\mathsf{K}_{\vartheta}(t - Y_{(j)}) = (\mathsf{b}_1 \mathsf{d}_{j\mathsf{k}})^{-1}\mathcal{K}((t - Y_{(j)})/\mathsf{b}_2 \mathsf{d}_{j\mathsf{k}})$ for $\mathsf{d}_{j\mathsf{k}}$ being the distance to the kth-nearest failure neighbor in the sample from the point $Y_{(j)}$. The $\mathsf{d}_{j\mathsf{k}}$ will be large (small) and the kernel will be flat (peaked) in data-sparse (-dense) regions; thus, the 3-parameter estimator is a variable kernel estimator. They developed a data-based algorithm with modified-likelihood criterion for bandwidth selection by employing the idea of cross-validation and showed via a simulation study that the performance of the data-based 3-parameter estimator is superior to that of the data-based 1-parameter estimator. Tanner[135] studied the asymptotic properties of the following **variable kernel estimator** of $h(t)$:

$$\hat{h}_{\mathsf{d}_{\mathsf{k}}}(t) = \frac{1}{2\mathsf{d}_{\mathsf{k}}} \sum_{j=1}^{n} \frac{\Delta_{(j)}}{n-j+1} \mathcal{K}\left(\frac{t - Y_{(j)}}{2\mathsf{d}_{\mathsf{k}}}\right), \quad (5)$$

where d_{k} is the distance to the kth-closest failure neighbor from t.

To tackle the problems of boundary effects near the endpoints of the support of $h(t)$ and a substantial increase in the variance from left to right over the range of abscissas where $h(t)$ is estimated, Müller and Wang[102] modified the kernel estimator $\hat{h}_{\mathsf{b}}(t)$ as follows:

$$\hat{h}_{\mathsf{b}_t}(t) = \frac{1}{\mathsf{b}_t} \sum_{j=1}^{n} \frac{\Delta_j}{n-j+1} \mathcal{K}_t\left(\frac{t - Y_{(j)}}{\mathsf{b}_t}\right), \quad (6)$$

which allows for variable degrees of smoothing at different time points and implementation of boundary kernels. Here the bandwidth $\mathbf{b}_t$ and the kernel $\mathcal{K}_t(\cdot)$ depend on the time point t, where the estimate of $h(t)$ is to be computed. $\mathcal{K}_t(\cdot)$ is a kernel if t is in the interior region; it is a polynomial boundary kernel if t is in the boundary regions. See [102] for details of construction of polynomial boundary kernels. Other specific boundary kernels have been considered by Gasser, Müller, and Mammitzsch[57], Müller[101], and Messer and Goldstein[99]. Additionally, removing boundary effects has been proposed by Müller[100], Hougarrd[73], Hougaard, Plum, and Ribel[74], and by Hall and Wehrly[67].

Liebscher[96] derived uniform strong convergence rates of kernel estimators of the density and hazard functions when the failure times form a stationary α-mixing sequence; his results represented an improvement over Cai's[28].

2.2. *Spline-based Estimation*

Let $\tilde{y}_1 < \tilde{y}_2 < \cdots < \tilde{y}_s$ denote the distinct uncensored and censored times, and let m_i and c_i be the uncensored and censored numbers, respectively, at $\tilde{y}_i$. The log-likelihood of $h(\cdot)$ can be expressed as

$$\ell(h) = \sum_{j=1}^{n} \left[\delta_j \log(h(y_j)) - \int_0^{y_j} h(u)du \right] \tag{7}$$

$$= \sum_{i=1}^{s} \left[m_i \log(h(\tilde{y}_i)) - (m_i + c_i) \int_0^{\tilde{y}_i} h(u)du \right]. \tag{8}$$

To get a nonnegative estimate of $h(t)$, by developing Anderson and Senthilselvan's approach[8] to estimating the baseline hazard function in the PH model, Senthilselvan[127] made the substitution $\xi(t) = \sqrt{h(t)}$ and applied the penalized likelihood technique that was introduced by Good and Gaskins[60] in the context of nonparametric probability density estimation, by adding the roughness penalty functional $\lambda \int_{\mathcal{I}} \{\xi'(u)\}^2 du$ to the log-likelihood $\ell(h)$ (8) to obtain the **penalized log-likelihood**

$$\ell_p(\xi) = \sum_{i=1}^{s} \left[2m_i \log(\xi(\tilde{y}_i)) - (m_i + c_i) \int_0^{\tilde{y}_i} \xi^2(u)du \right]$$

$$- \lambda \int_{\mathcal{I}} \{\xi'(u)\}^2 du. \tag{9}$$

Here λ is the smoothing parameter to be used throughout this chapter. It regulates the trade-off between smoothness and goodness-of-fit. The $\xi'(\cdot)$ is the first derivative of $\xi(\cdot)$. $\mathcal{I}$ is an interval in the positive real axis containing the closed interval $[\tilde{y}_0, \tilde{y}_s]$ for $\tilde{y}_0 = 0$. The maximum penalized likelihood estimate of $\xi(t)$ is a **hyperbolic spline function** (Schumaker, 1981) with knots at $\tilde{y}_i$, $i = 0, \ldots, s$, which is expressed as

$$\hat{\xi}(t) = a_{s-1} \exp(\omega_{s-1} u_{s-1}) + b_{s-1} \exp(-\omega_{s-1} u_{s-1}), \ t \in (\tilde{y}_0, \tilde{y}_s),$$

where (i) $a_0 = b_0 = 0$; (ii) $a_i = a_{i-1} \mu_{i-1}^+ \exp(\omega_{i-1} u_{i-1}) + b_{i-1} \mu_{i-1}^- \exp(-\omega_{i-1} u_{i-1}) - E_i/(2\omega_i)$, $i = 1, \ldots, s - 1$; (iii) $b_i = a_{i-1} \mu_{i-1}^+ \exp(\omega_{i-1} u_{i-1}) + b_{i-1} \mu_{i-1}^- \exp(-\omega_{i-1} u_{i-1}) + E_i/(2\omega_i)$, $i = 1, \ldots, s - 1$; (iv) $a_{s-1}^2 \exp(2\omega_{s-1} u_{s-1}) - b_{s-1}^2 \exp(-2\omega_{s-1} u_{s-1}) - 1/(\lambda \omega_{s-1}) = 0$ for $u_i = \tilde{y}_{i+1} - \tilde{y}_i$, $\mu_i^+ = (\omega_i + \omega_{i+1})/(2\omega_{i+1})$, $\mu_i^- = (\omega_i - \omega_{i+1})/(2\omega_{i+1})$ with $\omega_i = \sqrt{\sum_{j=i+1}^{s}(m_j + c_j)/\lambda}$, $i = 0, 1, \ldots, s-1$, and $E_i = m_i/\{\lambda[a_{i-1} \exp(\omega_{i-1} u_{i-1}) + b_{i-1} \exp(-\omega_{i-1} u_{i-1})]\}$, $i = 1, \ldots, s - 1$. Note that $\hat{\xi}(\cdot)$ is continuous on $[\tilde{y}_0, \tilde{y}_s]$, and the discontinuities of $\hat{\xi}'(\cdot)$ are at the time points $\tilde{y}_i$ with $m_i \neq 0$. Therefore, for a given value of λ, the estimate of $h(t)$ is $\hat{h}(t) = \hat{\xi}^2(t)$, $t \in \mathcal{I}$. The methods used to maximize $\ell_p(\cdot)$ (9) with respect to $\xi(\cdot)$ are similar to those in [117]. The proposed estimation method can be modified to estimate the intensity function of a nonstationary Poisson process. This method is not applicable to estimation from grouped data, for which the kernel estimates of Tanner and Wong[136] may be used.

Rosenberg[119] proposed a flexible parametric procedure to model $h(t)$ as a linear combination of cubic B-splines as follows:

$$h(t; \mathbf{a}) = \sum_{k=-3}^{K} \exp(\mathbf{a}_k) B_k(t), \ t \in [y_{min}, y_{max}] \tag{10}$$

in which using $\exp(\mathbf{a}_k)$ as coefficients insures that an estimate of $h(t)$ is nonnegative. Here $\mathbf{a} = (\mathbf{a}_{-3}, \ldots, \mathbf{a}_K)^{\mathrm{T}}$; K is the number of interior knots $\kappa_1 < \cdots < \kappa_K$, to be used throughout this chapter unless stated otherwise; and $B_k(t)$ are **cubic B-spline functions**[40] of t expressed as follows:

$$B_k(t) = (\kappa_{k+4} - \kappa_k) \sum_{\ell=k}^{k+4} \frac{(\kappa_\ell - t)_+^3}{\prod_{\substack{m \neq \ell \\ m=k,\ldots,k+4}} (\kappa_m - \kappa_\ell)}, \ k = -3, \ldots, K,$$

for u_+ equal to u if $u > 0$ and 0 if $u \leq 0$. This can be constructed by following the parameterization in Atkinson[12], letting $\kappa_0 = y_{min}$ and $\kappa_{K+1} = y_{max}$, and defining six arbitrary "slack" knots such that $\kappa_{-i} = \kappa_0 - i$, and

$\kappa_{K+1+i} = \kappa_{K+1} + i$, $i = 1, 2, 3$. Using the log-likelihood (7) corresponding to the model (10), one can have the log-likelihood $\ell(\mathbf{a}; K)$ as follows:

$$\ell(\mathbf{a}; K) = \sum_{i=1}^{n} \left\{ \delta_i \log(h(t; \mathbf{a})) - \sum_{k=-3}^{K} \exp(\mathbf{a}_k) \left[IB_k(y_i) - IB_k(y_{min}) \right] \right\}, \quad (11)$$

where

$$IB_k(t) = -\frac{\kappa_{k+4} - \kappa_k}{4} \sum_{\ell=k}^{k+4} \frac{(\kappa_\ell - t)_+^4}{\prod_{\substack{m \neq \ell \\ m=k,\dots,k+4}} (\kappa_m - \kappa_\ell)}.$$

For a given value of K, one can obtain an ML estimate $\hat{\mathbf{a}}$ of $\mathbf{a}$, hence the cubic B-spline estimates $h(t; \hat{\mathbf{a}})$ of $h(t)$ and $S(t; \hat{\mathbf{a}}) = \exp(-\int_{y_{min}}^{t} h(u; \hat{\mathbf{a}})du)$ of $S(t)$ by maximizing $\ell(\mathbf{a}; K)$ (11). Within the model framework, three methods (i.e., delta-method, profile likelihood, and bootstrap) can be used to calculate confidence intervals of $h(t)$ and $S(t)$. To avoid numerical difficulties when it occurs that $\mathbf{a}_k \to -\infty$ for some k, Rosenberg suggested adding a penalty term $-10^5 \sum_{k=-3}^{K} (-10 - \mathbf{a}_k)_+^3$ to $\ell(\mathbf{a}; K)$ (11). He also developed an automatic knot selection procedure by choosing the kth knot corresponding to the $k/(K+1)$ quantile of the uncensored failure times. The final model is the one that maximizes the Akaike information criterion[5], $AIC(K) = -2\ell(\hat{\mathbf{a}}; K) - 2(K + 4)$.

Cai, Hyndman, and Wand[27] proposed a `linear spline model`

$$\eta(t; \boldsymbol{\beta}_1, \boldsymbol{\beta}_2) = \beta_{10} + \beta_{11}t + \sum_{k=1}^{K} \beta_{2k}(t - \kappa_k)_+ \quad (12)$$

for the log-hazard function $\eta(t) = \log h(t)$, where $\boldsymbol{\beta}_1 = (\beta_{10}, \beta_{11})^{\mathrm{T}}$ and $\boldsymbol{\beta}_2 = (\beta_{21}, \dots, \beta_{2K})^{\mathrm{T}}$. The implementation chooses the kth interior knot κ_k approximately corresponding to the k sample quantile of the unique observed times y_i and sets $K = \min(\lfloor n/4 \rfloor, 30)$, where $\lfloor a \rfloor$ is the greatest integer less than or equal to a. See Ruppert (2002) for further reference on the selection of K. To remedy the situation that the estimate of $\eta(t)$ will be a somewhat wiggly piecewise linear function, Cai, Hyndman, and Wand treated the β_{2k}s as random effects and assumed they were independent and normally distributed with zero mean and finite variance σ^2, whose reciprocal acts as a smoothing parameter controlling the amount of smoothing. Let $\mathbf{Z}_1 = [1, y_i]_{1 \leq i \leq n}$ and $\mathbf{Z}_2 = [(y_i - \kappa_k)_+]_{1 \leq i \leq n; 1 \leq k \leq K}$. Let $\mathcal{H}(\boldsymbol{\beta}_1, \boldsymbol{\beta}_2)$ be the sum of cumulative hazards evaluated at the y_is. Let $\tilde{\ell}(\boldsymbol{\beta}_1, \boldsymbol{\beta}_2, \sigma) = \boldsymbol{\delta}^{\mathrm{T}}(\mathbf{Z}_1\boldsymbol{\beta}_1 + \mathbf{Z}_2\boldsymbol{\beta}_2) - \mathcal{H}(\boldsymbol{\beta}_1, \boldsymbol{\beta}_2) - \frac{1}{2\sigma^2}\boldsymbol{\beta}_2^{\mathrm{T}}\boldsymbol{\beta}_2$, where $\boldsymbol{\delta} = $

$(\delta_1, \ldots, \delta_n)^{\mathrm{T}}$. Cai, Hyndman, and Wand used the ML estimate of σ^2 as a natural, automatic smoothing parameter that maximizes the marginal log-likelihood $\ell(\sigma) = \log \int \exp(\tilde{\ell}(\beta_1, \beta_2, \sigma)) d\beta_2 d\beta_1 - K \log(\sigma)$. This is approximated by

$$\tilde{\ell}(\hat{\beta}_1(\sigma), \hat{\beta}_2(\sigma), \sigma) - \frac{1}{2}\log\left| - \tilde{\ell}''(\hat{\beta}_1(\sigma), \hat{\beta}_2(\sigma), \sigma) \right| - K \log(\sigma) \qquad (13)$$

by using Laplace's method to resolve the problem of the intractable $K + 2$-dimensional integral, where for fixed σ^2, $(\hat{\beta}_1(\sigma), \hat{\beta}_2(\sigma)) = \mathrm{argmax}_{\beta_1, \beta_2} \tilde{\ell}(\beta_1, \beta_2, \sigma)$, and $\tilde{\ell}''(\hat{\beta}_1(\sigma), \hat{\beta}_2(\sigma), \sigma)$ is the second-order partial derivatives of $\tilde{\ell}(\beta_1, \beta_2, \sigma)$ with respect to (β_1, β_2), evaluated at $(\hat{\beta}_1(\sigma), \hat{\beta}_2(\sigma))$. Once the ML estimate $\hat{\sigma}$ of σ is obtained by maximizing (13), we can have the estimate $(\hat{\beta}_1, \hat{\beta}_2) = (\hat{\beta}_1(\hat{\sigma}), \hat{\beta}_2(\hat{\sigma}))$ of (β_1, β_2), hence the penalized spline fit $\eta(t; \hat{\beta}_1, \hat{\beta}_2) = \hat{\beta}_{10} + \hat{\beta}_{11}t + \sum_{k=1}^{K} \hat{\beta}_{2k}(t - \kappa_k)_+$. Cai, Hyndman, and Wand also proposed a simpler alternative to obtain a mixed model-based estimate of $h(t)$ by approximating the cumulative hazard function via a quadrature formula in which the log-likelihood $\ell(\beta_1, \beta_2, \sigma)$ for $(\beta_1, \beta_2, \sigma)$ is approximately the log-likelihood corresponding to a Poisson mixed model that can be used to estimate $h(t)$. Given σ, the covariance matrix of $(\hat{\beta}_1, \hat{\beta}_2 - \beta_2)^{\mathrm{T}}$ can be approximated by $-(\tilde{\ell}''(\hat{\beta}_1, \hat{\beta}_2, \sigma))^{-1}$ via the likelihood theory, hence pointwise confidence intervals of the hazard estimate are available.

Cai and Betensky[26] have also used this mixed model approach to spline estimation of the baseline hazard function in the PH model for interval-censored data. Bloxom[21] proposed a constrained quadratic spline as an estimator of the hazard function by using a maximum penalized likelihood procedure. Whittemore and Keller[152] estimated the hazard function by using splines with a nonparametric ML procedure and extended the procedure to estimate the baseline hazard function in the PH model. O'Sullivian[106] proposed a fast algorithm for computation of fully automated or data-driven penalized likelihood estimators of log-density and log-hazard functions by using cubic B-spline approximations; the estimator of the log-hazard function can be generalized to obtain smooth estimators of the baseline hazard function in the PH model. Cox and O'Sullivian[33] described a general approach to the first-order asymptotic analysis of penalized likelihood and related estimators, of which O'Sullivian's hazard estimator[106] is a special case. In addition, see [45, 146, 65] for general treatments of splines.

2.3. *Other Smooth Estimation Methods*

Paralleling the approach to density estimation proposed by Olkin and Spiegelman[105], Kouassi and Singh[85] proposed the model

$$h_{\mathbf{w}_t}(t; \hat{\boldsymbol{\theta}}) = \mathbf{w}_t h(t; \hat{\boldsymbol{\theta}}) + (1 - \mathbf{w}_t)\hat{h}(t) \qquad (14)$$

for $h(t)$. Here the weight parameter $\mathbf{w}_t \in [0, 1]$ is unknown and depends on the time point t. The $\mathbf{w}_t$ is estimated by minimizing the mean squared error (MSE) of $h_{\mathbf{w}_t}(t; \hat{\boldsymbol{\theta}})$, and its estimator $\hat{\mathbf{w}}_t$ is then used in (14) to obtain the estimator $h_{\hat{\mathbf{w}}_t}(t; \hat{\boldsymbol{\theta}})$ for $h(t)$. $\hat{\boldsymbol{\theta}}$ is the ML estimator of the unknown parameter or parameter vector $\boldsymbol{\theta}$ in the parametric hazard model $h(t; \boldsymbol{\theta})$ that can be, e.g., Weibull with unknown shape and scale parameters, and $h(t; \hat{\boldsymbol{\theta}})$ is the parametric estimator of $h(t)$. The $\hat{h}(t)$ is any smooth nonparametric hazard estimator of $h(t)$. For technical simplicity, Kouassi and Singh took $\hat{h}(t)$ to be the kernel estimator $\hat{h}_b(t)$[116,136,157]. The $\hat{\mathbf{w}}_t$ provides some insight into which of the parametric or nonparametric estimators is more commensurate with the data; it is expected to be close to 1 when the parametric model is valid or close to 0 otherwise. The $h_{\hat{\mathbf{w}}_t}(t; \hat{\boldsymbol{\theta}})$ is a semiparametric estimator, because it is a combination of a parametric and nonparametric estimators. When the parametric model holds, the semiparametric hazard estimator $h_{\hat{\mathbf{w}}_t}(t; \hat{\boldsymbol{\theta}})$ converges to the true model at the same rate as the parametric hazard estimator; otherwise, it converges at the same rate as the nonparametric hazard estimator. The proposed method leads to a more precise hazard estimator in the sense that the MSE of the semiparametric estimator is smaller than those of its parametric and nonparametric competitors.

In addition, Patil[110] and Antoniadis, Grégoire, and Nason[10] estimated the hazard function $h(t)$ with wavelet methods.

3. Smooth Estimation of Hazard Function with Covariates

The linear PH model (2) is a popular regression tool for the analysis of censored failure time data, but the linearity assumption of the covariate effects may not be valid in practice. One can remedy the violation by means of various nonparametric regression techniques. Therefore, in this section we will first introduce some existing nonparametric regression techniques for modeling covariate effects in the PH model and then some semiparametric and nonparametric regression models for the conditional hazard functions as alternatives to the linear PH model. First, we introduce some notations to be used in the following sections. Let $(Y_i, \mathbf{X}_i, \Delta_i)$, $i = 1, \ldots, n$, be a sample of i.i.d. random variables, each having the same distribution as $(Y, \mathbf{X}, \Delta)$, where $\mathbf{X}$ is the p-vector of covariates. Let $(y_i, \mathbf{x}_i, \delta_i)$ be observed data. Let $t_{(1)} < \cdots < t_{(m)}$ be m ordered uncensored failure times and d_j be the number of observed failures at time $t_{(j)}$, $\mathcal{R}_j = \{i : Y_i \geq t_{(j)}\}$ the risk set at time $t_{(j)}^-$, just prior to time $t_{(j)}$, $j = 1, \ldots, m$.

3.1. *Local Polynomial PH Models*

Assume that the functional form of the covariate effects $\psi(\mathbf{x})$ (i.e., the logarithm of the relative risk) in the PH model is unspecified. Then, we refer to the conditional hazard model

$$h(t|\mathbf{x}) = h(t)\exp(\psi(\mathbf{x})) \tag{15}$$

as a nonparametric PH model. For simplicity of discussion, for the moment, we consider the univariate case; thus, the nonparametric PH model (15) becomes

$$h(t|x) = h(t)\exp(\psi(x)). \tag{16}$$

The log-likelihood corresponding to the model (16) is

$$\ell(h, \psi) = \sum_{i=1}^{n} \left\{ \delta_i \left[\log h(Y_i) + \psi(X_i)\right] - H(Y_i)\exp[\psi(X_i)] \right\}. \tag{17}$$

To estimate $\psi(x)$, Fan, Gijbels, and King[50] used the local polynomial regression technique[130,131,132,32,46,47,48,121]. They assumed that the pth derivative of $\psi(X)$ at the point x_0 exists and, by a Taylor's expansion, they modeled $\psi(X)$ as

$$\psi(X) \approx \mathbf{X}^*\boldsymbol{\beta}^*, \tag{18}$$

where $\mathbf{X}^* = (1, X - x_0, \ldots, (X - x_0)^p)$, and $\boldsymbol{\beta}^* = (\beta_0^*, \ldots, \beta_p^*)^{\mathrm{T}} = (\psi(x_0), \ldots, \psi^{(p)}(x_0)/p!)^{\mathrm{T}}$. We refer to the conditional hazard model

$$h(t|x) = h(t)\exp(\mathbf{x}^*\boldsymbol{\beta}^*) \tag{19}$$

as a local polynomial PH model.

To estimate $\boldsymbol{\beta}^*$, Fan, Gijbels, and King considered two cases – when the baseline hazard function is parameterized and when it is not. We will focus on the latter case. When $h(t)$ is not parameterized, they used the local polynomial model (18) with a local version of the log partial likelihood to find the $\boldsymbol{\beta}^*$ that maximizes the `local log partial likelihood`

$$\sum_{j=1}^{m} \mathsf{K}_{\mathrm{b}}(X_{\{j\}} - x_0)\left\{\mathbf{X}_{\{j\}}^*\boldsymbol{\beta}^* - \log\left[\sum_{i\in\mathcal{R}_j}\exp(\mathbf{X}_i^*\boldsymbol{\beta}^*)\mathsf{K}_{\mathrm{b}}(X_i - x_0)\right]\right\}, \tag{20}$$

where $\{j\}$ denotes the label of the individuals failing at time $t_{(j)}$, $j = 1, \ldots, m$, and $\mathsf{K_b}(u) = \mathsf{b}^{-1}\mathcal{K}(u/\mathsf{b})$ for $\mathcal{K}(\cdot)$ being a symmetric nonnegative kernel function and b a given bandwidth. Let $\hat{\boldsymbol{\beta}}^* = (\hat{\beta}_0^*, \ldots, \hat{\beta}_p^*)^{\mathrm{T}}$ maximize the local log partial likelihood (20). Then $\hat{\psi}^{(\nu)}(x_0) = \nu!\hat{\beta}_\nu^*$ is an estimator of $\psi^{(\nu)}(x_0)$. Note that the local log partial likelihood (20) does not involve the intercept $\beta_0^* = \psi(x_0)$ because it cancels out. Therefore, the function value $\psi(x_0)$ is not directly estimable. The identifiability of $\psi(x)$ is ensured by imposing the condition $\psi(0) = 0$. The function $\psi(x) = \int_0^x \psi'(u)du$ can be estimated by

$$\hat{\psi}(x) = \int_0^x \hat{\psi}'(u)du. \tag{21}$$

For practical implementation, Tibshirani and Hastie[143] suggested approximating the integration by the trapezoidal rule.

Fan, Gijbels, and King suggested the estimator $H(t; \hat{\boldsymbol{\theta}}) = \sum_{j=1}^m \hat{\theta}_j I(t_{(j)} \leq t)$ for the cumulative baseline hazard function $H(t)$. Here $\hat{\boldsymbol{\theta}} = (\hat{\theta}_1, \ldots, \hat{\theta}_m)^{\mathrm{T}}$, and $\hat{\theta}_j = [\sum_{i \in \mathcal{R}_j} \exp(\hat{\psi}(X_i))]^{-1}$, which is the Breslow-type estimator of the baseline hazard function[22,23] for θ_j in the nonparametric model $H(t; \boldsymbol{\theta}) = \sum_{j=1}^m \theta_j I(t_{(j)} \leq t)$ for $H(t)$ and can be obtained by maximizing $\ell(h, \psi)$, given in (17) with respect to $\boldsymbol{\theta} = (\theta_1, \ldots, \theta_m)^{\mathrm{T}}$. $H(Y_i; \boldsymbol{\theta})$ and $\hat{\psi}(X_i)$ replace $H(Y_i)$ and $\psi(X_i)$, respectively. One can employ a kernel smoothing technique to obtain an estimate of $h(t)$ via $h(t; \hat{\boldsymbol{\theta}}) = \int \mathsf{W_g}(t - x)dH(x; \hat{\boldsymbol{\theta}})$, where $\mathsf{W_g}(u) = \mathsf{g}^{-1}\mathcal{W}(u/\mathsf{g})$ for $\mathcal{W}$ being a given kernel function and g a given bandwidth. An alternative approach to estimating $H(\cdot)$ and $h(\cdot)$ is the locally approximated $H(t)$ and $h(t)$ as follows:

$$H(t) \approx \exp(\mathsf{b}_0 + \mathsf{b}_1(t - t_0)), \text{ and } h(t) \approx \exp(\mathsf{b}_0 + \mathsf{b}_1(t - t_0))\mathsf{b}_1, \tag{22}$$

where t is in a neighborhood of t_0. For a given estimator $\hat{\psi}(\cdot)$ such as the one in (21), the local version of the log-likelihood (17) corresponding to the local linear models (22) can be expressed as

$$\sum_{i=1}^n \mathsf{W_g}(Y_i - t_0)\Big\{\delta_i\Big[\mathsf{b}_0 + \mathsf{b}_1(Y_i - t_0) + \log \mathsf{b}_1 + \hat{\psi}(X_i)\Big]$$

$$- \exp[\mathsf{b}_0 + \mathsf{b}_1(Y_i - t_0)]\exp[\hat{\psi}(X_i)]\Big\}. \tag{23}$$

Let $\hat{\mathsf{b}}_0$ and $\hat{\mathsf{b}}_1$ maximize the local log-likelihood (23). Then $\hat{H}(t_0) = \exp(\hat{\mathsf{b}}_0)$, and $\hat{h}(t_0) = \exp(\hat{\mathsf{b}}_0)\hat{\mathsf{b}}_1$ are smoothed type estimators of $H(t_0)$ and $h(t_0)$, respectively. Consequently, one can have smoothed type estimators of $H(t|x)$ and $h(t|x)$. The above approaches are quite different from the local full likelihood procedure by Gentleman and Crowley[58] that used an iterative procedure.

When there is more than one covariate, one could use a multivariate Taylor's expansion to approximate $\psi(\cdot)$ locally with a pth-degree polynomial. This would lead to a straightforward generalization of the above results. However, a serious problem in multivariate situations is the curse of dimensionality, which was coined by Bellman[15]. A possible approach to tackling this problem is to consider, e.g., additive modeling[68,69,70,71], hazard regression models (low-order interaction models)[82,83], adaptive regression spline Cox models[91] that used the multivariate adaptive regression spline (MARS) technique[53], and functional analysis of variance (ANOVA) modeling[133,75].

Fan and Gijbels[49] have also used the local polynomial fitting procedure on the transformed censored data to estimate the mean regression function. Kim and Truong[81] used the local linear fitting to estimate the conditional survival, cumulative hazard, mean, and median functions by modifying the procedure of Beran[17], who employed local constant fitting to estimate the conditional survival and cumulative hazard functions as an alternative to the PH model. Wu and Tuma[155] considered a general class of local hazard models. Betensky, et al.[18,19] used the local likelihood method to estimate the baseline hazard function in the PH model for right- and interval-censored data.

3.2. *Additive PH Models*

As Friedman and Stuetzle[54], among others, pointed out, dimensionality problems incurred when using multidimensional smoothers. Friedman and Stuetzle proposed the projection pursuit regression technique as an alternative to multidimensional smoothing. An additive model[68,69,71] is a special case of a projection pursuit regression model in which exactly p directions are fixed at the coordinate directions. The additive model is less general than the projection pursuit model, but it is more easily interpretable. Therefore, Hastie and Tibshirani[70] proposed an additive model

$$\psi(\mathbf{x}; \mathsf{G}) = \sum_{j=1}^{p} g_j(x_j) \tag{24}$$

for $\psi(\mathbf{x})$ in the model (15), where $\mathsf{G} = (g_1, \ldots, g_p)$; the $g_j(\cdot)$s are unspecified smooth functions; and $g_j \in \mathcal{Q}_j$ that is the space of functions with square integrable second derivatives on Ω_j that is the domain of the jth covariate,

$j = 1, \ldots, p$. The conditional hazard model

$$h(t|\mathbf{x}) = h(t) \exp(\psi(\mathbf{x}; \mathsf{G})) \tag{25}$$

is referred to as an additive PH model. Let $\boldsymbol{\Psi} = (\psi(\mathbf{x}_1; \mathsf{G}), \ldots, \psi(\mathbf{x}_n; \mathsf{G}))^{\mathrm{T}}$. Then, the partial likelihood corresponding to the model (25) with Peto's (1972) approximation for ties is

$$PL(\boldsymbol{\Psi}) = \prod_{r=1}^{m} \frac{\exp\left(\sum_{i \in \mathcal{D}_r} \psi(\mathbf{x}_i; \mathsf{G})\right)}{\left(\sum_{i \in \mathcal{R}_r} \exp(\psi(\mathbf{x}_i; \mathsf{G}))\right)^{d_r}}, \tag{26}$$

where D_r is the set of indices of failures at $t_{(r)}$. To estimate $g_j(\cdot)$, Hastie and Tibshirani maximized the **penalized log partial likelihood**

$$\ell_p(\boldsymbol{\Psi}) = \ell(\boldsymbol{\Psi}) - \frac{1}{2} \sum_{j=1}^{p} \lambda_j \int g_j''(x)^2 dx, \tag{27}$$

where $\ell(\boldsymbol{\Psi}) = \log PL(\boldsymbol{\Psi})$ and $\lambda_j \geq 0$ are smoothing parameters. The first term in (27) measures the closeness of the fit to the data, and the second term penalizes the curvature of the fitted functions. One can establish the existence of a unique solution to this problem under certain conditions by using the arguments of O'Sullivan[107] extended to the additive model by Buja, Hastie, and Tibshirani[25]. Given that a unique solution exists, it can be seen that the solution must be a cubic spline for each j.

One can restrict the infinite-dimensional problem to a finite one by choosing a suitable basis. A convenient basis can result from considering the evaluations of the cubic splines $g_j(\cdot)$ at the observed points $x_{1j}, \ldots, x_{nj}$. The penalized log partial likelihood (27) then can be rewritten as

$$\ell_p(\boldsymbol{\Psi}) = \ell(\boldsymbol{\Psi}) - \frac{1}{2} \sum_{j=1}^{p} \lambda_j \mathbf{g}_j^{\mathrm{T}} \mathbf{K}_j \mathbf{g}_j, \tag{28}$$

where $\mathbf{K}_j$ are symmetric penalty matrices, and $\mathbf{g}_j = (g_j(x_{1j}), \ldots, g_j(x_{nj}))^{\mathrm{T}}$ is a vector of the values of g_j at $x_{1j}, \ldots, x_{nj}$. One may obtain (28) as the log posterior from a Bayesian model with independent priors $\mathbf{g}_j \sim N(\mathbf{0}, \mathbf{K}_j^{-1})$; the additive function solution lies in a reproducing kernel Hilbert space with $\sum_{j=1}^{p} \mathbf{K}_j^{-}$ equal to the reproducing kernel evaluated at $x_{1j}, \ldots, x_{nj}$. The curves $\mathbf{g}_j$ maximizing $\ell_p(\boldsymbol{\Psi})$ can be obtained by using the Newton-Raphson algorithm with the "Gauss-Seidel" method. In the statistical literature, the Gauss-Seidel method has become known as "backfitting," which was first proposed on more heuristic grounds using nonlinear smoothers[54]. Note that in the algorithm the functions are standardized to have a mean of zero, because any additive constant can be absorbed into $h(t)$. According to Gill, Murray, and Wright[59], if step size is optimized, the proposed algorithm is globally convergent.

When the x values are tied, fitted values will be required only at the unique values of a given covariate, so the tied values will reduce the parameter space. The algorithm handles the tied values correctly as long as the smoother returns the same estimated value for the same x values. This is the case for the cubic spline smoother, and other reasonable smoothers. Hastie and Tibshirani derived some approximate methods for inference and smoothing parameter selection through heuristic arguments. The proposed methodology may be applied in principle to time-dependent covariates, though substantial computational difficulties may arise.

O'Sullivan[107] proposed an algorithm for the PH model based on a conjugate gradient method in which the cubic B-spline representation was used for $\psi(\mathbf{x})$; the proposed algorithm is globally convergent. Sleeper and Harrington[129] have also used a liner combination of B-splines to approximate $\psi(\mathbf{x})$. Durrelman and Simon[41] used restricted cubic splines for $\psi(\mathbf{x})$.

In contrast to smooth additive functions for $\psi(\mathbf{x})$ by Hastie and Tibshirani[70], O'Sullivan[107], and Sleeper and Harrington[129], among others, LeBlanc and Crowley[91] modeled $\psi(\mathbf{x})$ by using the MARS technique[53]. The conditional hazard model is referred to as an adaptive regression spline PH model. The technique can automatically fit models with terms that represent nonlinear effects and interactions among covariates. LeBlanc and Crowley's method is related to the method by Gray[63] who used fixed knot splines in the PH model. However, their method adaptively selects locations and is restricted to piecewise linear functions of the covariates $\mathbf{x}$.

To ameliorate the curse of dimensionality, Huang, Kooperberg, Stone, and Truong[75] proposed a functional ANOVA model for $\psi(\mathbf{x})$ in which the overall effect of the covariates is modeled as a specified sum of a constant effect, main effects (functions of one covariate), and selected low-order interactions (functions of a few covariates). At the same time, the functional ANOVA model retains the flexibility of nonparametric modeling. This approach also can deal with the situation of time-dependent covariates. Stone, Hansen, Kooperberg, and Truong[133] gave a comprehensive review of one approach to functional ANOVA modeling. In addition, Wahba, Wang, Gu, Klein, and Klein[147] discussed ANOVA decompositions for smoothing spline models in a general context.

3.3. *Partially Linear PH Models*

In practice, if without loss of generality the first p_1 covariates of $\mathbf{x}$ are assumed to have linear effects and the functional forms of the other covariate effects are unknown and smooth, one can use the model $\sum_{j=1}^{p_1} \beta_j x_j + \sum_{j=p_1+1}^{p} g_j(x_j)$, considered by Gray (1992) for $\psi(\mathbf{x})$ in model (15) instead of the additive model (27), where the g_js are unknown smooth functions. To simplify this discussion, we will assume that the functional form of the pth covariate effect is unspecified. Gray[64] considered the **partially linear model**

$$\psi(\mathbf{x}; \boldsymbol{\beta}_1^*, g) = \mathbf{x}_1^* \boldsymbol{\beta}_1^* + g(x_p) \tag{29}$$

for $\psi(\mathbf{x})$, where $\mathbf{x}_1^* = (x_1, \ldots, x_{p-1})$, the first $p-1$ covariates for the linear terms, $\boldsymbol{\beta}_1^*$ is the vector of the associated parameters, and g is an unknown smooth function that gives the pth covariate effect on the outcome. Engle, Granger, Rice, and Weiss[43] were the first to consider the partially linear model. The conditional hazard model

$$h(t|\mathbf{x}) = h(t) \exp(\psi(\mathbf{x}; \boldsymbol{\beta}_1^*, g)) \tag{30}$$

is referred to as a partially linear or semiparametric additive PH model. Let $B_1(x_p), \ldots, B_{K+4}(x_p)$ be the cubic B-spline basis for the space of cubic splines with the prespecified interior knots $\kappa_1, \ldots, \kappa_K$. Gray[64] parameterized g as

$$g(x_p) = \theta_0 x_p + \sum_{k=1}^{K+2} \theta_k B_k(x_p), \tag{31}$$

where $\theta_0, \theta_1, \ldots, \theta_{K+2}$ are unknown parameters. Because the space of cubic B-splines includes the constant and linear functions, the constant is absorbed into $h(t)$, and the linear term is specified separately in (31), only $K + 2$ of the B-spline basis functions are used in (31). Therefore, any two of the $K + 4$ B-spline basis functions could be dropped, provided the resulting parameterization is of full rank. Let $\boldsymbol{\vartheta}_1 = (\theta_1, \ldots, \theta_{K+2})^{\mathrm{T}}$ and $\boldsymbol{\vartheta}_2 = (\theta_0, \boldsymbol{\vartheta}_1^{\mathrm{T}})^{\mathrm{T}}$. To investigate the effects of the covariate x_p, Gray considered two hypotheses about g: (i) the hypothesis of no effect, $g(x_p) = 0$, i.e., $\boldsymbol{\vartheta}_2 = \mathbf{0}$. (ii) the hypothesis of linear effect of x_p, $g(x_p) = \theta_0 x_p$, i.e., $\boldsymbol{\vartheta}_1 = \mathbf{0}$.

Constructing tests for hypothesis (ii) is exactly the same as that for hypothesis (i), so we will confine our discussion to testing hypothesis (i). To estimate $\boldsymbol{\beta}_1^*$ and g, Gray[64] maximized the **penalized log partial** likelihood

$$\ell_p(\boldsymbol{\beta}_1^*, \boldsymbol{\vartheta}_2) = \ell(\boldsymbol{\beta}_1^*, \boldsymbol{\vartheta}_2) - \frac{1}{2}\lambda \int g''(u)^2 du, \tag{32}$$

where $\ell(\boldsymbol{\beta}_1^*, \boldsymbol{\vartheta}_2)$ is the log partial likelihood; $\frac{1}{2}\lambda \int g''(u)^2 du = \frac{1}{2}\lambda \boldsymbol{\vartheta}_1^T \mathbf{K} \boldsymbol{\vartheta}_1 = \frac{1}{2}\lambda \boldsymbol{\vartheta}_2^T \mathbf{K}^* \boldsymbol{\vartheta}_2$ is a penalty function; $\mathbf{K}$ is a positive-definite matrix that is a function only of the knot locations; $\mathbf{K}^*$ is a $(K+3) \times (K+3)$ matrix with zeros in the first row and column and $\mathbf{K}$ is in the remainder of the matrix. To test hypothesis (i) by analogy with the usual (unpenalized) parametric likelihood procedures, Gray conducted three test statistics: a penalized quadratic score statistic, a Wald-type statistic, and a penalized likelihood ratio statistic that is similar to the deviance statistics discussed by Hastie and Tibshirani[70,71] and applied to this setting. The main difference is that the penalty function in the deviance is not included.

Within the fixed knot framework and assuming that the usual conditions are satisfied so that the standard asymptotic expansions hold for the unpenalized log partial likelihood[9,64] showed that under the null hypothesis the three test statistics all have the same asymptotic distribution, which is a linear combination of chi-squares. Imhof[76] and Davies[38,39] developed methods for calculating the distribution of a linear combination of chi-squares based on inverting the characteristic function. For the practical use of the proposed tests, the value of λ that gives the specified degrees of freedom of the proposed tests is used. The definition of degrees of freedom corresponds to Definition 3 of Buja, Hastie, and Tibshirani[25]. The proposed methodology can be extended for time-dependent covariate effects.

3.4. *Extended Hazard Regression Models*

Etezadi-Amoli and Ciampi[44] proposed the **extended hazard regression (EHR) model**

$$h(t|\mathbf{x}) = h(\exp(-\mathbf{x}\boldsymbol{\alpha})t)\exp(-\mathbf{x}\boldsymbol{\beta}) \tag{33}$$

for $h(t|\mathbf{x})$, where $h(u)$ is an unspecified baseline hazard function, and $\boldsymbol{\alpha}$ and $\boldsymbol{\beta}$ are vectors of regression parameters. It can be seen that the EHR model (33) includes the PH ($\boldsymbol{\alpha} = \mathbf{0}$) and AFT ($\boldsymbol{\alpha} = \boldsymbol{\beta}$) models as special cases. Let $u = \exp(-\mathbf{x}\boldsymbol{\alpha})y$. Etezadi-Amoli and Ciampi[44] modeled $h(u)$ with a quadratic spline with K knots denoted by $\boldsymbol{\kappa} = (\kappa_1, \ldots, \kappa_K)$ as follows:

$$h(u; \boldsymbol{\zeta}) = \sum_{l=0}^{2} \gamma_{0l} u^l + \sum_{k=1}^{K} \gamma_{1k}(u - \kappa_k)_+^2 \tag{34}$$

$$= \gamma_{0j}^* + \gamma_{1j}^* u + \gamma_{2j}^* u^2 \text{ for } u \in [\kappa_j, \kappa_{j+1}], \ j = 1, \ldots, K-1, \tag{35}$$

where $\boldsymbol{\zeta} = (\boldsymbol{\gamma}_0, \boldsymbol{\gamma}_1, \boldsymbol{\kappa})$ is the $(2K + 3)$-vector of parameters for $\boldsymbol{\gamma}_0 = (\gamma_{00}, \gamma_{01}, \gamma_{02})$, $\boldsymbol{\gamma}_1 = (\gamma_{11}, \ldots, \gamma_{1K})$, $\gamma_{0j}^* = \gamma_{00} + \sum_{k=1}^{j} \gamma_{1k} \kappa_k^2$, $\gamma_{1j}^* = \gamma_{01} - 2 \sum_{k=1}^{j} \gamma_{1k} \kappa_k$, and $\gamma_{2j}^* = \gamma_{02} + \sum_{k=1}^{j} \gamma_{1k}$. The log-likelihood corresponding to the EHR model (33) with the quadratic spline model (34) is

$$\ell(\boldsymbol{\alpha}, \boldsymbol{\beta}, \boldsymbol{\zeta}) = \sum_{i=1}^{n} \left\{ \delta_i [-\mathbf{x}_i \boldsymbol{\beta} + \log h(u_i; \boldsymbol{\zeta})] \right.$$

$$\left. - \exp(-\mathbf{x}_i(\boldsymbol{\beta} - \boldsymbol{\alpha})) - H(u_i; \boldsymbol{\zeta}) \right\}, \qquad (36)$$

where $H(u; \boldsymbol{\zeta}) = \int_0^u h(t; \boldsymbol{\zeta}) dt$ is a cumulative hazard function. Thus, once the estimate $(\hat{\boldsymbol{\alpha}}, \hat{\boldsymbol{\beta}}, \hat{\boldsymbol{\zeta}})$ of $(\boldsymbol{\alpha}, \boldsymbol{\beta}, \boldsymbol{\zeta})$ is obtained by maximizing $\ell(\boldsymbol{\alpha}, \boldsymbol{\beta}, \boldsymbol{\zeta})$, we can have the estimate of $h(t|\mathbf{x})$. Let $u_{\max}$ be the value of $u = \exp(-\mathbf{x}\hat{\boldsymbol{\alpha}})y$ corresponding to the maximum observed time. To ensure that $h(u; \boldsymbol{\zeta})$ must be nonnegative in $[0, u_{\max}]$ while estimating $(\boldsymbol{\alpha}, \boldsymbol{\beta}, \boldsymbol{\zeta})$, the following constraints are needed: (i) $\gamma_{00} \geq 0$; (ii) $h(u_{\max}; \boldsymbol{\zeta}) > 0$; (iii) $h(\kappa_k; \boldsymbol{\zeta}) \geq 0$, $k = 1, \ldots, K$; (iv) if the jth polynomial piece of (35) has an extremum in $[\kappa_j, \kappa_{j+1}]$, then

$$\gamma_{0j}^* - (\gamma_{1j}^*)^2 / 4\gamma_{2j}^* \geq 0; \qquad (37)$$

otherwise $h((\kappa_j + \kappa_{j+1})/2; \boldsymbol{\zeta}) \geq 0$. Notice that (37) is the value of $h(u; \boldsymbol{\zeta})$ at the extremum of the jth polynomial piece, provided it falls in $[\kappa_j, \kappa_{j+1}]$.

The subroutine GRG2 (Lasdon and Waren, Department of General Business, University of Texas at Austin, 1982) can be used for the numerically constrained optimization while maximizing $\ell(\boldsymbol{\alpha}, \boldsymbol{\beta}, \boldsymbol{\zeta})$ (36) subject to constraints (i) through (iv). The algorithm, which is based on the generalized reduced gradient method[3,89], is considered one of the best in regard to reliability and numerical stability of the solutions[123]. Within the framework of the EHR model, the likelihood ratio test can be used to determine the shape of the baseline hazard function, to determine the significance of the regression coefficients, and to discriminate between AFT and PH. Although several approaches to testing the PH assumption have been developed[11,142], the EHR model offers the unique advantage of permitting a comparison between PH and AFT.

3.5. *Hazard Regression*

Kooperberg, Stone, and Truong[82] developed an adaptive hazard regression (HARE) methodology to model the conditional log-hazard function $\eta(t|\mathbf{x}) = \log h(t|\mathbf{x})$ as an alternative to the various aforementioned PII models. Let $\mathbf{x} = (x_1, \ldots, x_p)$ range over the subset $\mathcal{X} = \mathcal{X}_1 \times \cdots \times \mathcal{X}_p$ of

$\mathbb{R}^p$ for x_i ranging over the subset $\mathcal{X}_i$ of $\mathbb{R}$, $i = 1, \ldots, p$. Let $1 \leq q < \infty$ and G a q-dimensional linear space of functions on $[0, \infty) \times \mathcal{X}$ such that $g(\cdot|\mathbf{x})$ is bounded on $[0, \infty)$ for $g \in G$. Let $\mathcal{B}_1, \ldots, \mathcal{B}_q$ be a basis of this space. They used the following linear combination of linear splines and their tensor products to develop the following HARE model:

$$\eta(t|\mathbf{x}; \boldsymbol{\Phi}) = \sum_{j=1}^{q} \phi_j \mathcal{B}_j(t|\mathbf{x}), \tag{38}$$

for $\eta(t|\mathbf{x})$, where $\boldsymbol{\Phi} = (\phi_1, \ldots, \phi_q)^{\mathrm{T}}$. The method is similar to the MARS technique[53]. It can be seen from (38) that the approach to modeling $\eta(t|\mathbf{x})$ does not depend on the validity of the basic assumption of the PH model that the conditional log-hazard function is an additive function of time and the vector of covariates. One can obtain the ML estimate $\hat{\boldsymbol{\Phi}}$ of $\boldsymbol{\Phi}$ by maximizing the log-likelihood corresponding to the HARE model (38) for $\eta(t|\mathbf{x})$

$$\ell(\boldsymbol{\Phi}) = \sum_{i=1}^{n} \left\{ \delta_i \eta(y_i|\mathbf{x}_i; \boldsymbol{\Phi}) - \int_0^{y_i} \exp[\eta(u|\mathbf{x}_i; \boldsymbol{\Phi})] du \right\}, \tag{39}$$

which is a concave function on $\mathbb{R}^q$. Consequently, the corresponding ML estimates of the conditional log-hazard function, hazard function, survival function, and density function are given by $\hat{\eta}(t|\mathbf{x}) = \eta(t|\mathbf{x}; \hat{\boldsymbol{\Phi}})$, $\hat{h}(t|\mathbf{x}) = h(t|\mathbf{x}; \hat{\boldsymbol{\Phi}}) = \exp(\eta(t|\mathbf{x}; \hat{\boldsymbol{\Phi}}))$, $\hat{S}(t|\mathbf{x}) = \exp(-\int_0^t \hat{h}(u|\mathbf{x}) du)$, and $\hat{f}(t|\mathbf{x}) = \hat{h}(t|\mathbf{x})\hat{S}(t|\mathbf{x})$, respectively.

To resolve the problem of choosing the linear space G (i.e., the selection of the final model), Kooperberg, Stone, and Truong[82] proposed an automatic procedure involving the ML method, stepwise addition using Rao statistic, stepwise deletion using Wald statistic, and the Bayes information criterion[126]. If the selected space is the space of constant functions, then the HARE model (38) has $q = 1$, $\mathcal{B}_1(t|\mathbf{x}) = 1$, and $\eta(t|\mathbf{x}; \boldsymbol{\Phi}) = \phi_1$, which means that the conditional distribution of T given $\mathbf{X} = \mathbf{x}$ is exponential with mean $\exp(-\phi_1)$ independent of $\mathbf{x}$. If none of the basis functions of the selected space depends on both t and $\mathbf{x}$, then the HARE model (38) is a PH model, hence the HARE models include PH models as a subclass. However, if any of the basis functions in the final model depends on both time and a covariate, a PH model might not be appropriate. Therefore, the presence or absence of interaction terms between time and covariates in the final model can be regarded as a check on the proportionality of the underlying conditional hazard model.

When the covariates are absent, the model (38) reduces to

$$\eta(t|\mathbf{\Phi}) = \sum_{j=1}^{q} \phi_j \mathcal{B}_j(t). \tag{40}$$

Kooperberg, Stone, and Truong[82] developed the approach hazard estimation with flexible tails (HEFT) to estimate the log-hazard function by using cubic splines. To allow for greater flexibility in the extreme tails, they incorporated two additional log terms into the fitted model for the log-hazard function. With inclusion of these two basis functions, HEFT can fit Weibull and Pareto distributions exactly; HEFT is useful as a preprocessor of HARE. They wrote programs in C for implementing HARE and HEFT and developed interfaces based on S[14,29]; the software is available from statlib [statlib@stat.cmu.edu] by requesting `hare from S or heft from S`.

Under suitable conditions, Kooperberg, Stone, and Truong[83] obtained the L_2 rate of convergence for a nonadaptive version of the proposed methodology. Kooperberg and Clarkson[84] extended the HARE methodology to accommodate interval-censored data, time-dependent covariates, and cubic splines. Gu[66] formulated a general procedure for penalized likelihood hazard estimation. When a covariate is present, the class of the conditional hazard models constructed via tensor-product splines includes the PH model and the model of Zucker and Karr[160] as special cases, and in the absence of the covariate, the estimate of the hazard function reduces to that of [106]. Gu's methodology is similar to the HARE methodology.

4. Discussion

We have reviewed some nonparametric regression techniques for estimation of the hazard or log-hazard functions. We also have discussed functional forms of the effects of the covariates in the PH model and some semiparametric or nonparametric regression models for the conditional hazard function as alternatives to the PH model. Although we have focused on nonparametric modeling of time-independent covariate effects in the PH model (Sec. 3), examining the PH assumption and modeling nonproportional hazards are also very important issues that have generated an extensive literature. See [115, 138, 124, 61, 56, 13, 113, 141, 62, 122, 72, 108, 6, 37] and those mentioned in the previous sections for details. In addition, the book[140] provided a detailed discussion of model building, testing for the PH models, and using SAS and S-Plus for these methodologies. The proportional odds regression model[16,158] is also an alternative to the PH model.

Li[95] gave a detailed review of the proportional odds regression model. It is commonly seen in survival analysis that estimated survival curves level off at a nonzero value after a certain time, even when many individuals are followed beyond that time. This type of data has heavy censoring at the end of the follow-up period. One can regard the population as consisting of two groups: individuals who are not susceptible to an event of interest, and individuals who are susceptible to the event if they are followed long enough. A number of parametric and semiparametric cure (or mixture) models for this type of heavily censored data have been proposed by Farewell[51], Yamaguchi[156], Kuk and Chen[86], Taylor[139], Chen, Ibrahim, and Sinha[30], Sy and Taylor[134], Peng and Dear[111], and Li and Taylor[93,94]. See [98] for a detailed introduction to cure models. Li, Taylor, and Sy[92] systematically studied the identifiability of cure models. Finally, see [104] for a detailed review of statistical methodologies used in survival analysis that were not discussed in this chapter.

Acknowledgments

This work was partially supported by Cancer Center Support Grant CA21765 from the National Institutes of Health and by the American Lebanese Syrian Associated Charities (ALSAC).

References

1. O.O. Aalen, Nonparametric inference for a family of counting processes, *Ann. Statist.*, **6** (1978), 701-726.
2. O.O. Aalen and H.K. Gjessing, Understanding the shape of the hazard rate: a process point of view, *Statist. sci.*, **16** (2001), 1-22.
3. J. Abadie and J. Carpentier, Generalization of the Wolf reduced gradient method to the case of nonlinear constratins, In: *Optimization*, (R. Fletcher Ed.), pp.37-47, Academic Press, New York, 1969.
4. M. Abrahamowicz, A. Ciampi, and J.O. Ramsay, Nonparametric desity ostimation for censored survival data: regression-spline approach, *Can. J. Statist.*, **20** (1992), 171-185.
5. H. Akaiki, *2nd International Symposium on Information Theory*, (B.N. Petrov and F. Csáki, Ed.), Budapest, Akademiai Kiado, 1973.
6. D.G. Altman and B.L. De Stavola, Practical problems in fitting a proportional hazards model to data with updated measurements of the covariates, *Statist. Med.*, **13** (1994), 301-341.
7. B. Altshuler, Theory for the measurement of competing risk in animal experiments, *Math. Biosci.*, **6** (1970), 1-11.
8. J.A. Anderson and A. Senthilselvan, Smooth estimates for the hazard function, *J. R. Stat. Soc.*, **B42** (1980), 322-327.

9. P.K. Andersen and R.D. Gill, Cox's regression model for counting processes: a large sample study, *Ann. Statist.*, **10** (1982), 1100-1120.

10. A. Antoniadis, G. Grégoire, and G. Nason, Density and hazard rate estimation for right-censored data by using wavelet methods, *J. R. Stat. Soc.*, **B61** (1999), 63-84.

11. F.J. Aranda-Ordaz, An extension of the proportional hazards model for grouped data, *Biometrics*, **39** (1983), 109-118.

12. K.E. Atkinson, *An introduction to numerical analysis*, 2nd ed., John Wiley, New York, 1989.

13. W.E. Barlow and R.L. Prentice, Residuals for relative risk Regression, *Biometrika*, **75** (1988), 65-74.

14. R.A. Becker, J.M. Chambers, and A.R. Wilks, *The New S Language*, Wadsworth, Pacific Grove, 1988.

15. R.E. Bellman, *Adaptive Control Processes*, Princeton University Press, 1961.

16. S. Bennett, Analysis of survival data by the proportional odds model, *Statist. Med.*, **2** (1983), 273-277.

17. R. Beran, Nonparametric regression with randomly censored survival data, Technical report, University of California, Berkeley, 1981.

18. R.A. Betensky, J.C. Lindsey, L.M. Ryan, and M.P. Wand, Local EM estimation of the hazard function for interval-censored data, *Biometrics*, **55** (1999), 238-245.

19. R.A. Betensky, J.C. Lindsey, L.M. Ryan, and M.P. Wand, A local likelihood proportional hazards model for interval censored data, *Statist. Med.*, **21** (2002), 263-275.

20. B. Bloxom, *Principals of modern psychological measurement: A festschrift in honor of Frederick M. Lord*, (H. Waiber and S. Messick, Ed.), pp.303-328, Lawrence Eribaum, NJ, 1983.

21. B. Bloxom, A constrained spline estimator of a hazard function. *Psychometrika*, **50** (1985), 301-321.

22. N.E. Breslow, Comment on "Regression and life tables" by D.R. Cox, *J. R. Stat. Soc.*, **B34** (1972), 216-217.

23. N.E. Breslow, Covariance analysis of censored survival data, *Biometric*, **30** (1974), 89-99.

24. N.E. Breslow and J. Crowley, A large sample study of life table and product limit estimates under random censorship, *Ann. Statist.*, **2** (1974), 437-453.

25. A. Buja, T. Hastie, and R. Tibshirani, Linear smoothers and additive models (with discussion), *Ann. Statist.*, **17** (1989), 453-555.

26. T. Cai and R.A. Betensky, Hazard regression for interval-censored data with penalized spline, *Biometrics*, **59** (2003), 570-590.

27. T. Cai, R.J. Hyndman, and M.P. Wand, Mixed model-based hazard estimation, *J. Computat. Graph. Statist.*, **11** (2002), 784-798.

28. Z. Cai, Kernel density and hazard rate estimation for censored dependent data, *J. Multivariate Anal.*, **67** (1998), 23-34.

29. J.M. Chambers and T.J. Hastie, *Statistical Models in S*, Wadsworth, Pacific Grove, CA, 1992.

30. M.H. Chen, Ibrahim, and D. Sinha, A new Bayesian model for survival data

with a surviving fraction. *J. Am. Stat. Assoc.*, **94** (1999), 909-919.

31. A. Ciampi and J. Etezadi-Amoli, A general model for testing the proportional hazards and the accelerated failure times hypothesis in the analysis of censored survival data with covariates, *Commun. Statist.-Theory Meth.*, **14** (1985), 651-667.

32. W.S. Cleveland, Robust locally weighted regression and smoothing scatterplots, *J. Am. Stat. Assoc.*, **74** (1979), 829-836.

33. D.D. Cox and F. O'Sullivan, Asymptotic analysis of penalized likelihood and related estimators, *Ann. Statist.*, **18** (1990), 1676-1695.

34. D.R. Cox, Regression models and life-tables (with discussion), *J. R. Stat. Soc.*, **B34** (1972), 187-220.

35. D.R. Cox, Partial likelihood, *Biometrika*, **62** (1975), 269-276.

36. D.R. Cox and D. Oakes, *Analysis of Survival Data*, Chapman and Hall, London, 1984.

37. D.M. Dabrowska, Smoothed Cox regression, *Ann. Statist.*, **25** (1997), 1510-1540.

38. R.B. Davies, Numerical inversion of a characteristic function, *Biometrika*, **60** (1973), 415-417.

39. R.B. Davies, The distribution of a linear combination of χ^2 random variables, *Appl. Statist.*, **29** (1980), 323-333.

40. C. de Boor, *A Practical Guide to Splines*, Springer-Verlag, New York, 1978.

41. S. Durrleman and R. Simon, Flexible regression models with cubic splines, *Statist. Med.*, **8** (1989), 551-561.

42. B. Efron, The efficiency of Cox's likelihood function for censored data, *J. Am. Stat. Assoc.*, **72** (1977), 557-565.

43. R.F. Engle, C.W.J. Granger, J. Rice, and A. Weiss, Semiparametric estimates of the relation between weather and electricity sales, *J. Am. Stat. Assoc.*, **81** (1986), 310-320.

44. J. Etezadi-Amoli and A. Ciampi, Extended hazard regression for censored survial data with covariates: a spline approximation for the baseline hazard function, *Biometrics*, **43** (1987), 181-192.

45. R.L. Eubank, *Spline Smoothing and Nonparametric Regression*, Marcel Dekker, New York, 1988.

46. J. Fan, Design-adaptive nonparametric regression, *J. Am. Stat. Assoc.*, **87** (1992), 998-1004.

47. J. Fan, Local linear regression smoothers and their minimax efficiencies, *Ann. Statist.*, **21** (1993), 196-216.

48. J. Fan and I. Gijbels, Variable bandwidth and local linear regression smothers, *Ann. Statist.*, **20** (1992), 2008-2036.

49. J. Fan and I. Gijbels, Censored regression: local linear approximations and their applications, *J. Am. Stat. Assoc.*, **89** (1994)., 560-570.

50. J. Fan, I. Gijbels, and M. King, Local likelihood and local partial likelihood in hazard regression, *Ann. Statist.*, **25** (1997), 1661-1690.

51. V.T. Farewell, The use of mixture models for the analysis of survival data with long-term survivors, *Biometrics*, **38** (1982), 1041-1046.

52. A. Földes and L. Rejtö, Strong uniform consistency for nonparametric sur-

vival curve estimators from randomly censored data, *Ann. Statist.*, **9** (1981), 122-129.

53. J.H. Friedman, Multivariate adaptive regression splines (with discussion), *Ann. Statist.*, **19** (1991), 1-141.

54. J.H. Friedman and W. Stuetzle, Projection pursuit regression, *J. Am. Stat. Assoc.*, **76** (1981), 817-823.

55. M. Fygenson and Y. Ritov, Monotone estimating equations for censored data, *Ann. Statist.*, **22** (1994), 732-746.

56. D. Gamerman and M. West, An application of dynamic survival models in unemployment studies, *Statistician*, **36** (1987), 269-274.

57. T. Gasser, H.G. Müller, and V. Mammitzsch, Kernels for nonparametric curve estimation, *J. R. Statist. Soc.*, **B47** (1985), 238-252.

58. R. Gentleman and J. Crowley, Local full likelihood estimation for the proportional hazards model, *Biometrics*, **47** (1991), 1283-1296.

59. P. Gill, W. Murray, and M. Wright, *Practical Optimization*, Academic Press, London, 1981.

60. I. J. Good and R.A. Gaskins, Nonparametric roughness penalties for probability densities, *Biometrika*, **58** (1971), 255-277.

61. S.M. Gore, S.J. Pocock, and G.R. Kerr, Regression models and nonproportional hazards in the analysis of breast cancer survival, *Appl. Statist.*, **33** (1984), 176-195.

62. R.J. Gray, Some diagnostic methods for Cox regression models through hazard smoothing, *Biometrics*, **46** (1990), 93-102.

63. R.J. Gray, Flexible methods for analyzing survival data using splines, with applications to breast cancer prognosis, *J. Am. Stat. Assoc.*, **87** (1992), 942-951.

64. R.J. Gray, Spline-based tests in survival analysis, *Biometrics*, **50** (1994), 640-652.

65. P.J. Green and B.W. Silverman, *Nonparametric Regression and Generalized Linear Models*, Chapman and Hall, London, 1974.

66. C. Gu, Penalized likelihood hazard estimation: a general procedure, *Statist. Sin.*, **6** (1996), 861-876.

67. P. Hall and T.E. Wehrly, A geometrical method for removing edge effects from kernel-type nonparametric regression estimators, *J. Am. Stat. Assoc.*, **86** (1991), 665-672.

68. T. Hastie and R. Tibshirani, Generalized additive models (with discussion), *Statist. Sci.*, **1** (1986), 297-318.

69. T. Hastie and R. Tibshirani, Generalized additive models: Some applications, *J. Am. Stat. Assoc.*, **82** (1987), 371-386.

70. T. Hastie and R. Tibshirani, Exploring the nature of covariate effects in the proportional hazards model, *Biometrics*, **46** (1990), 1005-1016.

71. T. Hastie and R. Tibshirani, *Generalized Additive Models*, Chapman & Hall, London, 1990.

72. T. Hastie and R. Tibshirani, Varying-coefficient models (with discussion), *J. R. Stat. Soc.*, **B55** (1993), 757-796.

73. P. Hougaard, A boundary modification of kernel function smoothing, with

application to insulin absorption kinetics, *CompStat*, (T. Havranek, A. Sidak and M. Novak, Ed.), pp. 31-36, Physica-Verlag Wien., 1988.

74. P. Hougaard, A. Plum, and U. Ribel, Kernel function smoothing of insulin absorption kinetics, *Biometrics*, **45** (1989), 1041-1052.

75. J.Z. Huang, C. Kooperberg, J. Stone, and Y.K. Truong, Functional ANOVA modeling for proportional hazards regression, *Ann. Statist.*, **28** (2000), 961-999.

76. J.P. Imhof, Computing the distribution of quadratic forms in normal variables, *Biometrika*, **48** (1961), 419-426.

77. Z. Jin, D.Y. Lin, L.J. Wei, and Z. Ying, Rank-based inference for the accelerated failure time model, *Biometrika*, **90** (2003), 341-353.

78. M.P. Jones, A class of semiparametric regression for the accelerated failure time model, *Biometrika*, **84** (1997), 73-84.

79. J.D. Kalbfleisch and R.L. Prentice, *The Statistical Analysis of Failure Time Data*, 2nd ed., John Wiley, New York, 2002.

80. E.L. Kaplan and P. Meier, Nonparametric estimation from incomplete observations, *J. Am. Stat. Assoc.*, **53** (1958), 457-481.

81. H.T. Kim and Y.K. Truong, Nonparametric regression estimates with censored data: local linear smoothers and their applications, *Biometrics*, **54** (1998), 1434-1444.

82. C. Kooperberg, C.J. Stone, and Y.K. Truong, Hazard regression, *J. Am. Stat. Assoc.*, **90** (1995), 78-94.

83. C. Kooperberg, C.J. Stone, and Y.K. Truong, The L_2 rate of convergence for hazard regression, *Scand. J. Statist.*, **22** (1995), 144-157.

84. C. Kooperberg and D.B. Clarkson, Hazard regression with interval-censored data, *Biometrics*, **53** (1997), 1485-1494.

85. D.A. Kouassi and J. Singh, A semiparametric approach to hazard estimation with randomly censored observations, *J. Am. Stat. Assoc.*, **92** (1997), 1351-1355.

86. A.Y.C. Kuk and C.H. Chen, A mixture model combining logistic regression with proportional hazards regression, *Biometrika*, **79** (1992), 531-541.

87. T.L. Lai and Z. Ying, Rank regression methods for left-truncated and right-censored data, *Ann. Statist.*, **19** (1991), 531-536.

88. T.L. Lai and Z. Ying, Large sample theory of a modified Buckley-James estimator for regression analysis with censored data, *Ann. Statist.*, **19** (1991), 1370-1402.

89. L.S. Lasdon, A.D. Waren, A. Jain, and M. Ratner, Design and testing of generalized reduced gradient code for nonlinear programming, *ACM Trans. Math. Softw.*, **4** (1978), 34-50.

90. J.F. Lawless, *Statistical Models and Methods for Lifetime Data*. 2nd ed. John Wiley, New York, 2003.

91. M. LeBlanc and J. Crowley, Adaptive regression splines in the Cox model, *Biometrics*, **55** (1999), 204-213.

92. C.S. Li, J.M.G. Taylor, and J.P. Sy, dentifiability of cure models, *Statist. & Probab. Lett.*, **54** (2001), 389-395.

93. C.S. Li and J.M.G. Taylor, Smoothing covariate effects in cure models,

Commun. Statist.-Theory Meth., **31** (2002), 477-493.

94. C.S. Li and J.M.G. Taylor, A semi-parametric accelerated failure time cure model, *Stat. Med.*, **21** (2002), 3235-3247.

95. C.S. Li, Failure-time model, *Encyclopedia of Biopharmaceutical Statistics*, (S.C. Chow, Ed.), pp.1-8, Marcel Dekker, New York, 2004.

96. E. Liebscher, Kernel density and hazard rate estimation for censored data under α-mixing condition, *Ann. Inst. Statist. Math.*, **54** (2002), 19-28.

97. T.A. Louis, Nonparametric analysis of an accelerated failure time model, *Biometrika*, **68** (1981), 381-390.

98. R.A. Maller and Z. Zhou, *Survival Analysis with Long-term Survivors*, John Wiley, New York, 1996.

99. K. Messer and L. Goldstein, A new class of kernels for nonparametric curve estimation, *Ann. Statist.*, **21** (1993), 179-195.

100. H.G. Müller, Boundary effects in nonparametric curve estimation models, *CompStat*, (T. Havranek, A. Sidak and M. Novak, Ed.), pp.84-89, Physica-Verlag Wien., 1984.

101. H.G. Müller, Smooth optimum kernel estimators near endpoints, *Biometrika*, **78** (1991), 521-530.

102. H.G. Müller and J.L. Wang, Hazard rate estimation under random censoring with varying kernels and bandwidths, *Biometrics*, **50** (1994), 61-76.

103. W. Nelson, Theory and applications of hazard plotting for censored failure data, *Technometrics*, **14** (1972), 945-965.

104. D. Oakes, Biometrika centenary: survival analysis, *Biometrika*, **88** (2001), 99-142.

105. I. Olkin and C.H. Spiegelman, A semiparametric approach to density estimation, *J. Am. Stat. Assoc.*, **82** (1987), 858-865.

106. F. O'Sullivan, Fast computation of fully automated log-density and log-hazard estimators, *SIAM J. Sci. Statist. Comput.*, **9** (1988), 363-379.

107. F. O'Sullivan, Nonparametric estimation of relative risk using splines and cross-validation, *SIAM J. Sci. Statist. Comput.*, **9** (1988), 531-542.

108. F. O'Sullivan, Nonparametric estimation in the Cox model, *Ann. Statist.*, **21** (1993), 124-145.

109. W.J. Padgett and D.T. McNichols, Nonparametric density estimation from censored data, *Commun. Statist.-Theory Meth.*, **13** (1984), 1581-1611.

110. P. Patil, Nonparametric hazard rate estimation by orthogonal wavelet methods, *J. Statist. Plan. and Inference*, **60** (1997), 153-168.

111. Y. Peng and K.B.G. Dear, A nonparametric mixture model for cure rate estimation, *Biometrics*, **56** (2000), 237-243.

112. R. Peto, Contribution to the discussion of paper by D.R. Cox, *J. R. Stat. Soc.*, **B34** (1972), 205-207.

113. A.N. Pettitt and I.B. Daud, Investigating time dependence in Cox's proportional hazards model, *Appl. Statist.*, **39** (1990), 313-329.

114. R.L. Prentice, Linear rank tests with right censored data, *Biometrika*, **65** (1978), 167-179.

115. R.L. Prentice and J.D. Kalbfleisch, Hazard rate models with covariates, *Biometrics*, **35** (1979), 25-39.

116. H. Ramlau-Hansen, Smoothing counting process intensities by means of kernel functions, *Ann. Statist.*, **11** (1983), 453-466.

117. C. Reinsch, Smoothing by spline function, *Numer. Math.*, **10** (1967), 177-183.

118. Y. Ritov, Estimation in a linear regression model with censored data, *Ann. Statist.*, **18** (1990), 303-328.

119. P.S. Rosenberg, Hazard function estimation using B-splines, *Biometrics*, **51** (1995), 874-887.

120. D. Ruppert, Selecting the number of knots for penalized splines, *J. Computat. Graph. Statist.*, **11** (2002), 735-757.

121. D. Ruppert and M.P. Wand, Multivariate locally weighted least squares regression, *Ann. Statist.*, **22** (1994), 1346-1370.

122. M. Schemper, Cox analysis of survival data with non-proportional hazard functions, *Statistician*, **41** (1992), 455-465.

123. K. Schittkowski, *Nonlinear Programming Codes*, Lecture Notes in Economics and Mathematical Systems, Springer-Verlag, New York, 1980.

124. D. Schoenfeld, Partial residuals for the proportional hazards regression model, *Biometrika*, **69** (1982), 239-241.

125. L.L. Schumaker, *Spline Functions: Basic Theory*, John Wiley, New York and London, 1981.

126. G. Schwarz, Estimating the dimension of a model, *Ann. Statist.*, **6** (1978), 461-464.

127. A. Senthilselvan, Penalized likelihood estimation of hazard and intensity functions, *J. R. Statist. Soc.*, **B49** (1987), 170-174.

128. N.D. Singpurwalla and M.Y. Wong, Estimation of the failure rate-a survey of nonparametric methods PartI: non-bayesian methods, *Commun. Statist.-Theory Meth.*, **12** (1983), 559-588.

129. Y.A. Sleeper and D.P. Harrington, Regression splines in the Cox model with application to covariate effects in liver disease, *J. Am. Stat. Assoc.*, **65** (1990), 941-949.

130. C.J. Stone, Consistent nonparametric regression, *Ann. Statist.*, **5** (1977), 595-645.

131. C.J. Stone, Optimal rates of convergence for nonparametric estimators, *Ann. Statist.*, **8** (1980), 1348-1360.

132. C.J. Stone, Optimal global rates of convergence for nonparametric regression, *Ann. Statist.*, **10** (1982), 1040-1053.

133. C.J. Stone, M.H. Hansen, C. Kooperberg, and Y.K. Truong, Polynomial splines and their tensor products in extended linear modeling (with discussion), *Ann. Statist.*, **25** (1997), 1371-1470.

134. J.P. Sy and J.M.G. Taylor, Estimation in a Cox proportional hazards cure model, *Biometrics*, **56** (2000), 227-236.

135. M.A. Tanner, A note on the variable kernel estimator of the hazard funcction from randomly censored data, *Ann. Statist.*, **11** (1983), 994-998.

136. M.A. Tanner and W.H. Wong, The estimation of the hazard function from randomly censored data by the kernel method, *Ann. Statist.*, **11** (1983), 989-993.

137. M.A. Tanner and W.H. Wong, Data-based nonparametric estimation of the hazard function with applications to model diagnostics and exploratory analysis, *J. Am. Stat. Assoc.*, **79** (1984), 174-182.

138. J.D. Taulbee, A general model for the hazard rate with covariables, *Biometrics*, **35** (1979), 439-450.

139. J.M.G. Taylor, Semi-parametric estimation in failure time mixture models, *Biometrics*, **51** (1995), 899-907.

140. T.M. Therneau and P. Grambsch, *Modeling Survival Data: Extending the Cox Model*, Springer-Verlag, New York, 2000.

141. T.M. Therneau, P.M. Grambsch, and T.R. Fleming, Martingale-based residuals for survival models, *Biometrika*, **77** (1990), 147-160.

142. R. Tibshirani and A. Ciampi, A family of proportional- and additive-hazaeds models for survival data, *Biometrics*, **39** (1983), 141-147.

143. R. Tibshirani and T. Hastie, Local likelihood estimation, *J. Am. Stat. Assoc.*, **82** (1987), 559-567.

144. A.A. Tsiatis, A large sample study of Cox's regression model, *Ann. Statist.*, **9** (1981)., 93-108.

145. A.A. Tsiatis, Estimating regression parameters using linear rank tests for censored data, *Ann. Statist.*, **18** (1990), 354-372.

146. G. Wahba, *Spline Models for Obsvervational Data*, SIAM, Philadelphia, 1990.

147. G. Wahba, Y. Wang, C. Gu, R. Klein, and B. Klein, Smoothing spline anova for exponential families, with application to the Wisconsin epidemiological study of diabetic retinopathy, *Ann. Statist.*, **23** (1995), 1865-1895.

148. G.S. Watson and M.R. Leadbetter, Hazard analysis I, *Biometrika*, **51** (1964), 175-184.

149. G.S. Watson and M.R. Leadbetter, Hazard analysis II, *Sankhya*, **A26** (1964), 101-116.

150. L.J. Wei, Z. Ying, and D.Y. Lin, Linear regression analysis of censored survival data based on rank tests, *Biometrika*, **77** (1990), 845-851.

151. J. Wellner, Asymptotic optimality of the product limit estimator, *Ann. Statist.*, **10** (1982), 595-602.

152. A.S. Whittemore and J.B. Keller, Survival estimation using splines, *Biometrics*, **42** (1986), 495-506.

153. W.H. Wong, Theory of partial likelihood, *Ann. Statist.*, **14** (1986), 88-123.

154. L.L. Wu, Issues in smoothing empirical hazard rates, *Sociol. Methodol.*, **19** (1989), 127-159.

155. L.L. Wu and N.B. Tuma, Local hazard models, *Sociol. Methodol.*, **20** (1990), 141-180.

156. K. Yamaguchi, Accelerated failure-time regression models with a regression model of surviving fraction: an application to the analysis of 'permanent employment' in Japan, *J. Am. Stat. Assoc.*, **87** (1992), 284-292.

157. B.S. Yandell, Nonparametric inference for rates with censored survival data, *Ann. Statist.*, **11** (1983), 1119-1135.

158. S. Yang and R.L. Prentice, Semiparametric inference in the proportional odds regression model, *J. Am. Stat. Assoc.*, **94** (1999), 125-136.

159. Z. Ying, A large sample study of rank estimation for censored regression data, *Ann. Statist.*, **21** (1993), 76-99.

160. D.M. Zucker and A.F. Karr, Nonparametric survival analysis with time-dependent covariate effects: A penalized partial likelihood approach, *Ann. Statist.*, **18** (1990), 329-353.

UNIT IV

MATHEMATICAL MODELS
FOR DISEASES

CHAPTER 12

EIGENSLOPE METHOD FOR SECOND-ORDER PARABOLIC PARTIAL DIFFERENTIAL EQUATIONS AND THE SPECIAL CASE OF CYLINDRICAL CELLULAR STRUCTURES WITH SPATIAL GRADIENTS IN MEMBRANE CAPACITANCE

Lloyd Lee Glenn[a] and Jeff Knisley

The Institute for Quantitative Biology,
East Tennessee State University,
P.O. Box 70658, Johnson City, TN 37614, USA
E-mail: [a]glennl@etsu.edu

Boundary value problems in PDEs usually require determination of the eigenvalues and Fourier coefficients for a series, the latter of which are often intractable. A method was found that simplified both analytic and numeric solutions for Fourier coefficients based on the slope of the eigenvalue function at each eigenvalue (eigenslope). Analytic solutions by the eigenslope method resulted in the same solutions, albeit in different form, as other methods. Numerical solutions obtained by calculating the slope of the eigenvalue function at each root (hand graphing, Euler's, Runge-Kutta, and others) also matched. The method applied to all classes of separable PDEs (parabolic, hyperbolic, and elliptical), orthogonal (Sturm-Liouville) or non orthogonal expansions, and to complex eigenvalues. As an example, the widespread assumption of uniform capacitance was tested. An analytic model of cylindrical brain cell structures with an exponential distribution of membrane capacitance was developed with the eigenslope method. The stimulus-response properties of the models were compared under different configurations and shown to fit to experimental data from dendritic neurons. The long-standing question was addressed of whether the amount of variation of membrane capacitance measured in experimental studies is sufficient to markedly alter the vital neuron characteristic of passive signal propagation. We concluded that the degree of membrane capacitance variation measured in cells does not alter electrical responses at levels that are physiologically significant. The widespread assumption of uniform membrane capacitance is likely to be a valid approximation.

1. Introduction

Mathematical and statistical models are often the only resort when an important problem is not amenable to known experimental or empirical methods. Often, the model is expressed analytically as boundary value problem in a linear partial differential equation (PDE) or system of PDEs, and solving the PDE requires the construction of a Fourier series, which in turn requires solving for both eigenvalues and Fourier coefficients. The eigenvalue problem is not always so difficult and needs to be solved first before the Fourier coefficients can be determined. The `Fourier coefficient` problem can be an obstacle to the development and solution of more realistic models.

An array of methods have been developed to identify Fourier coefficients, each of which usually applies to a narrow set of PDEs and boundary conditions. The methods include the classic method of integration[1,2,3], the modified orthogonality relation[4,5], the technique of residues derived from the theory of functions of a complex variable[6,7,8,9,10,11], and others. Often, the Fourier coefficients of the resulting solutions are unwieldy for all but the simplest of boundary conditions[9,11]. The analytic methodology is consequently restricted to specialized subsets of researchers invested in the mathematics of a specialized subsets of boundary value problems in particular PDEs.

The present communication helps removes some of these restrictions using a more general method that is often more tractable than other approaches. The `eigenslope` method[12] can be used for analytically and numerically solving those parabolic, hyperbolic, and elliptical PDEs that have solutions expressed as an orthogonal or non orthogonal Fourier series with either real or imaginary eigenvalues. As stated above, the method has the advantage that it not only provides a new approach to the solution of such models, but also helps clarify the biophysical meaning and significance of the Fourier coefficients. It applies at least to any second order linear PDE in which variables can be separated.

2. Overview of the Eigenslope Method

Is there a simple relationship between Fourier coefficients and eigenvalues? Or is the relationship a complex mathematical relationship that differs for each different PDE or set of boundary values? The answer is that the relationship is simple. *The Fourier coefficient for a given eigenvalue is inversely proportional to the product of the eigenslope and eigenvalue, where*

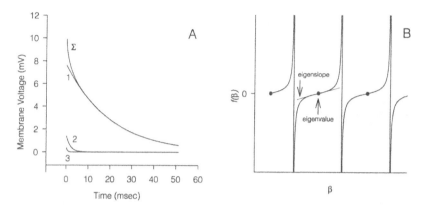

Fig. 1. Definition of eigenslope with an example of multiexponential decay of voltage across a membrane. The decay rate of the exponentials (inverse of time constant) are equal to the eigenvalue, and the initial voltages (at $t = 0$) are proportional to the inverse of the eigenslope. A: The voltage decay (Σ) is composed of the sum of simple exponential decays (1, 2, 3, ...). B: Example of transcendental eigenvalue function associated with multiexponential decay in A. Eigenvalues are the roots (zero crossings) and the eigenslope is the slope of the curve at the zero crossing. Vertical lines show where eigenvalue function goes to $\pm\infty$. From Glenn and Knisley[12] by permission.

*the **eigenslope** is defined to be the slope of the eigenvalue function at the given eigenvalue*[12].

The eigenslope is shown in Fig. 1. We consider a `Fourier series` solution common in electrical engineering and neurobiology of the form:

$$V(t) = \sum_{i=1}^{\infty} C_i \, e^{-\beta_i t}.$$

The solution for V (which later will represent membrane voltage) for any set of initial value and boundary conditions is an infinite series of simple exponentials, each with a time constant of $1/\beta_i$, the first three terms of which are plotted in Fig. 1A. The eigenvalues β_i are obtained from an eigenvalue function

$$f(\beta) = 0$$

plotted in Fig. 1B, where the eigenvalues are the points where the eigenvalue function intercepts the abscissa. The eigenslope is then defined as the first derivative of the equation, or

$$df(\beta)/d\beta$$

at each eigenvalue. To reiterate, the `eigenslope` has a simple inverse relation to the Fourier coefficients (C), diagrammatically depicted as

$$C_i = \frac{k}{\beta_i f'(\beta_i)}$$

where k is independent of β_i. Note that the Fourier coefficients can be obtained numerically, analytically, or even *graphically* — by measurement of the plotted slope with ruler and protractor.

The intractability of Fourier coefficients in all but the most simple boundary conditions is probably the reason why the simple relation between Fourier coefficients and the eigenslope has not been heretofore recognized, or at least widely recognized. One of the authors (L.G.) reviewed 45 PDE textbooks, 28 research compendia on 2nd order PDEs, as well as several hundred articles on PDEs in mathematics, physics, engineering, and mathematical biology. No previous work could be found that mentioned the relation between the eigenslope or the relation of the first derivative of the eigenvalue function to Fourier coefficients. Accordingly, our work on this topic is described here.

3. Derivation of the Eigenslope Method

Let λ_i be a sequence of distinct positive eigenvalues for the Fourier series

$$V(x,t) = \sum_{i=1}^{\infty} A_i \phi_i(x) e^{-\lambda_j t}$$

where the A_i are the Fourier coefficients and the ϕ_i are trigonometric or exponential eigenfunctions. As is typical in neuroscience applications, we assume that $\sum |\lambda_k|^{-1} = \infty$ and $\sum |\lambda_k|^{-2} < \infty$. Although separation of variables with modified orthogonality conditions can be used when the boundary conditions are sufficiently simple, more realistic models usually require solution by Laplace transforms and the method of residues[6,7,11]. The Laplace transform of $V(x,t)$ is

$$\hat{V}(x,p) = \sum_{i=1}^{\infty} \frac{A_i \phi_i(x)}{p + \lambda_j}$$

It follows that there exists $g(p,x)$ and $h(p)$ that are analytic in p such that

$$\hat{V}(x,p) = \frac{g(x,p)}{h(p)} \tag{1}$$

where $h(-\lambda_j) = 0$ and $h'(-\lambda_j) \neq 0$, for all $j = 1, 2, \ldots$ and where $g(x,p)$ is also second differentiable in x with $g(x, -\lambda_j) \neq 0$ for all $j = 1, 2, \ldots$ and for all x (for example, define $g(x,p) = h(p)\hat{V}(x,p)$ where

$$h(p) = \prod_{j=1}^{\infty} \left(1 + \frac{p}{\lambda_j}\right) e^{-p/\lambda_j}$$

comes from Hadamard's theorem[6]). It follows that

$$A_i \phi_i(x) = \lim_{p \to -\lambda_j} \frac{(p + \lambda_j) g(x,p)}{h(p)} = \frac{g(x, -\lambda_j)}{h'(-\lambda_j)}. \tag{2}$$

If $g_1(x,p)$ and $h_1(p)$ are analytic and also satisfy (1), then define $m(p)$ such that $h_1(p) = m(p) h(p)$ for all p and $m(-\lambda_j) \neq 0$ for all $j = 1, 2, \ldots$. Since $h_1'(\lambda_j) = m(-\lambda_j) h'(-\lambda_j)$, the limit (2) holds for any ratio of the form (1).

In particular, it follows that the A_n are given by

$$\hat{V}(x,p) = \frac{-1}{pf(x,p)}$$

where $f(x, -\lambda_j) = 0$ for all j. We say that $f(x,p)$ is the *eigenvalue function* for the problem. It follows that

$$A_i \phi_i(x) = \frac{1}{\lambda_j \left[\frac{\partial f}{\partial p}(x, -\lambda_j)\right]}.$$

For each fixed x, we say that $f_p(x, -\lambda_j)$ is the **eigenslope** of the eigenvalue function.

Analytically, the eigenslope approach provides a new approach to finding the coefficients (A_i), namely, by differentiation of the eigenvalue equation. Numerically, it provides a new method for determining the coefficients by finding the slope of the eigenvalue function at each eigenvalue by standard numeric methods. Conceptually, the eigenslope shows that eigenvalues and Fourier coefficients are related by a very simple relation. Next, the eigenslope method is used to develop, solve, and verify a model that addresses the significance of non uniform cell membrane capacitance in electrotonic signal propagation.

4. Application of the Eigenslope Method to Cellular Models With Propagation

Cell membranes are key building blocks of all cells, and regardless of cell type, the membranes have the hallmark electrical property of a constant capacitance of approximately $1\mu F$ per cm^{2}[13,14,15,16]. The existence of an electrical capacitance across cell membranes is vital to cell life[17,18]. Capacitance is used as a mechanism for rapid biological signaling and for integration of electrical signals over time and space[3]. Capacitance-dependent synaptic integration is also the basis of central nervous system function (thought, sensation, perception, behavior, etc.). Until recently, models of cellular integration have assumed a constant membrane capacitance over the cell, usually of $1\mu F$ per cm^2. Although there is a wide agreement that cell membranes have an average membrane capacitance near $1\mu F$ per cm^2, recent experimental work has led to questions about the assumption that membrane capacitance is constant over the surface of a cell[19]. Membrane capacitance is dependent on ion channel density[20,21,22,23] (but see Gentet et al[24].), and evidence has been mounting that ion channels are often distributed unevenly in cells[25,26,27,28,29]. The consequences of capacitative non uniformities in the passive propagation of electrical potentials in cylindrical membrane processes (such as axons, dendrites, and muscle fibers) are not known. In fact, the simplifying assumption that membrane capacitance is fixed has been made in almost all analytic and computational models of neurons and other cells to date (see reviews by Rall[3], Lindsay et al[30]., and Glenn and Knisley[9]). No systematic studies have been conducted to test this assumption, so one of us (J.K.) used the eigenvalue method to develop models in space and time of cylinder-shaped brain cells with longitudinally graded membrane capacitance specifically with an exponential increment with distance from the end of the cylinder. The hypothesis tested was that there are no biologically-significant differences between membrane cylinders with a homogeneous membrane capacitance and those with a exponentially-graded capacitance, provided that the spatial variation in capacitance is within the range of that estimated in experimental studies.

4.1. Definition of the General Model

A membrane cylinder with spatially-graded capacitance can be modeled by the cable equation

$$\frac{\partial^2 V}{\partial X^2} - R_m C_m(X)\frac{\partial V}{\partial t} - V = 0, \quad 0 < X < L \tag{3}$$

where $V(X,t)$ is membrane potential, R_m is the specific membrane resistance in ohms, C_m is the specific membrane capacitance in farads, L is the electrotonic length of the equivalent cylinder, and X is the electronic distance from the origin (electronic units are dimensionless and by convention, dimensionless units are denoted by uppercase variables)[52]. Note that C_m is a function of X and varies with distance from origin, which is the end of the cylinder. We assume sealed-end boundary conditions

$$\frac{\partial V}{\partial X}(L,t) = 0 \tag{4}$$

$$\frac{\partial V}{\partial X}(0,t) = 0. \tag{5}$$

Typically, the cell is saturated to a **steady state** using a somatic current source with a constant magnitude of I^{stim}, and then the current source is switched off (actually, it is switched to a voltage recorder). Thus, the initial condition for (3) - (5) is the steady state of equations (3) and (5) subject to the modified boundary condition

$$\frac{\partial V}{\partial X}(L,t) = \gamma I^{stim}.$$

Separation of variables with $V(X,t) = \phi(X)T(t)$ yields

$$\phi'' + (\alpha R_m C_m(X) - 1)\phi = 0$$

and

$$T' = -\alpha T.$$

The solution is of the form[8,9,10,11]

$$V(X,t) = \sum_{n=0}^{\infty} A_n \phi_n(X) e^{-\alpha_n t}$$

where the $\alpha_n > 0$ are the eigenvalues, the A_n are the Fourier coefficients and the ϕ_n are the separated solutions or eigenfunctions of equations (3) - (5). We normalize the eigenfunctions so that $\phi_n(0) = 1$. At the proximal end of the cylinder,

$$V(0,t) = \sum_{n=0}^{\infty} A_n e^{-\alpha_n t}.$$

On $\mathcal{L}^2[0,L]$, we define the inner product with weight $\tau(X)$ by

$$\langle f,g \rangle = \int_0^L f(X)\,g(X)\,\tau(X)\,dX.$$

From Sturm-Liouville theory[2] we have orthogonality of the eigenfunctions and

$$A_n e^{-\alpha_n t} = \frac{\langle V(\cdot,t),\phi_n \rangle}{\langle \phi_n,\phi_n \rangle}$$

which can be used to estimate the A_n once the eigenvalues and eigenfunctions are known. The Fourier coefficients can be estimated using the method of residues, as shown below.

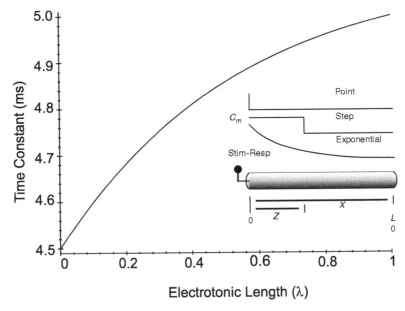

Fig. 2. Dependence of decay time (τ) on electronic length (L) in the exponential model with a 10% origin-to-terminal capacitance change. Inset diagram summarizes the three models developed, including the stimulus and response (I^{stim}, V_m) and the longitudinal capacitance distribution in the point, step, and exponential models.

Saturation to a **steady state** by a constant current stimulus prior to voltage recording implies that the initial potential distribution for (3) - (5) is the steady state distribution V^{ss} of the system

$$\frac{d^2V^{ss}}{dX^2} - V^{ss} = 0, \quad 0 < X < L$$

$$\frac{dV^{ss}}{dX}(L) = 0$$

$$G^\infty \frac{dV^{ss}}{dX}(0) = I^{stim}$$

where G^∞ is the input conductance. The solution is given by

$$V^{ss}(X) = \frac{-I^{stim}\cosh(L-X)}{G^\infty \sinh(L)}. \tag{6}$$

It follows that the A_n are given by

$$A_n = \frac{\langle V^{ss}, \phi_n \rangle}{\langle \phi_n, \phi_n \rangle}.$$

This approach was used to solve for three models of non uniform capacitance: (1) point change in capacitance, (2) step change in capacitance, and (3) exponentially graded capacitance. The three models are diagrammed in the inset of Fig. 2.

4.2. Definition of Fundamental Point and Stepped Models

The solutions to point capacitance and stepped `capacitance` models were first determined as a reference point for the final exponential model. If $C_m = C_m(L)$ and $C_s = C_m(0)$ (i.e., C_s is capacitance at the soma), then

$$C_m(X) = \begin{cases} C_s & \text{if } 0 \leq X \leq Z \\ C_m & \text{if } Z < X \leq L \end{cases}$$

for any Z between 0 and L. By previous methods[7,10,11], the Laplace transform of the transient at $X = 0$ is

$$W(0) = \frac{I^{stim}}{G^\infty s b_s} \frac{b_s + b_m \tanh(b_s Z) \tanh(b_m(L-Z))}{b_m \tanh(b_m(L-Z)) + b_s \tanh(b_s L)}, \tag{7}$$

where $b_s = \sqrt{sR_mC_s + 1}$ and $b_m = \sqrt{sR_mC_m + 1}$. If we assume that $\rho = G^\infty \tanh(L)/Z$ is constant with respect to Z, then (7) is given by

$$W(0) = \frac{I^{stim}}{b_s} \frac{b_s + b_m \tanh(b_s Z) \tanh(b_m(L-Z))}{G^\infty b_m \tanh(b_m(L-Z)) + \rho b_s \tanh(b_s Z) \coth(L)/Z}.$$

It is easy to show that the point membrane capacity model (in Fig. 2) defined by (7) is a limiting case of the varying capacity model when $C_m(X)$ is the step function. In the limit as $Z \to 0$, the transient $W = W(0)$ becomes

$$W = \frac{I^{in}}{G^\infty \sqrt{sR_mC_m + 1} \tanh L \sqrt{sR_mC_m + 1} + \rho \coth L (sR_mC_s + 1)}$$

which is the solution for the voltage for a membrane cylinder with a different point membrane capacity at the origin.

4.3. Definition of an Exponentially-Graded Model

The weakness of fundamental models in which membrane `capacitance` changes are at a point or are stepped, of course, is that the discontinuity at the point of change that is unlikely to be biologically realistic. An exponentially graded model, on the other hand, has a smooth, continuous change in membrane capacitance, and thus meets the minimum requirement for biologically realism of continuity.

Unfortunately, the cable equation (3) cannot be solved in general. The same waveform can be well-approximated by more than one multi-exponential[11], so numerical solutions to (3) - (5) are limited in their applicability to the problem of parameter identification. There are certain choices for $C_m(X)$ for which closed form solutions are possible, but for such choices of $C_m(X)$, it has not been possible to find closed form solutions for the eigenvalues and Fourier coefficients except in special cases. However, many choices for $C_m(X)$ lead to closed form expressions for the Laplace transform of the solution. From the Laplace transform solutions, the eigenvalues and Fourier coefficients can be determined using the theory of residues from complex analysis[1,6,31].

In particular, such a solution is possible if $C_m(X)$ represents the exponentially graded membrane capacitance given by

$$C_m(X) = \frac{\mu}{(1 + Me^{-2X})^2}$$

where for the ratio parameter $\varepsilon = C/C_m$ we have

$$M = \frac{1 - \sqrt{\varepsilon}}{\sqrt{\varepsilon} - e^{-2L}}$$

$$\mu = C(1 + M)^2.$$

In Fig. 2, the relation between τ and L is shown for $\varepsilon = 0.9$, $R_m C_m = 0.005$. Note how cylinders with an electrotonic length greater than one, and a 10% exponential gradient in capacitance produce a decay time that is very close to that of the uniform capacitance model (in which $\tau = 0.005\ ms$).

The Laplace transform of (3) is

$$\hat{V}'' - (sRC(X) + 1)\hat{V} = -C_m(X)V^{ss} \tag{8}$$

which has a solution of the form

$$\hat{V}(X) = W(X) - \frac{V^{ss}(X)}{s},$$

where the transient W satisfies the homogeneous equation associated with (8). The Laplace transform of the transient is given by

$$W(X) = \sqrt{Me^{-2x} + 1}\left(D_1\left(M + e^{2x}\right)^{\sqrt{s\mu+1}/2} + D_2\left(M + e^{2x}\right)^{-\sqrt{s\mu+1}/2}\right)$$

as can be verified by substitution. The sealed end boundary condition at $X = L$ yields

$$D_2 = D_1 \frac{\left(\sqrt{s\mu + 1} - Me^{-2L}\right)}{\left(\sqrt{s\mu + 1} + Me^{-2L}\right)} \left(M + e^{2L}\right)^{\sqrt{s\mu + 1}}$$

which is combined with the other boundary condition to yield a transient at $X = 0$ where $W = W(0)$ of

$$W = \frac{I^{stim} (M + 1)}{G^\infty s} \frac{\left(\frac{M+1}{M+e^{2L}}\right)^{\sqrt{s\mu+1}} + \frac{\left(\sqrt{s\mu+1} - Me^{-2L}\right)}{\left(\sqrt{s\mu+1} + Me^{-2L}\right)}}{D\left(\sqrt{s\mu + 1} + M\right)}, \qquad (9)$$

where

$$D = \left(\frac{\sqrt{s\mu+1} - M}{\sqrt{s\mu+1} + M}\right) \left(\frac{M+1}{M+e^{2L}}\right)^{\sqrt{s\mu+1}} - \frac{\left(\sqrt{s\mu+1} - Me^{-2L}\right)}{\left(\sqrt{s\mu+1} + Me^{-2L}\right)}.$$

Table 1. Example of eigenvalues and Fourier coefficients produced by a model with a step change in membrane capacitance with distance and a model with exponential spatial variation in membrane capacitance for a voltage response at $X=0$ to a current pulse stimulus at $X=0$ for a membrane cylinder with a length of $L = 1$. Amplitude coefficients are reported as a fraction of steady state. Z is the distance from the origin for a step change in membrane capacity (Fig. 2, inset) (*Note:* The first two Fourier coefficients were computed numerically using the eigenslope method (Knisley and Glenn 1997), and then verified using analytical expressions. The eigenvalues were found using a bisection method, and the slopes at the eigenvalues were found by the divided difference method (see Equation 4 in Section 7.1 of Kincaid and Cheney 1991). The τ_0 and τ_1 were computed for the point capacitance model with $C_s = 0.9\mu F$, $C_m = 1\mu F$, $R_m = 5,000\Omega$, $I_i = 1$, and $rho = 0.5, 1, 2, 3$.)

Model	τ_0(ms)	A_0	τ_1(ms)	A_1
Exponential	4.8222	0.7551	0.4334	0.1481
$Z = 0.2$	4.9000	0.7543	0.4355	0.1465
$Z = 0.3$	4.850	0.7524	0.4304	0.1497
$Z = 0.4$	4.801	0.7515	0.4282	0.1522

Since the eigenvalues of (9) are negative, the exponents in (9) are imaginary, complex exponentials and De Moivre's formula, transform (9) into the eigenvalue function

$$\frac{\sqrt{\alpha R_m C_m - 1} + M \tan\left(\sqrt{\alpha R_m C_m - 1}\ln\left(\sqrt{M+1}\right)\right)}{\sqrt{\alpha R_m C_m - 1}\tan\left(\sqrt{\alpha R_m C_m - 1}\ln\left(\sqrt{M+1}\right)\right) - M}$$

$$= \frac{\sqrt{\alpha R_m C_m - 1} + M e^{2L}\tan\left(\sqrt{\alpha R_m C_m - 1}\ln\left(\sqrt{M + e^{-2L}}\right)\right)}{\sqrt{\alpha R_m C_m - 1}\tan\left(\sqrt{\alpha R_m C_m - 1}\ln\left(\sqrt{M + e^{-2L}}\right)\right) - M e^{2L}}.$$

When M is chosen such that $\sqrt{\alpha_n \mu - 1} \neq M$, the coefficients A_n are of the form

$$A_n = \frac{-2I^{stim}(M+1)}{G^\infty \alpha_n f(\alpha_n)\mu\left(\sqrt{\alpha_n\mu - 1} - M\right)}.$$

$$\left(\cos\left(\sqrt{\alpha_n\mu - 1}\ln\left(\frac{M+1}{M+e^{2L}}\right)\right)\right) +$$

$$i\sin\left(\sqrt{\alpha_n\mu - 1}\ln\left(\frac{M+1}{M+e^{2L}}\right)\right) + \left(\frac{i\sqrt{\alpha_n\mu - 1} - Me^{-2L}}{i\sqrt{\alpha_n\mu - 1} + Me^{-2L}}\right)\right), \quad (10)$$

where $f(\alpha_n)$ is given by

$$f(\alpha_n) =$$

$$\frac{\cos\left(\sqrt{\alpha_n\mu - 1}\ln\left(\frac{M+1}{M+e^{2L}}\right)\right) + i\sin\left(\sqrt{\alpha_n\mu - 1}\ln\left(\frac{M+1}{M+e^{2L}}\right)\right)}{i\sqrt{k_j\mu - 1}}\ln\left(\frac{M+1}{M+e^{2L}}\right)$$

$$-\frac{2M}{i\sqrt{\alpha_n\mu - 1}}\frac{\left(M^2 e^{-2L} - \alpha_n\mu + 1\right)\left(1 - e^{-2L}\right)}{\left(i\sqrt{\alpha_n\mu - 1} - M\right)^2\left(i\sqrt{\alpha_n\mu - 1} + Me^{-2L}\right)^2}.$$

The Fourier coefficients were subsequently obtained from the eigenvalue function by the **eigenslope** method[12], and confirmed to numerically match the above solution. Examples of the eigenvalues and **Fourier coefficients** for the above models are shown in Table 1.

4.4. *Biophysical Representation*

The eigenvalues in this model correspond biophysically to the decay rates of the series of superimposed exponential decays reflected by the ends of the cylindrical cells. The Fourier coefficients represent the effective (distributed) membrane capacitance. That is, the coefficients correspond to the total amount of charge storage at steady-state, for each of the reflected exponential decays. The **eigenslope** relation indicates that steady-state amplitude of each reflected and superimposed decay is an inverse function of its decay rate and effective membrane capacitance.

Table 2. Eigenvalues and Fourier coefficients for decomposed experimental waveform (voltage responses to current step) and for model with exponentially-distributed membrane capacitance. Experimental data came from a selected spinal motoneuron from Glenn and others (1987). Amplitude coefficients are reported as a fraction of the steady state value, $V = 0.01266$

	Experimental Data	Model Prediction	Deviation
τ_0	5.28 ms	5.28 ms	0%
τ_1	0.787 ms	0.866 ms	10%
A_0	0.4779	0.4826 ms	1%
A_1	0.3791	0.2891 ms	-23.7%

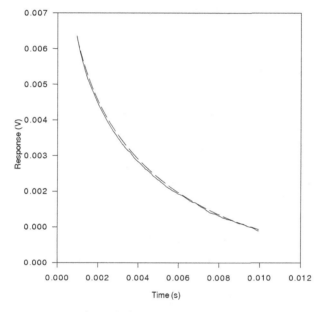

Fig. 3. Experimental data (solid line) fit with a recording from the exponentially varying membrane capacity model (dashed line), from 1 ms to 10 ms.

5. Comparison of Model Responses to Experimental Responses

The question addressed was whether a single membrane cylinder model with sealed ends and a point or exponential distribution of C_m could account for the voltage response of single quasi-cylindrical cells to a current pulse. Experimental data from studies on spinal motoneurons (stimulation and response determined at X = 0) were used for this purpose. The values of C, R_m, C_m, and L were chosen from empirical studies on

spinal motoneurons[24,32,33,34,35]. The multiexponential decomposition algorithm described in Knisley and Glenn[36] was used to estimate τ_0, τ_1, A_0,
and A_1 for representative experimental response data from a series of spinal
motoneurons taken from the study of Glenn et al[32]. Fig. 3 shows the results
of a best fit procedure between the experimental voltage recording and the
theoretical response in the exponential model. Table 2 shows the first two
eigenvalues and initial amplitudes for the two waveforms. The parameters
for the best fit under the above assumption were $C_m = 1\mu F$, $C = 0.34\mu F$,
$R_m = 7,000\Omega$, $L = 1.55$, and $V^{ss} = 0.01266$.

Voltage transients produced by constant current pulses in the soma of
neurons are more closely approximated the exponential model than a point
or stepped model. In experimental waveforms analyzed, $A0$ varied from 34%
to 75% of the steady state value and had only rarely come close to 90%
of steady state. The point capacitance model could not produce responses
consistent with experimentally-derived curves of electrotonic responses in
the neurons. The stepped model produce similar responses to the neurons
within the range $0.4 < Z < .6$, and thus a stepped capacitance change could
account for the empirical findings under this condition. The range condition
has an interesting correlation: It is also the range under which response of
the step model most closely approximated the exponential model (Table 1),
arguing indirectly for the greater applicability of the exponential model.

6. The Constant Membrane Capacitance Assumption

6.1. Errors Produced by Assumption of Constant C_m

In this section, the exponential model developed with the eigenslope
method will finally be applied to the long-standing problem of whether
or not the assumption of constant capacitance is justified. The response
of a membrane cylinder with constant C_m was compared to a cylinder with
an exponential gradient in C_m under the conditions that the average C_m
is the same in both models and the variation in C_m is within the range
measured in recent studies. As shown in the responses of Fig. 4 and in
measurements of decay rate derived from those responses in Table 3, a 2%
gradient in membrane capacitance causes about a 1.0% error in the time to
decay to 90% of the initial value, a 0.5% error in time to 50% decay, and a
0.3% error in time to 90% decay. A 10% gradient causes about a 7% change
in time to decay to 90% of the initial value, a 3.5% error in time to 50%
decay, an a 2.4% error in time to 90% decay.

Table 3. Change in decay times in membrane cylinders with exponentially distributed non uniformity in C_m. The C_m was decreased across $[0, L]$ by 2% to 20%, decreased across $[0, L]$ from -2% to -20%, and made constant (0%). In all cases, the average C_m across $[0, L]$ remained constant (see 0%) at $R_m C_m = 0.01$ s. Other parameters: $L = 1$, $I^{stim} = G^{\infty}$

Percentage Increase in C_m	90% Decay Time (ms)	50% Decay Time (ms)	10% Decay Time (ms)
20%	0.12772	3.98	18.87
10%	0.14597	4.16	19.66
5%	0.15519	4.25	20.04
2%	0.15628	4.29	20.24
0%	0.15693	4.31	20.30
−2%	0.15744	4.33	20.51
−5%	0.15883	4.37	20.70
−10%	0.15948	4.41	21.06
−20%	0.15987	4.52	21.63

6.2. *Discussion*

The hypothesis tested by the mathematical models was that biologically-significant differences between membrane cylinders with a homogeneous membrane capacitance and those with a heterogeneous exponentially-graded membrane `capacitance` do not affect passive responses, provided that the variation in capacitance is within the range estimated in experimental studies. The hypothesis was accepted. An exponential spatial variation in membrane capacitance at experimentally measured levels (5%) produces an error of 1.5% in the time it takes the voltage response to a step stimulus to decay to 50% of its initial value (Table 3), as compared to the assumption of a uniform membrane capacitance. This is a relatively small difference. Moreover, although the evidence is limited (see discussion below), the maximum that capacitance changes with distance is closer to 2%. This produces a 0.5% error in the same. Therefore, for most models of cells with a non uniform distribution of sodium channels or other channels, we conclude that the assumption of uniform membrane capacitance is largely a valid approximation.

The property of capacitance stems from the close proximity of two electrically conducting structures surfaces with the space between them filled by a poorly conducting medium. The membrane that envelops cells basically consists of a thin lipid bilayer that incorporates proteins, many of which span the membrane. The membrane capacitance stems from conductive extracellular fluid being separated by the inner hydrophobic layer of the cell membrane, which forms the poorly conducting structure required

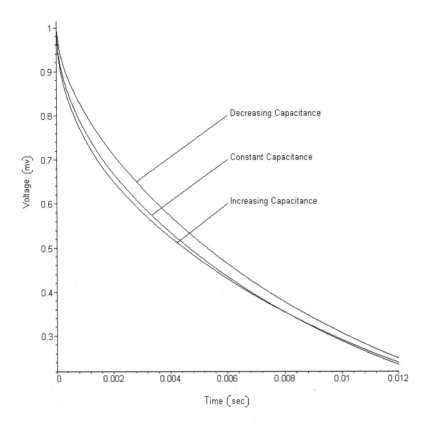

Fig. 4. Effect of C_m non uniformity of 20% on passive voltage responses of a membrane cylinder. Average C_m over the cylinder was the same in all three models, but it decreased exponentially with distance in the upper curve (from $1.1\mu F$ at $X = 0$ to 0.9 at $X = L = 1$), was constant in the middle curve, and increased exponentially with distance in the lower curve (from 0.9 F at $X = 0$ to 1.1 at $X = L = 1$). Other parameters: $L = 1$, $R_m = 10^4 \Omega - cm$, $I^{stim} = G^\infty$

for the electrical property of capacitance. The capacitance of the membranes depends on the thickness of the membrane, the number of carbons in the lipid chain that comprises the membrane, the electrical properties of the non polar, electrically-insulating interior of the bilayer membrane (dielectric constant), the location and density of non polar residues of the proteins embedded in the membrane[19,37,38], and the size and time course of ion channel gating currents.

Studies in spinal neurons, brain neurons, cell migration, cardiac muscle cells, egg fertilization, and others[39,40,41,42,43,44] have been in agreement that ion channels are not generally uniformly distributed over the surface of cell membranes. The question is unsettled, however, of whether or not the membrane capacitance changes according to the density of ion channels in the membrane. Thurbon *et al*[19]. suggests that non uniformities in membrane capacitance are caused by ion channel proteins. Ion channel proteins could theoretically alter membrane capacitance by changing both the thickness and dielectric constant of the membrane. However, Gentet *et al*[24]. found no major changes in membrane capacitance from 0.9 μF per cm^2 in kidney cells transfected with a plasmid that added glycine receptors to the membrane. On the other hand, both theoretical work[22,23] and experimental work[20,21] found membrane capacitance to be dependent on the density of sodium or potassium channels in squid axon and pituitary nerve terminals. In models of the squid giant axon, Schmid[22] concluded that "The membrane capacity at rest exhibits a bell-shaped dependence on the ion channel density." The greatest changes in membrane capacitance are attributed to gating currents, which are minute currents in the channel proteins themselves, associated with conformation changes between the open and closed states. For the squid giant axon[45], the change in membrane capacitance due to sodium channel gating currents ranged up to 0.15 μF per cm^2, which is a 15% difference. Kilic and Lindau[21] found the maximum capacitance change around 0.10μF in pituitary nerve endings, which is a 3% difference in pituitary capacitance, however the average was lower at 0.03μF, which is a 1% difference. Thus, although the evidence is very limited, the maximum possible capacitance change would appear to be 15%, and a more likely value would be between 1% and 5%.

6.3. *Clinical Significance*

The capacitance across cell membranes is just as vital and central of a building block of living function as is protein synthesis, chemical receptors, and DNA. Given its fundamental biomedical importance, alterations in membrane capacitance are accordingly a factor in the pathogenesis of a great variety of disorders, such as asbestos toxicity[46], seizures[47], metal poisoning[48], and hearing loss[49]. The heart beat itself, and its shape and timing, are dependent on membrane capacitance[50]. Despite its universality and importance in maintenance of a healthy state, membrane capacitance remains difficult to measure and manipulate. This has forced researchers in thousands of studies in the past 40 years to resort to mathematical models that assume a uniform capacitance in the face of increasing evidence that it is not uniform. Using on the eigenslope method, the present study is the first to show that the simplifying assumption of uniform capacitance in neurons has not appreciably affected the findings in previous studies. So, our present understanding of how brain cells propagate signals and operate in health and in neurological and psychiatric conditions requires no modification at present due to the recent discovery of non uniformities in the cellular distribution of membrane capacitance.

7. Conclusion

The question is often asked of why analytic theory is important when differential equations can be solved numerically relatively quickly with computational methods. The answer is that mathematical analytics provides understanding of the underlying structure of the solution, and not just a set of numbers called the numerical solution. Understanding flows most naturally from simple geometrical insights. The eigenslope is such a case of a simple geometric relation between eigenvalues and Fourier coefficients within each eigenfunction.

The eigenslope method (1) simplifies the concept of Fourier coefficients and eigenfunctions, (2) provides a new method of solving for Fourier coefficients analytically based simply on differentiating the eigenvalue function, and solving for the slope at each eigenvalue, (3) enables manual graphical or numerical determination of Fourier coefficients by the Runge-Kutta method[51] without first having the analytic solution, and (4) provides an easy, independent method of validating analytical solutions numerically.

The `eigenslope` method was used derive the solutions for an analytic mathematical model of membrane cylinders (such as tube- or fiber-shaped cells or cylindrical processes such as dendrites) with exponentially-varying membrane capacitance. Solved models are provided for point, stepped, and exponential changes in capacitance with distance along a membrane cylinder. Comparison of the passive voltage responses of the three models to impulse stimuli and curve fitting of the responses to experimental voltage responses curve data from neurons led to the exponential model to be the selected model. Variation in the membrane capacitance of the exponential model of 5%, which is the range of capacitance variation found experimentally by others, produced only a 1.5% change in the half-time of the responses to impulses.

The widespread assumption of uniform membrane capacitance over the surface of a cells is thus a valid approximation, in the sense that the degree of non uniformity found in cells is unlikely to significantly affect electrical stimulus responses, electrotonic length estimates, and signal propagation.

Acknowledgements

The authors would like to thank the reviewers and the editors for their many exceptional suggestions. In particular, we would like to thank the reviewers whose insights led to a more satisfactory derivation of the eigenslope method itself. This research was supported in part by the National Science Foundation under Grant No. 0126682.

References

1. Z. Zauderer, *Partial Differential Equations of Applied Mathematics*, Wiley-Interscience, New York, 1983.
2. I. Stackgold, *Greens Functions and Boundary Value Problems*, Wiley-Interscience, New York, 1979.
3. W. Rall, Core conductor theory and cable properties of neurons, In: *The Nervous System II*, (J. Brookhart and V. B. Mountcastle, Eds.), pp. 39-97, Amer. Physiol. Soc., Bethesda, 1977.
4. R. V. Churchill, Expansions in series of non-orthogonal functions, *Am. Math. Soc. Bull.*, **48** (1942), 143-149.
5. D. Durand, The somatic shunt model for neurons, *Biophys. J.*, **46** (1984), 645-653.
6. J. B. Conway, *Functions of One Complex Variable*, 2nd. Ed., Springer-Verlag, New York, 1978.
7. G. W. Bluman and H. C. Tuckwell, Techniques for obtaining analytical solutions for Rall's model neuron, *J. Neurosci. Meth.*, **20** (1987), 151-166.
8. L. L. Glenn and J. R. Knisley, Methods in the mathematical and computational analysis of multipolar neurons with tapering dendrites, In: *Mathematical Modeling in the Neurosciences: From Ionic Channels to Neural Networks*, (R. R. Poznanski, Ed.), Harwood Academic Publishers, New York, 1999.
9. L. L. Glenn and J. R. Knisley, Voltage Transients in Branching Multipolar Neurons with Tapering Dendrites and Sodium Channels, In: *Modeling in the Neurosciences: From Biological Systems to Neuromimetic Robotics*, 2nd Edition, (K. Lindsay, R. Poznanski, J. Rosenberg and O. Sporns, Eds.), Taylor and Francis, London, 2005.
10. G. Major, J. D. Evans and J. J. Jack, Solutions for transients in arbitrarily branching cables: I. voltage recording with a somatic shunt, *Biophys. J.*, **65** (1993), 423-449.
11. G. Major and J. D. Evans, Solutions for transients in arbitrarily branching cables: IV. Nonuniform electrical parameters, *Biophys. J.*, **66** (1994), 615-634.
12. L. L. Glenn and J. R. Knisley, Use of Eigenslopes to Estimate Fourier Coef-

ficients for Passive Cable Models of the Neuron, *Neurosci. Res. Comm.*, **21** (1997), 187-194.

13. K. S. Cole, *Membranes, Ions and Impulses*, Univ. Calif. Press, Berkeley, 1968.

14. J. Jamieson, H. D. Boyd and E. M. McLachlan, Simulations to Derive Membrane Resistivity in Three Phenotypes of Guinea Pig Sympathetic Postganglionic Neuron, *J. Neurophysiol.*, **89** (2003), 2430-2440.

15. S. A. Lewis, Everything you wanted to know about the bladder epithelium but were afraid to ask, *Am. J. Physiol. Renal. Physiol.*, **278** (2000), F867-F874.

16. A. Roth and M. Hauser, Compartmental models of rate cerebellar Purkinje cells based on simultaneous somatic and dendritic patch-clamp recordings, *J. Physiol.*, (London) **72** (2001), 445-472.

17. C. Porth, *Pathophysiology, concepts of altered health states*, 5th Ed., Lippincott, Philladelphia, 1998.

18. K. McCance and S. Huether, *Pathophysiology*, 4th Ed., Mosby, St. Louis, Mo, 2001.

19. D. Thurbon, H. R. Luscher, T. Hofstetter and S. J. Redman, Passive electrical properties of ventral horn neurons in rate spinal cord slices, *J. Neurophysiol.*, **80** (1998), 2485-502.

20. F. Bezanilla and E. Perozo, D. M. Papazian, E. Stefani, Molecular basis of gating charge immobilization in Shaker potassium channels, *Science*, **254** (1991), 679-83.

21. G. Kilic and M. Lindau, Voltage-dependent membrane capacitance in rat pituitary nerve terminals due to gating currents, *Biophys. J.*, **80** (2001), 1220-1229.

22. G. Schmid, *Am. Physiol Soc. Conf.*, Los Angeles, California, March 21-25, 2005.

23. G. Schmid, I. Goychuk and P. Hnggi, Gating charge effects on nerve excitation, Deutsche Physikalische Gesellshaft Conf., Regensburg, Germany, March 8-12,2004.

24. L. J. Gentet, G. J. Stuart and J. D. Clements, Direct measurement of specific membrane capacitance in neurons, *Biophys. J.*, **79** (2000), 314-20.

25. E. J. Ramcharan and M. R. Matthews, Autoradiographic localization of functional muscarinic receptors in the rat superior cervical sympathetic ganlion reveals an extensive distribution over non-synaptic surfaces of neuronal somata, dendrites, and nerve endings, *Neuroscience*, **71** (1996), 797-832.

26. Y. S. Fu, G. F. Tseng and H.S Yin, Extrinsic inhibitory innervation to rubral neurons in rat brain-stem slices, *Exp. Neurology.*, **137** (1996), 142-150.

27. R. Miles, K. Toth, A. I. Gulyas, N. Hajos and T. F. Freund, Difference between somatic and dendritic inhibition in the hippocampus, *Neuron*, **16** (1996), 815-823.

28. E. De Schutter and J. M. Bower, An active membrane model of the cerbellar purkinje cell. i. simulation of current clamps in slice, *J. Neurophysiology*, **71** (1994), 375-400.

29. K. A. Starr and J. R. Wolpaw, Synaptic terminal coverage of primate triceps surae motoneurons, *J. Comp. Neurology*, **345** (1994), 345-358.

30. K. Lindsay, J. Ogden, D. M. Halliday and J. R. Rosenberg, An introduction to the principles of neuronal modeling, In Modern Techniques in Neuroscience Research, (U. Windhorst and H. Johansson, Eds.), pp. 213-306, Springer-Verlag, Berlin, 1999.

31. C. Lanczos, *Applied analysis*, Prentice Hall, Englewood Cliffs, NJ, 1961.

32. L. L. Glenn, B. G. Samojia and J. F. Whitney, Electrotonic parameters of cat spinal alpha motoneurons evaluated with an equivalent cylinder model that incorporates non-uniform membrane resistivity, *Brain Res.*, **435** (1987), 398-402.

33. J. W. Fleshman, I. Segev and R. E. Burke, Electrotonic architecture of type-identified alpha motoneurons in the cat spinal cord, *J. Neurophysiol.*, **60** (1988), 60-85.

34. J. D. Clements and S. J. Redman, Cable properties of cat spinal motoneurons measured by combining voltage clamps, current clamp, and intracellular staining, *J. Physiol.*, (London) **409** (1989), 63-87.

35. M. G. Maltenfort and T. M. Hamm, Estimation of the electrical parameters of spinal motoneurons using impedance measurements, *J. Neurophysiol.*, **92** (2004), 1433-1444.

36. J. R. Knisley and L. L. Glenn, A linear method for the curve fitting of multiexponentials, *J. Neurosci. Meth.*, **67** (1996), 177-183.

37. J. Risbo, K. Jorgensen and M. M. Sperotto and O. G. Mourtisen, Phase behaviour and permeability properties of phospholipid bilayers containing a short-chain phospholipid permeability, *Biochim. Biophys. Acta*, **1329** (1997), 85-96.

38. R. Pethig, *Dielectric and Electronic Properties of Biological Materials*, Wiley, Chichester, 1979.

39. R. E. Hice and W. J. Moody, Fertilization alters the spatial distribution and the density of voltage-dependent sodium current in the egg of the ascidian Boltenia villosa, *Dev. Biol.*, **127** (1988), 408-420.

40. L. M. Masukawa, A. J. Hansen and G. Shepherd, Distribution of single-channel conductances in cultured rat hippocampal neurons, *Cell. Mol. Neurobiol.*, **11** (1991), 231-243.

41. M. Siegel, E. Marder and L. F. Abbott, Activity-dependent current distributions in model neurons, *Proc. Natl. Acad. Sci.*, **91** (1994), 11308-11312.

42. Y. E. Korchev, Y. A. Negulyaev, C. R. Edwards, I. Vodyanoy and M. J. Lab, Functional localization of single active ion channels on the surface of a living cell, *Nat. Cell. Biol.*, **2** (2000), 616-619.

43. A. Schwab, Function and spatial distribution of ion channels and transporters in cell migration, *Am. J. Physiol. Renal Physiol.*, **280** (2001), F739-747.

44. S. R. Williams and G. J. Stuart, Voltage- and site-dependent control of the somatic impact of dendritic IPSPs, *J. Neurosci.*, **23** (2003), 7358-7367.

45. J. M. Fernandez, F. Bezanilla and R. E. Taylor, Distribution and kinetics of membrane dielectric polarization. II. Frequency domain studies of gating currents, *J. Gen. Physiol.*, **79** (1982), 41-67.

46. E. Dopp, L. Jonas, B. Nebe, A. Budde and E. Knippel, Dielectric changes in membrane properties and cell interiors of human mesothelial cells in vitro

after crocidolite, *Environ. Health. Perspect.*, **108** (2000), 153-158.

47. F. Amzica and D. Neckelmann, Membrane capacitance of cortical neurons and glia during sleep oscillations and spike-wave seizures, *J. Neurophysiol.*, **82** (1999), 2731-2746.

48. A. N. Chanturiya and H. V. Nikoloshina, Correlations between changes in membrane capacitance induced by changes in ionic environment and the conductance of channels incorporated into bilayer lipid membranes, *J. Membr. Biol.*, **137** (1994), 71-77.

49. J. Santos-Sacchi and E. Navarrete, Voltage-dependent changes in specific membrane capacitance caused by prestin, the outer hair cell lateral membrane motor, *Pflugers Arch.*, **444** (2002), 99-106.

50. M. Sunagawa, M. Yamakawa, M. Shimabukuro, N. Higa, N. Takasu and Y. Kosugi, Effect of Sodium Channel Blocker, Pilsicainide Hydrochloride, on Net Inward Current of Atrial Myocytes in Thyroid Hormone Toxicosis Rats, *Thyroid*, **15** (2005), 3-11.

51. D. Kincaid and W. Cheney, *Numerical Analysis, Mathematics of Scientific Computing*, Brooks/Cole Publ. Co., Pacific Grove, 1991.

52. H. C. Tuckwell, *Introduction to theoretical neurobiology: volume 1 linear cable theory and dendritic structure*, Cambridge University Press, New York, 1988.

CHAPTER 13

MATHEMATICAL MODELLING OF NON-INVASIVE PRESSURE SUPPORT VENTILATION: INVESTIGATION OF TIDAL VOLUME INSTABILITY

Sahattaya Rattanamongkonkul[a], Yongwimon Lenbury[b]
John R. Hotchkiss[c] and Philip S. Crooke[d]

[a]*Department of Mathematics, Burapha University, Chonburi, Thailand*
[b]*Department of Mathematics, Mahidol University, Bangkok, Thailand*
[c]*Department of Critical Care Medicine,*
University of Pittsburgh School of Medicine, Pittsburgh, PA, USA
[d]*Department of Mathematics, Vanderbilt University, TN, USA*

A mathematical model for non-invasive pressure support ventilation (NIPSV) is presented. The model consists of two differential equations describing the volume in a one-compartment lung. In this study, we used the model to simulate spontaneously breathing patients with obstructive lung disease undergoing pressure support ventilation at 22 cmH$_2$O, and PEEP of 5 cmH$_2$O. NIPSV can give rise to unintended instability with potential adverse effect. Tidal volume instability is defined as a situation when the tidal volume, delivered over 100 consecutive breaths, creates a coefficient of variation higher than 10%, or a skipped breath occurs. To explore the tidal volume instability, we investigated the variability of tidal volume (V_T) delivery during NIPSV under combinations of respiratory resistance, $R = 10, 15, 20$ and 25 cmH$_2$O/L/s, compliance, $C = 0.06, 0.08, 0.10$ and 0.12 L/cmH$_2$O, and frequency, $f = 14, 16, 18, 20$, and 22 breaths/min at inspiratory flow cut-off levels of 5% to 80%, and pressure triggering levels of 1, 3, 5, 10 and 15 cmH$_2$O. We discovered that lower pressure sensitivity, higher lung compliance, higher flow resistance, and higher breathing frequency increasing the likelihood of instability.

1. Introduction

Non-invasive pressure support ventilation (NIPSV) is an assisted mode of ventilation that is increasingly used in clinical medicine[20,16,27,28,18,25]. Recently, it has been utilized in the treatment of respiratory failure as an alternative to endotracheal intubation. NIPSV provides a safe and effective way to improve alveolar ventilation and oxygenation in patients with many forms of acute respiratory failure[24]. For instance, in patients with acute exacerbation of chronic obstructive pulmonary disease (COPD) and hypercapnic respiratory failure, adding noninvasive ventilation to standard therapy could decrease the need for endotracheal intubation[9,12,8], and reduce mortality[8]. In mechanically ventilated patients, endotracheal intubation is the single most important predisposing factor for developing nosocomial bacterial pneumonia and infections[13,17] and increases the risk for sinusitis. Endotracheal intubation also injures the compressed tracheal mucosa, inducing inflammation, oedema and submucosal hemorrhage. These conditions constitute the pathological basis of other complications, such as airway stenosis[13]. The recent development of noninvasive methods of ventilation has resulted from a desire to avoid complications of invasive mechanical ventilation during acute respiratory failure. NIPSV is also used in a growing population with sleep apnea.

In NIPSV, the patient determines the inspiratory rate, time, volume and flow for the pressure support ventilation. Volume delivered to the patient during NIPSV will be variable and related to pulmonary compliance, resistance, inspiratory time, and flow rate. The patient triggers the ventilator; the ventilator delivers a flow up to a level of ventilatory support, for example 10 cmH_2O, depending on the desired minute volume. The patient continues the breath for as long as desired, and flow cycles off when the patient's inspiratory flow rate falls below a certain percentage of their peak inspiratory flow (usually 25%). Tidal volumes may vary, just as they do in normal breathing. NIPSV can be implemented with or without positive end expiratory pressure (PEEP). On newer ventilators it is possible to adjust the rate of pressurization and the point at which the ventilator cycles off (as a percentage of peak flow). For many patients such adjustments are unnecessary, but in a significant fraction they can make a crucial difference.

The inspiratory flow cut-off (the criteria for terminating inspiratory pressure application) can affect patient-ventilator synchrony by causing a neural-mechanical dyssynchrony. This is most often manifested as prolonged inspiration, requiring active termination by the patient. Prolonged inspiratory time can also lead to ineffective inspiration (triggering) efforts by the patient. These effects are masked by positive pressure breath, prevent triggering of the ventilator, and further contribute to patient-ventilator asynchrony. There are also some limitations related to the specific triggering algorithms. These include low sensitivity, resulting in delayed or failed triggering efforts. Excessive sensitivity may cause auto-triggering that can give rise to hyperventilation and gas trapping.

Asynchrony is a term that denotes conflict between the patient and the ventilator[14,10,23]. In many cases, failure to synchronize is due to inadequate flow delivery from the ventilator. A number of technological solutions have been proposed to solve the problem[1,22,15,11,29,21]. One of the more commonly used is pressure augmentation[19,1,22,6,26,15,11,21].

Patients at risk of elevated `auto-PEEP`, which occurs when there is insufficient time for exhalation and the next ventilator breath stacks on the previous breath, typically are characterized by high minute ventilation, high respiratory rate, short expiratory times, and airway obstruction. Auto-PEEP can cause severe hyperinflation, discomfort and ventilator asynchrony. Patients with high levels of auto-PEEP may fail to trigger the ventilator. This is because auto-PEEP represents an inspiratory threshold load that the patient must first overcome before a ventilator breath can be triggered. Accordingly, the ventilator fails to sense the patient's effort. Such unintended instability in the level of ventilatory support can lead to dyspnea and/or complicate weaning. Moreover, the stability of tidal volume (V_T) may be related to the coordination of patient's effort with the pressure trigger level (P_{sen}). The effect of trigger levels on the stability of tidal volume has not be studied. To explore the potential for such variability in NIPSV, we investigate the roles of compliance (C), resistance (R), frequency (f), the inspiratory flow cut-off (α), and `pressure trigger level` (P_{sen}) on the stability of ventilation support.

2. Mathematical Model

We first consider a `mathematical model` for the respiratory system consisting of two ordinary differential equations, each describing a different phase of a breathing cycle. To obtain differential equations for inspiration and expiration volumes, we employ a "conservation of pressure" that states that the applied pressure (P_{vent}) is the sum of resistive ($P_{resistive}$), elastic ($P_{elastic}$), and residual pressures ($P_{residual}$), assuming that inertial losses are negligible. That is,

$$P_{vent} = P_{resistive} + P_{elastic} + P_{residual}.$$

In their study, Crooke[3] proposed linear and nonlinear mathematical models for noninvasive ventilation, addressing pressure support ventilation (PSV) applied to a one-compartment lung (Figure 1) with a constant compliance C. One can then write the following set of `differential equations` for the *nth* breath:

Inspiration

$$R_i \left(\frac{dV_i^{(n)}}{dt} \right)^\epsilon + \frac{V_i^{(n)}}{C} + P_{ex}^{(n-1)} = P_{set}, \quad \tau_{tot}^{(n-1)} \le t \le \tau_{tot}^{(n-1)} + t_i^{(n)} \tag{1}$$

$$V_i^{(n)}(0) = 0$$

Expiration

$$R_e \left(\frac{dV_e^{(n)}}{dt} \right)^\epsilon + \frac{V_e^{(n)}}{C} + P_{ex}^{(n)} = P_{peep}, \quad \tau_{tot}^{(n-1)} + t_i^{(n)} \le t \le \tau_{tot}^{(n)} \tag{2}$$

$$V_e^{(n)}(t_{tot}^{(n)}) = 0$$

where ϵ is either 1 or 2 and $n = 1, 2, \cdots$. $V_i^{(n)}(t)$ denotes the inspiratory lung volume during nth breath, $V_e^{(n)}(t)$ the expiratory lung volume during nth breath, $P_{ex}^{(n)}$ the end expiratory pressure at the end of nth breath, $t_i^{(n)}$ the length of inspiratory time of nth breath, $t_e^{(n)}$ the length of expiratory time of nth breath, P_{set} the applied ventilator pressure during inspiration, P_{peep} the applied ventilator pressure during expiration, R_i the inspiratory resistance, R_e the expiratory resistance, D the inspiratory time fraction, $D = \frac{t_i}{t_{tot}}$, and f the number of breaths per minute. Here $\tau_{tot}^{(n)}$, $n = 1, 2, \ldots$ is the actual time at the end of the nth breath. That is, we assume that each breath is of length $t_{tot}^{(n)} = 60k/f$, where k is a positive integer, and $t_i^{(n)} + t_e^{(n)} = t_{tot}^{(n)}$. In this notation,

$$\tau_{tot}^{(n)} = t_{tot}^{(1)} + t_{tot}^{(2)} + \ldots + t_{tot}^{(n)}.$$

In the expression, $t_{tot}^{(n)} = 60k/f$, if $k > 1$, then this indicates skipped breaths. If there are no skipped breaths during the nth breath, then $t_{tot}^{(n)} = 60/f$. If there is one skipped breath during the nth breath, then $t_{tot}^{(n)} = 120/f$; if two skipped breaths, then $t_{tot}^{(n)} = 180/f$; etc.

In equations (1) and (2), the resistive pressure, $P_{resistive}$, is $R_i \left(\frac{dV_i^{(n)}}{dt} \right)^\epsilon$ and $R_e \left(\frac{dV_e^{(n)}}{dt} \right)^\epsilon$, respectively, the elastic pressure, $P_{elastic}$, is $\frac{V_i^{(n)}}{C}$ and $\frac{V_e^{(n)}}{C}$, the residual pressure, $P_{residual}$, is the end-expiratory pressure, $P_{ex}^{(k)}$, $k = n-1, n$. The ventilator pressure, P_{vent}, is the applied ventilator pressure. That is,

$$P_{vent} = \begin{cases} P_{set} & \text{during inspiration} \\ P_{peep} & \text{during expiration} \end{cases}$$

During expiration, the applied airway pressure to the mask and airway pressure is fixed and is denoted by the symbol P_{peep}. The PEEP pressure may be zero. In [3], it was assumed that the pressure drop due to the leak in the face mask is

$$P_{mask} = R_m Q_{mask}$$

where R_m is a resistance factor and Q_{mask} is the flow through the leak.

Using conservation of mass, the total flow from the ventilator at any time during inspiration (Q_{vent}) is equal to the sum of the flow into the lung and flow out through the mask leak (to the atmosphere):

$$Q_{vent} = Q_{mask} + Q_{lung}.$$

The flow into the lung, Q_{lung}, was assumed to be equal to the instantaneous rate of change of the volume of the lung, $\frac{dV_i}{dt}$.

The flow from the ventilator $Q_{vent}(t)$ is determined by the equation:

$$Q_{vent}^{(n)}(t) = \frac{P_{set}}{R_m} + \frac{1}{R_i}\left(P_{set} - P_{ex}^{(n-1)} - \frac{V_i^{(n)}(t)}{C}\right) \tag{3}$$

for $\tau_{tot}^{(n-1)} \leq t \leq \tau_{tot}^{(n-1)} + t_i^{(n)}$. To determine the end-expiratory pressure, we set $V_i^{(n)}(\tau_{tot}^{(n-1)} + t_i^{(n)}) = V_e^{(n)}(\tau_{tot}^{(n-1)} + t_i^{(n)})$ and solve for $P_{ex}^{(n)}$.

3. The Linear Lung Model

We now consider a ventilator connected to a patient. The ventilator applies a constant pressure P_{set} until the flow Q into the patient drops to specified fraction α of the initial flow. At this point inspiration ends and the patient starts expiration. The differential equations for the relative lung volume during nth breath with $\epsilon = 1$ are:

Inspiration

$$R_i\left(\frac{dV_i^{(n)}}{dt}\right) + \frac{V_i^{(n)}}{C} + P_{ex}^{(n-1)} = P_{set}, \quad \tau_{tot}^{(n-1)} \leq t \leq \tau_{tot}^{(n-1)} + t_i^{(n)} \tag{4}$$

$$V_i^{(n)}(0) = 0$$

Expiration

$$R_e \left(\frac{dV_e^{(n)}}{dt} \right) + \frac{V_e^{(n)}}{C} + P_{ex}^{(n)} = P_{peep}, \quad \tau_{tot}^{(n-1)} + t_i^{(n)} \le t \le \tau_{tot}^{(n)}$$
$$V_e^{(n)}(\tau_{tot}^{(n)}) = 0 \tag{5}$$

for $n = 1, 2, 3, \dots$.

In our study, we restrict our analysis to settings where there is no leakage by the mask *i.e.*, $R_m \to \infty$. In this case, equation (3) becomes

$$Q_{vent}^{(n)}(t) = \frac{1}{R_i} \left(P_{set} - P_{ex}^{(n-1)} - \frac{V_i^{(n)}(t)}{C} \right), \quad \tau_{tot}^{(n-1)} \le t \le \tau_{tot}^{(n-1)} + t_i^{(n)}. \tag{6}$$

The inspiratory time, $t_i^{(n)}$, is determined by the ventilator cut-off. If we assume that the ventilator cuts off at some predetermined fraction of the initial flow, $Q_{vent}^{(n)}(\tau_{tot}^{(n-1)})$, which we denote by α, $0 < \alpha < 1$, then, since we assume that $V_i^{(n)}(\tau_{tot}^{(n-1)}) = 0$, the inspiratory time during the *n*th cycle can be computed as

$$t_i^{(n)} = CR_i \log \left(\frac{P_{set} - P_{ex}^{(n-1)}}{K^{(n)} R_i} \right) \quad n = 1, 2, 3, \dots \tag{7}$$

to which there is a possible solution of $Q_{vent}^{(n)}(t_i^{(n)}) = \alpha Q_{vent}^{(n)}(\tau_{tot}^{(n-1)}) \equiv K^{(n)}$.

4. Model Simulations

The inspiratory initial value problem (4) can be solved for $V_i^{(n)}(t)$, yielding

$$V_i^{(n)}(t) = C \left(1 - e^{k_i(t - \tau_{tot}^{(n-1)})} \right) \left(P_{set} - P_{ex}^{(n-1)} \right) \tag{8}$$

where $k_i = \frac{1}{CR_i}$. We may also solve the expiratory initial value problem (5) for $V_e^{(n)}(t)$, obtaining

$$V_e^{(n)}(t) = C \left(1 - e^{k_e(\tau_{tot}^{(n)} - t)} \right) \left(P_{peep} - P_{ex}^{(n)} \right) \tag{9}$$

where $k_c = \frac{1}{CR_e}$. Finally, we determine $P_{ex}^{(n)}$ by setting $V_i^{(n)}(\tau_{tot}^{(n)} + t_i^{(n)}) = V_e^{(n)}(\tau_{tot}^{(n)} + t_i^{(n)})$ and obtain:

$$P_{ex}^{(n)} = \frac{e^{-k_i t_i^{(n)}}}{e^{k_e\left(t_i^{(n)}+\tau_{tot}^{(n-1)}\right)}-e^{k_e\tau_{tot}^{(n)}}}\left(-e^{k_e\tau_{tot}^{(n)}+k_i t_i^{(n)}}P_{peep}\right.$$

$$+ e^{(k_i+k_e)t_i^{(n)}+k_e\tau_{tot}^{(n-1)}}\left(P_{peep}-P_{set}\right) \tag{10}$$

$$\left.+ e^{k_e\left(t_i^{(n)}+\tau_{tot}^{(n-1)}\right)}\left(P_{set}+\left(e^{k_i t_i^{(n)}}-1\right)P_{ex}^{(n-1)}\right)\right).$$

This gives iteratively defined expressions for the inspiratory and expiratory volumes and the end-expiratory pressure.

The problem is to compute $V_i^{(n)}(t)$, $V_e^{(n)}(t)$, $P_{ex}^{(n)}$ for $n = 1, 2, 3, \ldots$. This requires that we have a starting point for $P_{ex}^{(n)}$, namely, $P_{ex}^{(0)}$. This can be done by letting $P_{ex}^{(-1)} = 0$ and $t_{tot}^{(0)} = t_{tot} = 60/f$. Then equation (10) becomes:

$$P_{ex}^{(0)} = \frac{e^{-k_i t_i^{(0)}}}{e^{k_e t_i^{(0)}}-1}\left(-e^{-k_i t_i^{(0)}}P_{peep}+e^{(k_i+k_e)t_i^{(0)}}\left(P_{peep}-P_{set}\right)+e^{k_e t_i^{(0)}}P_{set}\right) \tag{11}$$

where $t_e^{(0)} = t_{tot} - t_i^{(0)}$, and $t_i^{(0)}$ is any number in the interval $(0, t_{tot}^{(0)})$, for example, $t_i^{(0)} = \frac{60D}{f}$.

At the end of each breath, the patient's trigger pressure P_{trig} is compared against the end expiratory pressure P_{ex}. If $P_{trig} > P_{ex}$, then the ventilator turns "ON" for another breath. If $P_{trig} < P_{ex}$, then the ventilator stays "OFF" for one breath or more until $P_{trig} > P_{ex}$. We assume that $P_{trig} = P_{peep} + P_{sen}$, where P_{sen} is the sensitivity setting of the ventilator.

In Figure 2 for illustrative purposes, we simulated our model for fifteen breaths with the following parameter values: $C = 0.1$ L/cmH$_2$O, $R_i = R_e = 20$ cmH$_2$O/L/s, $P_{set} = 22$ cmH$_2$O, $P_{peep} = 5$ cmH$_2$O, $P_{sen} = 15$ cmH$_2$O, $t_{tot} = 6$ s, $f = 20$ breaths/min, $\alpha = 0.3$. The ventilator sensitivity, P_{sen}, in the ICU is usually between $1 - 5$ cmH$_2$O. At the first breath $(n = 1)$, $t_{tot} = \frac{60}{f} = 3$, we calculate thaat $P_{ex} = 12.8$ and $P_{trig} = P_{peep} + P_{sen} = 20 > P_{ex} = 12.8$. Therefore, the ventilator is triggered. At the fourteenth breath, $P_{ex} = 21.1 > P_{trig}$. Therefore, the ventilator fails to be triggered and we have a prolonged expiration at the end of which we calculate that $P_{ex} = 6.5$. At the end of this long breath, $P_{trig} > P_{ex}$ and $P_{ex}^{(14)} = 6.5$, with $t_{tot}^{(14)} = \frac{2 \cdot 60}{f} = 6$. Thus, a skipped breath has occurred at this point. In other words, we have expiration occuring for an additional 3 seconds.

5. Instability Study

Our lung model was used to simulate spontaneously breathing patients with obstructive lung disease ventilated with PSV using the following parameters: $R_i = R_e = 20$ cmH$_2$O/L/s, $P_{set} = 22$ cmH$_2$O, $P_{peep} = 5$ cmH$_2$O, $D = 0.75$, $C = 0.6, 0.08, 0.10,$ and 0.12 L/cmH$_2$O, $f = 14, 16, 18, 20,$ and 22 breaths/min, over a range of flow cut-off settings from 5% to 80% of peak inspiratory flow ($0.05 \leq \alpha \leq 0.80$), and pressure triggering levels of 1, 3, 5, 10 and 15 cmH$_2$O. Instability is said to occur if the tidal volume (V_T) coefficient of variation (CV) is greater than 10% where $CV = 100 \left(\frac{SD}{Mean} \right)$, or there is a positive integer i such that $t_{tot}^{(i)} \neq t_{tot}^{(j)}$, if $i \neq j$ which defines "skipped breaths."

Figure 3 shows the tidal volume coefficient of variation (CV) computed from the lung volume, calculated from our mathematical model (4)-(5) over 100 consecutive breaths. In Figure 3(a), CV is greater than 10% if $0.08 < \alpha < 0.09$ and $0.31 < \alpha < 0.36$. At these points, the tidal volume V_T is unstable. In Figure 3(b-d), skipped breaths are seen to occur for $0.08 < \alpha < 0.09$ and $0.31 < \alpha < 0.36$. For example, at $\alpha = 0.36$, there are 65 breaths with $t_{tot}^{(} n) = \frac{120}{f}$ and 35 breaths with $t_{tot}^{(n)} = \frac{60}{f}$. At these points, V_T is unstable. Figure 3(e) shows the volume wave form for $\alpha = 0.20$, for which CV $< 10\%$ and there is no skipped breath, that is, for all n, $t_{tot}^{(n)} = \frac{120}{f}$, so that V_T is stable. Figure 3(f) shows the volume wave form for $\alpha = 0.35$, for which CV $> 10\%$, so that V_T is unstable. There is an $i = 14$ such that $t_{tot}^{(14)} = 6 \neq 3 = t_{tot}^{(j)}$, $j = 1, 2, ..., 13$.

We plotted the flow cut-off, α, against lung compliance C in Figure 4 in which P_{sen} is 1.0 and 15.0 cmH$_2$O. It is observed here that lower values of P_{sen} gives rise to more unstable regions at higher cut-off values. Moreover, instability is greater with a higher compliance. Figures 5 and 6 show that increasing respiratory frequency, resistance or compliance exacerbates the instability of ventilatory support.

6. Comparison of Model Simulation with Experimental Data

A comparison of model simulations and experimental data with $C = 0.08$ L/cmH$_2$O, $P_{set} = 22$ cmH$_2$O, $P_{peep} = 5$ cmH$_2$O, $t_{tot} = 6$ s, $P_{sen} = 15$ cmH$_2$O, $f = 20$ breaths/min, $R_i = R_e = 15$ cmH$_2$O/L/s, is shown in Figure 7. In this figure, the tidal volume coefficient of variation (CV) computed from the lung volume calculated from our mathematical model (4)-(5) over 100 consecutive breaths. It is then plotted against the flow cut-off α. The simulation result yields consistently higher C than experimentally observed, but predicts the rise in CV, becoming higher than 10%, in the proximity of flow cut-off value of 0.2 which compares well with the laboratory data.

In [4], factors creating instability during pressure support ventilation were studied by using a mechanical test lung (Hans-Rudolph) with adjustable resistance, compliance, and triggering frequency. Ventilatory patterns were examined using PSV over a range of flow cut-off settings from 5% to 45% of peak inspiratory flow. Instability was defined as a tidal volume (V_T) delivered with a coefficient of variation greater than 10%. They found that tidal volume delivery becomes unstable with clinically relevant combinations of inputs. For each frequency, the region above the line is associated with stable tidal volume delivery and region below the line is unstable (Figure 8). Increasing resistance shifted the area of instability giving rise to a system more prone to variable delivery of support. Both Figures 5 and 8 indicate that the region of unstable flow cut-off values enlarges as the breathing frequency increases.

7. Discussion and Conclusion

Although pressure support ventilation has been used for many years in different clinical settings, there have been relatively few investigations of the dynamical behavior of this mode of ventilation[3]. A major limitation in the employment of noninvasive ventilation, where PSV is frequently applied, is lack of patient tolerance. It has been reported that up to 30% of patients with chronic obstructive pulmonary disease (COPD) fail a trial of noninvasive ventilation for reasons which are often unclear although the number varies[3]. Since PSV should be capable of providing a level of inspiratory assistance that is adequate for most relaxed COPD patients, it is likely that intolerance of NIV may be related to the adverse patient-ventilator interactions, namely, ventilator dyssynchrony[5]. Unstable inspiratory support may require active patient effort to terminate inspiration, or inspiration may be spontaneously terminated prematurely. Moreover, breath-to-breath variations in auto-PEEP will require different levels of patient effort to trigger the ventilator. These phenomena may lead to failure of PSV.

Earlier studies[5,2,3] have revealed that application of pressure support ventilation in the context of **mask leaks**, can lead to significant breath to breath variability in the duration of inspiratory support, to oscillations in end expiratory lung volume, and to unstable tidal volumes. Although an adequate seal can usually be obtained, leaks frequently develop between the mask and the patient's face. The leakage likely contributes to instability since the inspiratory phase of pressure support terminates when flow falls to a predetermined fraction of peak inspiratory flow[5]. Instabilities predicted by the above mentioned studies were found to be entirely independent of patient's effort or volition.

Our study highlights the complex dynamic behaviors that occur even in the absence of a mask leak. Although the mathematical model we employed is a simple one-compartment linear system, the model simulations, in which we allowed the total breathing time t_{tot} to vary from one breath to another (in the case of skipped breaths), agree with experimental observations, illuminating factors that influence patient ventilator synchrony and tolerance. Regions of variable (unstable) V_T delivery are related to respiratory frequency, resistance and compliance, pressure sensitivity, and pressure triggering levels.

As can be seen in Figure 4, for fixed frequency, pressure sensitivity and resistance, elevated compliance C increases the unstable flow cut-off values, enlarging the region of instability. Figure 4 also indicates that lower pressure sensitivity exacerbates the V_T instability. On the other hand, for a fixed pressure sensitivity, P_{sen}, and resistance, increasing respiratory frequency results in larger region of V_T instability for each pressure triggering level.

Figure 6 indicates that higher flow resistance leads to greater V_T instability. It pushes the curve for each pressure triggering level further to the left and higher, and therefore enlarging the region of instability. At a low resistance level of 15 cmH$_2$O/L/s, with $P_{sen} = 5$ cmH$_2$O, and $f = 14$ breaths/min as in Figure 6(a), stability is predicted for all pressure triggering levels if $C < 0.8$.

Previous results indicated that the stability of support during PSV depends critically on complex dynamic interactions. As we have shown here, many of the determinants of instability are amenable to both mathematical analysis and clinical manipulation. This fact suggests clear potential for mathematical analysis to guide and improve patient care.

Acknowledgments

The authors, Rattanamongkonkul and Lenbury, would like to thank the Thailand Research Fund and the National Research Council of Thailand for the financial support. All of the authors are indebted to Dr. Li Chen for data that she collected from the mechanical lung experiments at Regions Hospital in St. Paul, MN.

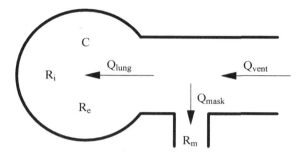

Fig. 1.   Face mask-lung diagram.

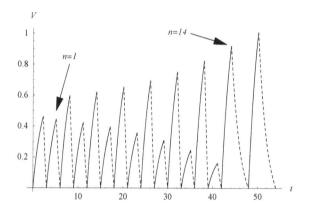

Fig. 2.   Volume waveform: $C = 0.1$ L/cmH$_2$O, $R_i = R_e = 20$ cmH$_2$O/L/s, $P_{set} = 22$ cmH$_2$O, $P_{peep} = 5$ cmH$_2$O, $P_{sen} = 15$ cmH$_2$O, $t_{tot} = 6$ s, $f = 20$ breaths/min., 20 consecutive breaths, $\alpha = 0.35$. The solid curves correspond to the inspiration volume and the dotted curves correspond to the expiration volume.

References

1. T. Bunburaphong, H. Imanaka, M. Nishimura, R.M. Kacmarek, Performance characteristics of bilevel pressure ventilators: A lung model study, *Chest*, **111** (1997), 50-60.
2. L. Chen, A.B. Adams, J.R. Hotchkiss, The nature of unstable ventilatory support during PSV in a lung model of obstructive disease, *the AARC Conferences* (Abstracts), 2001.
3. P.S. Crooke, J.R. Hotchkiss, J.J. Marini, Linear and nonlinear mathematical models for noninvasive ventilation, *Math. Comp. Mod.*, **35** (2002), 1297-1313.
4. D.J. Dries, J. Ong, L. Chen, A.B. Adams, J.J. Marini, J.R. Hotchkiss, Factor creating instability during pressure support ventilation, *The American*

Association for the Surgery of Trauma, (Abstracts), 2001.

5. G.D. Ferreyra, G. Montiel, D. Ferrante, Patient-ventilator synchrony: Pressure support (PS) and proportional assist ventilation (PAV), (Abstract), *ATS 97th International Conference*, May 18-23, 2001, San Francisco, USA.

6. S. Grasso, F. Puntillo, L. Mascia, G. Ancona, T. Fiore, F. Bruno, A.S. Slutsky, V.M. Ranieri, Compensation for increase in respiratory workload during mechanical ventilation, Pressure-support versus proportional-assist ventilation, *Am. J. Respir Crit. Care Med.*, **161** (2000), 819-826.

7. J.R. Hotchkiss, A.B. Adams, D.J. Dries, J.J. Marini, P.S. Crooke, Dynamic behavior during noninvasive ventilation. chaotic support? *Am J Respir Crit Care Med.*, **163** (2001), 374-378.

8. S.K. Keenan, P.D. Kernerman, D.J. Cook, C.M. Martin, D. McCormack, W.J. Sibbald, The effect of noninvasive positive pressure ventilation on mortality in patients admitted with acute respiratory failure: a meta-analysis, *Crit Care Med.* **25** (1997), 1685-1692.

9. N. Kramer, T.J. Meyer, J. Meharg, R.D. Cece, N.S. Hill, Randomized, prospective trial of noninvasive positive pressure ventilation in acute respiratory failure, *Am J Respir Crit Care Med.*, **151** (1995), 1799-1806.

10. P. Leung, A. Jubran, M.J. Tobin, Comparison of assisted ventilator modes on triggering, patient effort, and dyspnea, *Am J Respir Crit Care Med.*, **155**(6) 1997, 1940-1948.

11. N.R. MacIntyre, Evidence-based guidelines for weaning and discontinuing ventilatory support: A collective task force facilitated by the American college of chest physicians; the American association for respiratory care; and the American college of critical care medicine, *Chest*, **120** (2001), 375S-396S.

12. G.U. Meduri, R.E. Turner, N. Abou-Shala, E. Tolley, Wunderink RG. Noninvasive positive pressure ventilation via face mask: first-line intervention in patients with acute hypercapnic and hypoxemic respiratory failure, *Chest*, **109** (1996), 179-193.

13. G.U. Meduri, *Noninvasive ventilation*, In: *Physiological Basis of Ventilatory Support*, (J.J.Marini and A. Slustky, Eds.), pp. 921-998, Series on Lung Biology in Health and Disease, Marcel-Dekker, Inc., New York, 1998.

14. J. Munoz, J.E. Guerrero, J.L. Escalante, R. Palomino, C.B. De La, Pressure controlled ventilation versus controlled mechanical ventilation with decelerating inspiratory flow, *Crit Care Med.*, **21**(8) (1993), 1143-1148.

15. G. Musante, A. Schulze, T. Erhardt, R. Everett, N. Claure, P. Schaller, E. Bancalari, Proportional assist ventilation decreases thoracoabdominal asynchrony and chest wall distortion in preterm infants, *Pediatr Res.*, **49**(2) (2001), 175-180.

16. S. Nava, N. Ambrosino, F. Rubini, C. Fracchia, C. Rampulla, G. Torri, E. Calderini, Effect of nasal pressure support ventilation and external PEEP on diapragmatic activity in patients with severe stable COPD, *Chest*, **103** (1993), 143-150.

17. K. Nourdine, P. Combes, M.J. Carton, P. Beuret, A. Cannamela, J.C. Ducreux, Does noninvasive ventilation reduce the ICU nosocomial infection risk?: a prospective clinical survey, *Intens Care Med.*, **25** (1999), 567-573.

18. R. Porta, L. Appendini, M. Vitacca, L. Bianchi, C.F. Donner, R. Poggi, N. Ambrosino, Mask proportional assist versus pressure support ventilation in patients in clinically stable condition with chronic ventilatory failure - clinical investigations - Statistical Data Included, *Chest*, **122** (2002), 479-488.

19. V.M. Ranieri, R. Giuliani, L. Mascia, S. Grasso, V. Petruzzelli, N. Puntillo, G. Perchiazzi, T. Fiore, A. Brienza, Patient-ventilator interaction during acute hypercapnia: pressure support vs. proportional assist ventilation, *J Appl Physiol*, **81** (1996), 426-436.

20. L.J. Restrick, N.C. Fox, G. Braid, E.M. Ward, E.A. Paul, J.A. Wedzicha, Comparison of nasal pressure support ventilation with nasal intermittent positive pressure ventilation in patients with nocturnal hypoventilation, *Europ. Resp. J.*, **6** (1993), 364-370.

21. J.D. Schipke, G. Heusch, A.P. Sanii, E. Gams, J. Winter, Static filling pressure in patients during induced ventricular fibrillation, *Am J Physiol Heart Circ Physiol.*, **285** (2003), H2510-H2515.

22. A. Schulze, P. Schaller, Assisted mechanical ventilation using resistive and elastic unloading, *Semin Neonatal*, **2** (1997), 105-114.

23. M.J. Tobin, A. Jubran, F. Laghi, Patient-ventilator interaction, *Am J Respir Crit Care Med.*, **163**(5) (2001), 1059-1063.

24. A. Torres, R. Aznar, J.M. Gatell, P. Jimenez, J. Gonzalez, A. Ferrer, R. Celis, R. Rodriguez-Roisin, Incidence, risk and prognosis factors of nosocomial pneumonia in mechanically ventilated patients, *Am Rev Respir Dis.*, **142** (1990), 523-528.

25. A. Valipoura, W. Cozzarinib, O.C. Burghubera, Non-invasive pressure support ventilation in patients with respiratory failure due to severe acute cardiogenic pulmonary edema, *Respiration*, **71** (2004), 144-151.

26. M. Vitacca, E. Clini, M. Pagani, L. Bianchi, A. Rossi, N. Ambrosino, Physiologic effects of early administered mask proportional assist ventilation in patients with chronic obstructive pulmonary disease and acute respiratory failure, *Crit Care Med.*, **28** (2000), 1791-1797.

27. M. Vitacca, F. Rubini, K. Foglio, S. Scalvini, S. Nava, N. Ambrosino, A protocol for initiation of nasal positive pressure ventilation, *Am J Crit Care*, **2** (1993), 54-60.

28. M. Wysocki, L. Tric, M.A. Wolff, J. Gertner, H. Millet, B. Herman, Noninvasive pressure support ventilation in patients with acute respiratory failure, *Chest*, **103** (1993), 907-913.

29. Q. Ye, C. Wang, Z. Tong, K. Huang, C. Jiang, X. Weng, Proportional assist ventilation: methodology and therapeutics on COPD patients compared with pressure support ventilation, *Chin Med J (Engl).*, **115**(2) (2002), 179-183.

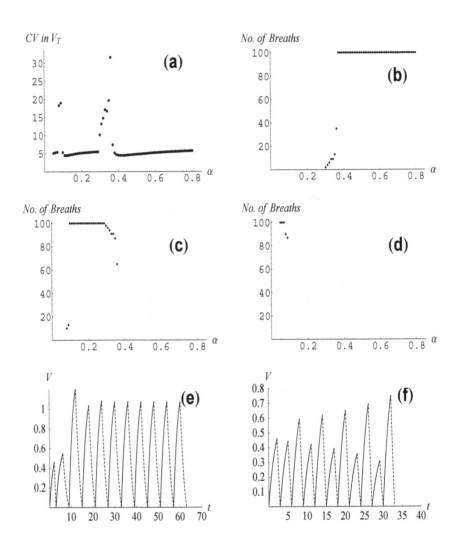

Fig. 3. Linear model simulations with $C = 0.1$ L/cmH$_2$O, $R_i = R_e = 20$ cmH$_2$O/L/s, $P_{set} = 22$ cmH$_2$O, $P_{peep} = 5$ cmH$_2$O, $P_{sen} = 15$ cmH$_2$O, $t_{tot} = 6$ s, $f = 20$ breaths/minute: (a) Scattergram of coefficients of variation against flow cut-off; (b) Scattergram of number of breaths (out of a possible 100 breaths) against flow cut-off for $t_{tot} = 60/f$; (c) Scattergram of number of breaths against flow cut-off for $t_{tot} = 120/f$; (d) Scattergram of number of breaths against flow cut-off for $t_{tot} = 180/f$; (e) volume waveform for $\alpha = 0.20$; (f) volume waveform for $\alpha = 0.35$.

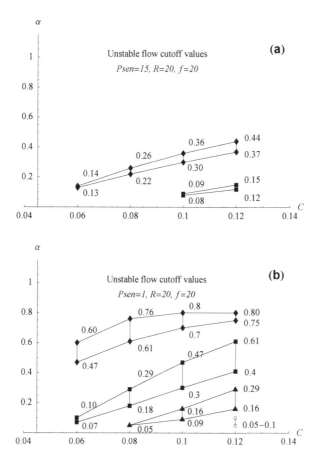

Fig. 4. Unstable flow cut-off values: $C = 0.06$, 0.08, 0.10 and 0.12 L/ cmH$_2$O, $R_i = R_e = 20$ cmH$_2$O/L/s, $P_{set} = 22$ cmH$_2$O, $P_{peep} = 5$ cmH$_2$O, $t_{tot} = 6$ s, $f = 20$ breaths/minute: (a) $P_{sen} = 15$ cmH$_2$O; (b) $P_{sen} = 1$ cmH$_2$O. The diamonds ($\blacklozenge - \blacklozenge$) indicate unstable flow cut-off region in which t_{tot} changes from $t_{tot} = 60/f$ to $t_{tot} = 120/f$. The boxes ($\blacksquare - \blacksquare$) indicate unstable flow cut-off region in which t_{tot} changes from $t_{tot} = 120/f$ to $t_{tot} = 180/f$. The triangles ($\blacktriangle - \blacktriangle$) indicate unstable flow cut-off region in which t_{tot} changes from $t_{tot} = 180/f$ to $t_{tot} = 240/f$, and the dots ($\circ - \circ$) indicate unstable flow cut-off region in which t_{tot} changes from $t_{tot} = 240/f$ to $t_{tot} = 300/f$.

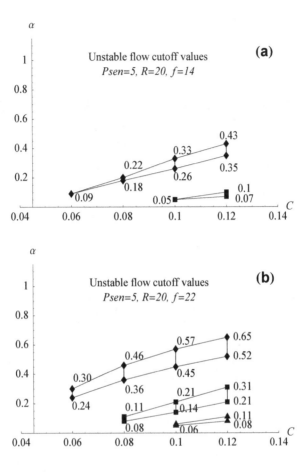

Fig. 5. Unstable flow cut-off values: $C = 0.06$, 0.08, 0.10 and 0.12 L/cmH$_2$O, $R_i = R_e = 20$ cmH$_2$O/L/s, $P_{set} = 22$ cmH$_2$O, $P_{peep} = 5$ cmH$_2$O, $t_{tot} = 6$ s, $P_{sen} = 5$ cmH$_2$O, (a) $f = 14$ breaths/minute; (b) $f = 22$ breaths/minute. The diamonds ($\blacklozenge - \blacklozenge$) indicate unstable flow cut-off region in which t_{tot} changes from $t_{tot} = 60/f$ to $t_{tot} = 120/f$. The boxes ($\blacksquare - \blacksquare$) indicate unstable flow cut-off region in which t_{tot} changes from $t_{tot} = 120/f$ to $t_{tot} = 180/f$. The triangles ($\blacktriangle - \blacktriangle$) indicate unstable flow cut-off region in which t_{tot} changes from $t_{tot} = 180/f$ to $t_{tot} = 240/f$.

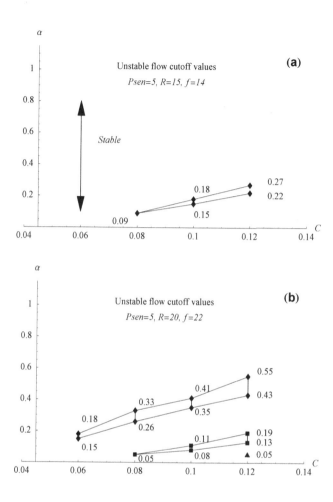

Fig. 6. Unstable flow cut-off values: $C = 0.06$, 0.08, 0.10 and 0.12 L/cmH$_2$O, $P_{set} = 22$ cmH$_2$O, $P_{peep} = 5$ cmH$_2$O, $t_{tot} = 6$ s, $f = 14$ breaths/min, $P_{sen} = 5$ cmH$_2$O, (a) $R_i = R_e = 15$ cmH$_2$O/L/second; (b) $R_i = R_e = 25$ cmH$_2$O/L/s. The diamonds ($\blacklozenge - \blacklozenge$) indicate unstable flow cut-off region in which t_{tot} changes from $t_{tot} = 60/f$ to $t_{tot} = 120/f$. The boxes ($\blacksquare - \blacksquare$) indicate unstable flow cut-off region in which t_{tot} changes from $t_{tot} = 120/f$ to $t_{tot} = 180/f$. The triangles ($\blacktriangle - \blacktriangle$) indicate unstable flow cut-off region in which t_{tot} changes from $t_{tot} = 180/f$ to $t_{tot} = 240/f$.

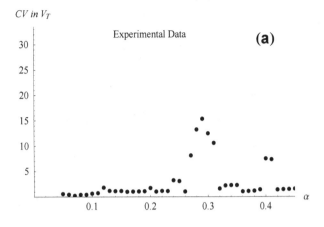

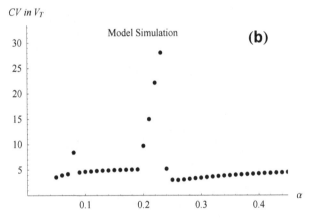

Fig. 7.   Scattergram of coefficients of variation against flow cut-off with $C = 0.08$ L/cmH$_2$O, $P_{set} = 22$ cmH$_2$O, $P_{peep} = 5$ cmH$_2$O, $t_{tot} = 6$ s, $f = 20$ breaths/min, $P_{sen} = 15$ cmH$_2$O, $R_i = R_e = 25$ cmH$_2$O/L/s, and $0 \leq \alpha \leq 45$: (a) experimental data; (b) model simulation.

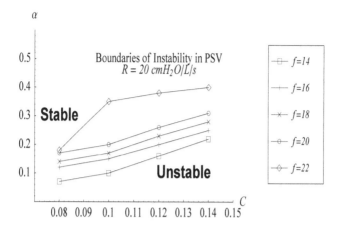

Fig. 8. Boundaries of instability in PSV where resistance $= 20$ cmH$_2$O/L/s, $f =$ 14, 16, 18, 20, and 22 breaths/min (figure taken from Dries *et al.*, 2001).

CHAPTER 14

MATHEMATICAL MODELS ON THE GROWTH
OF SOLID TUMORS

Zachariah Sinkala

Department of Mathematical Sciences, Middle Tennessee State University,
P.O. Box 34, Murfreesboro, Tennessee 37132, USA
E-mail: zsinkala@mtsu.edu

This paper discusses mathematical models dealing with the growth of solid tumors. Tumor growth is a very complex process, involving many different phenomena, which occur at different scales: subcellular, cellular, and extracellular scales. We survey models that address the problem at: subcellular scale, cellular scale, and extracellular scale. Then after we discuss multi-scale models and unification of models results from different scales.

1. Introduction

Cancer research has become increasingly important. This is because malignant neoplasms are the 2nd leading cause of death in the United States of America, and rank among top killers worldwide. Each year billions of dollars from government and private funding sources are spent on cancer research. In order to develop effective treatments, it is important to identify the mechanisms responsible for cancer growth, how they interact, and how can most easily be manipulated to eradicate (manage) the disease.

In order to gain such insight, it is usually necessary to perform large amounts of time consuming and intricating experiments but not always. Through the development and solutions of mathematical models that describe different aspects of solid tumor growth will provide insight into the complex mechanisms that control tumor growth and, hence suggest directions for new therapies. Thus, applied mathematics has potential to prevent excessive experimentation and also to provide biologists with complementary and valuable insight into the mechanisms that control the development of solid tumors.

The paper is organized as follows. In Section 2, we will discuss different stages of solid tumor. In Section 3, we discuss multistep transformation to cancer. In Section 4, we discuss experiments on cancer *in vitro* which are useful to estimate model parameters. Extracellular scale models, cellular scale models, and subcellular scales are discussed in Sections 5, 6, and 7 respectively. We discuss models dealing with capsule formation in section 8. The unifying results obtained from models at different scales and models which couple different scales are discussed in section 9. In Section 10, we will make conclusions and outlook.

2. Different stages of solid tumor

Cancerous tumors originate from mutation of one or more cells which usually undergo rapid uncontrolled growth thereby impairing the functioning of normal tissue. There is a large body of evidence proving that all the cells within a tumor mass are derived from a single cell. Even though all the cells within a tumor mass may be derived from a single cell, this does not mean that all the cells in a tumor are genetically identical. Tumor cells are more unstable than normal cells, meaning they mutate[1,27] at a much higher rate, they repair themselves much less effectively and they have ceased to respond to normal growth regulatory mechanism. Therefore, the cells within a tumor are different even from one another.

First, a piece of the DNA strand must be significantly mutated and the mutations must slip through the repair mechanisms. These mutations may take place over generations of cells. For example, one generation may have one mutation; the next may not have any. A subsequent generation may have another and so on, until the "cancer mutation" have occurred. The tumor cells respond both through induced alterations in physiology and metabolism and through altered gene and protein expression[12,28]

Due to these mutations, the cell must gain the ability to proliferate and thus lose its normal function. In a sense, the major purpose of the cell must be to divide.

There are probably only a limited number of alterations that will allow a cell to lose its functions and divide out of control. Some alterations affect nothing, others may cause a minor change that is not really threatening to the cell, and others can outrightly kill the cell. So, to become cancerous, the cell must maintain its ability to divide without causing any damage to limit its ability to survive.

If a cell becomes bent on dividing, the cell will just continue dividing and crowd out other cells within the area. In some fortunate cases an individuals own immune system may actually stop the growth of the tumor. The immune system may recognize that the cells within the tumor are not normal. If this happens, the immune cells may destroy the tumor. This may take place a number of times throughout an individuals life without them ever being affected.

If a tumor goes unnoticed and begins to grow, lack of nutrients can eventually limit its growth. If nutrients are not continuously supplied, the tumor cells cannot metabolize. In this case, at the very least, no new growth can occur. If a tumor becomes unable to grow and unable to support some of its functions and cell death occurs, the tumor may go into a dormant state. In this case it cannot spread. Once the tumor reaches this limiting size, and if it is unable to get more nutrients, it will stay in this dormant state and may eventually die off. Researchers are trying to develop tests that will determine whether for example an individuals breast and prostate tumors will remain dormant or spread. In that way, patients in the future could be spared unnecessary treatments.

There are many different cancers and there are many different components involved in the development of cancer making each person's cancer quite unique. Further, each type of cancer (e.g., breast, colon or prostate) does not necessarily behave like other cancers. For these reasons, there is no one "cure for cancer." Rather there will be lots of interventions and cures that are developed through a systematic approach and understanding. Researchers are constantly looking for ways to develop screening tools to identify cancers at their earliest phases so that they can be treated with surgery; however, each organ needs its own individual screening tool. For example, colon cancer is screened through a variety of techniques including colonoscopy. Cervical cancer is screened through the Pap test, which examines scrapings of cells from the cervix and discovers cells in the early stages of change. The mammogram is used to determine the presence of breast cancer hopefully at an early stage, but may not detect cells in the earliest phases of abnormal cell development prior to becoming cancerous.

The first stage growth of cancer is called Avascular. In the avascular state tumor growth, it has no blood vessels and relatively harmless. Its nutrients, oxygen and glucose are obtained and it eliminates waste products via diffusion. Cells in the center starve while Cells on the periphery thrive. Cells in the interior are quiescent, but not dead and do not divide. The growth of the avascular tumor is limited to a few *mm* in diameter. In response to an externally supplied nutrient, avascular tumors adopt a well defined, radially symmetric spatial structure.

Further tumor development, the genetic instability causes continued malignant alterations, invasion, angiogenesis, metastatic spread, resulting in a large biologically complex tumor. In fact, many of the later manifestations of malignancy, including invasion and angiogenesis, are thought to be enhanced, if not precipitated, by the stressful microenvironment which develops in the initial, avascular tumor nodule. Consequently, a better understanding of the regulation of the growth and malignant development of avascular avascular tumors would be beneficial; insights in such systems would also be valuable in understanding the heterogeneous microenvironments found within larger tumors[27].

The second stage of characteristics of cancer is Angiogenesis. This is formation of new blood vessels from the existing vasculature. Hypoxia is a condition in which there is a decrease in the oxygen supply to a tissue. In cancer treatment, the level of hypoxia in a tumor may help predict the response of the tumor to the treatment. Hypoxia is known to induce a chemical cascade which stimulates endothelial cells to aggregate, proliferate, and migrate towards the tumor.

The third stage of cancer characteristics is blood supply acquired. This is called the vascular tumor growth. The vascular tumor is made of 50% cells, 10% blood vessels, 40% extra cellular matrix (ECM) is basically connective tissue. The ECM is made of three major classes of biomolecules: structure proteins (collagen and elastin), specialized proteins and Proteoglycans.

3. The multistep transformation to cancer

The usual perspective on cancer progression is that it is a form of somatic evolution where certain mutations give one cell a selective growth advantage[15]. Tumor initiation in an organism (Oncogenesis) is thought to require several independent, rare mutation events to occur in the lineage of one cell[57]. Kinetic analyses have shown that four to six rate-limiting stochastic mutational events are required for the formation of a tumor[5,56]. Hanahan and Weinberg[33] proposed the following six attributes that a normal cell must acquire to become a cancer cell: (i) self-sufficiency in growth signals, (ii) insensitivity to anti-growth signals, (iii) evasion of apoptosis, (iv) limitless replicative potential, (v) sustained angiogenesis, and (vi) tissue invasion and metastasis.

Hanahan and Weinberg define genetic instability as an "enabling characteristics" that facilitates the acquisition of other mutations due to defects. Spencer et al[65] foresee cancer research developing into logical sciences, where the molecular and clinical complexities of the disease will be understood in terms of a few underlying principles.

4. Experiments

4.1. *MTS experiments*

Multicellular tumor spheroid (MTS) experiments as an *in vitro* tumor model can provide data on the duration of the cell cycle, growth rate, chemical diffusion, *etc*[26,27].

Tumor growth requires the transport of nutrients, for example oxygen, and glucose, from and waste products to the surrounding tissue. These nutrients regulate cell mitosis, cell death, and potentially cell mutation. MTS experiments have the great advantages of precisely controlling the external environment while maintaining the cells in the `spheroid` microenvironment[27,28]. Suspended in culture, tumor cells grow into a spheroid, in a process that closely mimics the growth characteristics of early stage tumors. MTS exhibits three distinct phases of growth:

(1) an initial phase during which individual cells form small clumps that subsequently grow quasi-exponentially;
(2) a layering phase during which the cell-cycle distribution within the spheroids changes, leading to formation of a necrotic core, accumulation of quiescent cells around the core, and sequestering of proliferating cells at the periphery; and
(3) a plateau phase during which the growth rate begins to decrease and the tumor ultimately attains a maximum diameter.

In order to understand the underlying dynamics of cell growth within a spheroid, Chandrasekar et al.[19] studied the spatial-temporal distribution of the cells spheroids cultured from cell line. They found that the size of the spheroids and their growth rates were dependent on the cell number, the proliferation was mostly limited to out most region as the spheroids grew in size, and the number of dead cells increased with age and size as well.

Mechanical effects from the surrounding environment as well as that generated internally by cellular growth play an important role in regulating tumor growth. Evidence that cell stress affects proliferation is provided by Helmlinger et al.[34]. By culturing spheroids in gels of different stiffness, it was demonstrated that the stress exerted on tumor cells by their surrounding affects its equilibrium size. High stress is observed to down-regulate cell proliferation and promote cell death[38].

5. Extracellular scale models

The macroscopic (extracellular) scale refers to phenomena which are typical of continuum systems: cell migration, convection, diffusion (of chemical factors, nutrients), phase transition (from free to bound cells and vice versa) detachment of cells and formation of metastases, and so on. The avascular stage of growth is characterized by:

(i) Small and occult lesions (1-2mm in diameter),

(ii) Formation of a necrotic core of dead tumor cells where a process of destroying cellular debris may take place,

(iii) Formation of an outer region of proliferating tumor cells and of an intermediate region of quiescent cells,

(iv) Production of chemical factors, among which several growth inhibitory factors, generally called GIF, and growth promoting factors, called GPF, by the tumor mass, thus controlling the mitosis,

(v) Dependence of the tumor cells mitotic rate on the GIF and GPF concentration,

(vi) Non-uniformities in the proliferation of cells and in the consumption of nutrients, which filter through the surface of the spheroid and diffuse in the intracellular space.

Since at this stage the tumor is not surrounded yet by capillaries, this phase can be observed and studied in laboratory by culturing cancer cells. On the other hand, the tumor angiogenic phase is characterized by:

(i) Secretion of tumor angiogenesis factors promoting the formation of new blood vessels (VEGF, FGF and others) as described in Bussolino et al.[13]

(ii) Degradation of basement membrane by several enzymes. **Endothelial** cells are then free to proliferate and migrate towards the source of the angiogenic stimulus,

(iii) Recruitment of new blood vessel that supply the tumor (neovascularization) and increase of tumor progression,

(iv) Aberrant vascular structure, abnormal blood flow, with continuous growth of new tumor blood vessels.

A macroscopic description of the system should focus on these features and aim at giving their evolution in time. Obviously, the macroscopic behavior depends on phenomena occurring at the cellular level, e.g. proliferation, death, activation and inhibition of single cells, interaction between pairs of cells, etc. The evolution of macroscopic observable can be described by models developed in the framework of continuum **phenomenologic** theories, e.g. those of continuum mechanics. These models are generally stated in terms of partial differential equations.

We will start by reviewing the different extracellular models. Over the last ten years a number of important advancement have been made in the development of mathematical models to simulate the growth and extracellular scale behavior of solid malignant tumors, for example see the recent reviews by Araujo and McElain[4].

Extracellular scale models deal with phenomena typical of continuous systems, such as cell migration, convection, diffusion. Evolving from the early chemical diffusion and differential equation models of Burton[14] and Greenspan[30], descriptions of tumor growth has been presented more recently using different approaches have been developed to describe the features of avascular tumor growth. Some of these models Continuum including those using classical growth models such as **logistic** or **Gompertz** models[52,53], a universal growth models of tumors[22,31,32], and partial differential equations models, for example see, Bellomo et al[10]; Byrne and Chaplain[15]; Owen and Sherratt[59]; Mallet[50];Pettet et al.[61]. The common feature of these mathematical model on tumor growth is that they have assumed that the tumor cells are of the same type for the simplicity of closing the system of mass balance equations. Further extensions of these models used a continuum, extracellular framework in one space dimension[67,69,70]. None of these rate models (empirical ordinary differential equations) can simulate the evolution of tumor structure, or predict the effect of chemicals on tumor structure.

Mechanical effects from the surrounding environment as well as that generated internally by cellular growth play an important role in regulating tumor growth. The resulting gel-like structure lends itself towards **proelastic** assumptions in that the tissue is assumed to consist of points of localized flow and fluid injection in an otherwise elastic medium. In this case a poroelastic model[56] can be used to model neoplastic environment in solid tumor. The poroelastic model is used to predict stress and pressure in the tumor and ECM. Verifiable computational models with likely become part of arsenal of techniques used to better understand tumor evolution and treatment strategies in near future. Continuum based models can be used to predict the evolution of tumors boundary time and this knowledge may in turn help estimate the effect that various methods of treatment, for example, chemotherapy and ultrasound, may have on the tumor behavior as well as on the ECM and ultimately on the host. A continuous based mathematical model can also be used how hypoxia is a promoter of angiogenesis. A model taking account of the main components, that is, tumor size, vessel density, oxygen concentration, anti-angiogenic factors and pro-angiogenic factors could predict the likelihood of angiogenesis of different configurations. Thus the model can be validated against experimental measurements.

6. Cellular scale models of growth of solid tumors

The cellular scale refers to the main (interactive) activities of the cells: activation and proliferation of tumor cells and competition with immune cells. More specifically, one has

(i) Fast proliferation of tumor cells, which are often degenerated endothelial cells, takes place when an environmental cell loses its death program and/or starts undergoing mitosis without control.

(ii) Competition with the immune system starts when tumor cells are recognized by immune cells, resulting either in the destruction of tumor cells or in the inhibition and depression of the immune system.

(iii) After differentiation tumor cells undergo a process of maturation, which makes them more and more proliferative and aggressive toward the environment and the immune system. Tumor cells can be additionally activated towards proliferation by nutrient supply from the environment.

(iv) Activation and inhibition of the immune cells in their competition with tumor cells are regulated by **cytokine** signals. These interactions, developed at the cellular level, are ruled by processes which are performed at the subcellular scale.

(v) Activation and inhibition of cells belonging to the tumor and to the immune system can also be induced by a properly addressed medical treatment.

A model developed at the microscopic scale defines the time evolution of the physical state of a single cell. Often these models are stated in terms of ordinary differential equations. On the other hand, if we aim to describe the evolution of a system comprising a large number of cells, then the system of ordinary differential equations (one for each cell) can be replaced by a kinetic equation on the statistical distribution of the state of all cells. The application of methods of mathematical kinetic theory to model the competition between tumor and immune cells was initiated by Bellomo and Forni[9].

Cellular models[39,51] deal with interaction between cells, which is of course strongly related to what happens at the subcellular level. Cellular Automata models that treat cells as single points on a lattice, for example, the LGCA model of Alarcon et al.[2], Dormann and Deutsch[23]. They adopt local rules specifying adhesion, pressure (cells are pushed towards regions of low cell density) and couple the LGCA to a continuum chemical dynamics. Their two-dimensional simulations produce a layered structure that resembles a cross-section of an MTS.

6.1. *Cellular Potts model*

The cellular `Potts` model is a more sophisticated Cellular Automata model, which describes individual cells as extended objects of variable shapes. The cellular Potts model can be applied to model tumor growth. Any cellular scale model of tumor growth must consider cell-cell adhesion, `chemotaxis`, cell dynamics including cell growth, cell division and cell mutation, as well as the reaction-diffusion of chemicals: nutrients and waste products, and eventually, angiogenesis factors and hormones. In additional to differential adhesion and chemotaxis, cellular models can include the reaction-diffusion dynamics for relevant chemicals:

$$\frac{\partial C_0}{\partial t} = D_0 \nabla^2 C_0 - a(x), \tag{1}$$

$$\frac{\partial C_n}{\partial t} = D_n \nabla^2 C_n - b(x), \tag{2}$$

$$\frac{\partial C_w}{\partial t} = D_w \nabla^2 C_w + c(x), \tag{3}$$

where C_0, C_n, and C_w are concentrations of oxygen, nutrients (glucose), and metabolic wastes (lactate), their initial values are a_0, b_0 and c_0 respectively. D_0, D_n, and D_w are their respective diffusion constants; are metabolic rates of the cell located at x; and c is the coefficient of the metabolic waste production.

$$a = a_0 \frac{C_0 - C_0^T}{C_0^O - C_0^T},$$

$$b = b_0 \frac{C_n - C_n^T}{C_n^O - C_n^T},$$

and

$$c = c_0 \frac{a/a_0 - b/b_0}{2}$$

where C^O is the "optimal concentration, and C^T is the "threshold" concentration. The "optimal" concentration is $0.28mM$ for oxygen and is 5.5 for glucose. Each cell follows its own cell cycle, which depends sensitively on its local environment. It is assumed that the target volumes are twice the initial volumes. The volume constraints in the total energy allows cell volumes to stay close to the target volume, thus describing cell growth. If the nutrient concentration falls below a threshold or waste concentration exceeds its threshold, the cell stops growing and become quiescent: alive but not growing. When the nutrient concentration drops lower or waste increases further, the quiescent cell may become necrotic. Only when the cell reaches the end of its cycle and its volume reaches a target volume will the cell divide. The mature cell splits its longest axis into two daughter cells, which may inherit all the properties of the mother cell or undergo a mutation with a defined probability.

The simulation data show that the early exponential stage of tumor growth slows down when quiescent cells appear. Other measurements also qualitatively reproduce experimental data from multicellular spheroids grown *in vitro*. These simulations model a monoclonal cell population (The cells that are derived from a single common ancestor cell are part of a single clone. For example, all leukemias, lymphomas, and myeloma are the result of the malignant transformation of a single cell and are monoclonal diseases.) in accordance with MTS experiments. However, including cellular heterogeneity as for example in the model of Kansas et al.[40] is straightforward. Model extensions will incorporate genetic and epigenetic cell heterogeneity (A factor that changes the phenotype without changing the genotype). The CPM allows easy implementation of cell differentiation as well as additional signal molecules. Cellular automation models describe cell-cell and cell-environment interactions by *phenomenological* local rules, allowing simulation of solid growth of tumors.

7. Subcellular models on growth of solid tumors

The subcellular scale refers to the main activities within the cells or at the cell membrane. Among an enormous number of phenomena one can focus on

(i) Aberrant activation of signal transduction pathways that control cell growth and survival,
(ii) Genetic changes, distortion in the cell cycle and loss of apoptosis,
(iii) Response of the cellular activity to the signals received,
(iv) Absorption of vital nutrients. A large amount of literature related to the above features can be found.

Several interesting papers are cited in the review paper by Lustig and Behrens (2003), focusing on the dependence of cancer development on the aberrant activation of signal pathways that control cell growth and survival.

Subcellular scale models deal with models concerning the intra-celllular origin of cancer, which involves genetic changes and distortion in the cell cycle. They refer to the origins of unlimited and inappropriate cell proliferation, loss of apoptosis, and the production, release and recognition of messenger substances such as interleukins.

Micro environment study of multicellular tumor spheroids is a good place to start. There is some data evidence that growth inhibitors are due to small protein factors[21,38]. The desire to understand tumor complexity has given rise to mathematical models to describe the tumor microenvironment. New mathematical models for avascular tumor growth and development that spans three distinct scales can be developed. At the cellular level, a lattice Monte Carlo model describes cellular dynamics (proliferation, adhesion, and viability). At the subcellular level, a network regulates the expression of proteins that control the cell cycle. At the extracellular level, reaction-diffusion equations describe the chemical dynamics (nutrient, waste, growth promoter, and inhibitor concentrations). Reaction diffusion equation coupled with an integro differential equation describing tumor radius response to externally supplied nutrient.

Data from experiments with multicellular spheroids are used to determine the parameters of the simulations. Starting with a single tumor cell, these models produce an avascular tumor that quantitatively mimics experimental measurements in multicellular spheroids. Based on the simulations, these models predict: 1), the microenvironmental conditions required for tumor cell survival; and 2), growth promoters and inhibitors have diffusion coefficients, corresponding to molecules. Using the same parameters, the model also accurately predicts spheroid growth curves under different external nutrient supply conditions.

In the cellular automaton, a layered tumor has formed, comprised of necrotic "cell" material, quiescent and proliferating tumor cells.

8. Capsule is a key prognostic indicator

The formation of a capsule of dense, fibrous extracellular matrix around a solid tumor is a key prognostic indicator in a wide range of cancers. However, the cellular mechanisms underlying capsule formation remain unclear. The dormant state is ended by invasion into surrounding tissue. Tumor `encapsulation` is the cascade of events that result in the formation of a multi-layered sheath of epithelium surrounding a tumor. A multilobular tumor is one in which lobes of different sizes are separated by strands of connective tissue.

8.1. Capsule composition and importance

Two complementary theories have been postulated in order to explain the mechanism of capsule formation[7,8]. One hypothesized mechanism is the *expansive growth hypothesis,* which suggests that a capsule may form by the rearrangement of existing extracellular matrix without new matrix production. Berenblum[11] observed that tumors growing within the lumen of a hollow organ, or on the surface of the body, do not become encapsulated, a finding that Berenblum suggests confirms the hypothesis that capsules can only be formed in situations where a tumor can exert pressure on surrounding tissue. According to the expansive growth hypothesis, the appearance of fibrous capsule is essentially a passive phenomena, and the capsular collagen is derived from mature, pre-existing collagen rather than being newly deposited. The aggregation of connective tissue represents the cumulative effect of a series of lower level interactions at the interface of the expanding tumor and the connective tissue. The implication of this hypothesis was proposed studied by Perumpanani at el[60]. The `macrocellular` scale model consists of conservation equations for tumor cells and extracellular matrix and exhibit traveling wave solutions in which a pulse of extracellular matrix, corresponding to a capsule, moves in parallel with the advancing front of the tumor. Their model consists of conservation equations for the densities of tumor cells and extracellular matrix, denoted $u(x,t)$ and $c(x,t)$, respectively, where t and x denote time and space in a one-dimensional spatial domain:

$$\frac{\partial u}{\partial t} = f(u) + \frac{\partial}{\partial x}\left[h(c)\frac{\partial u}{\partial x}\right], \qquad (4)$$

$$\frac{\partial c}{\partial t} = k \frac{\partial}{\partial x} \left[ch(c) \frac{\partial u}{\partial x} \right]. \tag{5}$$

where the term $f(u)$ represents cell division and death; $f(0)$ must clearly be zero, and for simplicity Sherratt assumed that the cell density was rescaled so that $u = 1$ is the equilibrium level within the tumor, implying $f(1) = 0$. Random cell movement was assumed, and kinetics of extracellular matrix are neglected, in keeping with expansive growth hypothesis, so that the extracellular matrix density only changes because of convection with the cells. This convection does not imply large-scale movement of intact matrix by a cell; rather it is the net result of local matrix movement and remodeling during cell movement. This will increase with local matrix density and is represented in the model as kc, and the function $h(c)$ represent the reduction in cell motility at high matrix density.

Another hypothesis, foreign body hypothesis is derived from the notion that capsule formation is an attempt by the body localize the tumor and assumes that, when stress, normal cells begin to secrete collagen or other fibrous components of ECM. This view is essentially of an active process where the body mounts a response akin to inflammation to create a fibrous barrier. Ewing's[25] work suggested that the encapsulated tumors may; thus be shielded from cellular attack. Similarly, Enneking's[24] work suggests that the hosts attempt to encapsulate and contain tumors. Barr et al[8] gave a detail review of the mechanism of encapsulation and also suggested a compromise hypothesis embodying both of the above mechanisms.

The major differences between the foreign body hypothesis and the expansive growth hypothesis is that the latter is a passive process, where the former is an active response of the host. Since it is difficult to discriminate the two hypotheses using experimental techniques, mathematical modeling provides a natural approach for testing and comparing the assumptions and the consequences associated with each of them. Jackson and Byrne[37] developed a mechanical approach to study both hypotheses.

9. Coupling and unifying different scales

9.1. *Unification of model results of different scales*

The problem of relationships between the various scales of description seems to be the most important problems of the mathematical modeling of complex systems, for example modeling of solid tumor growth. The following strategy can be applied. One starts with the deterministic extracellular scale model for which the identification of parameters by an experiment is easier. Then one provides the theoretical framework for modeling at cellular scale in such way that the corresponding models at extracellular scale and cellular prediction should be close. If the cellular scale model is designed properly, one may hope it covers not only the extracellular behavior of the system in question, but also some of its cellular scale features. The cellular model by its nature is richer and it describes a larger variety of phenomena. In a similar manner the subcellular scale model should be richer than cellular and extracellular scale models.

This survey refers to a general framework for a program for finding transitions between the different scales of descriptions, interacting entities (cellular, subcellular), statistical description of test entity, and macroscopic scale (extracellular).

In mathematical terms the links of the following mathematical structures was developed for various situations of biological interest[43,44,45,46,47]:

(1) The micro-scale of stochastically interacting entities (cells, individuals,..), in terms of continuous linear semigroups of Markov operators (continuous stochastic semigroups)[48];

(2) The meso-scale of statistical entities in terms of continuous nonlinear semigroups related to the solutions of bilinear Boltzamann-type nonlocal kinetic equations[49];

(3) The macroscopic scale of densities of interacting entities (in terms of dynamical systems related to bilinear reaction-diffusion-chemotaxis equations.

Lachowicz[46] deals with the mathematical theory of a large class of reaction-diffusion systems (with small diffusion) and then generalized to include reaction-diffusion-chemotaxis systems. This was motivated by a particular model of tissue invasion by solid tumor reaction-diffusion equations with a chemotaxis-type term[30,55]. The model is quite general and can be applied to a large class of systems at the macroscopic level including the Keller-Segel-type systems.

There is a huge literature related to the rigorous derivation of chemotaxis equations from cellular scale models[54]. Stevens[66] proved that for sufficiently large numbers of particles the dynamics of an interacting particles system can be approximated by the solutions of chemotaxis systems.

Later, Lachowicz proposed a more general approach in the sense that it can be applied to large class of models at the macroscopic scale. Moreover it relates the three scales of descriptions. The methods may lead to new and more accurate modeling of complex process, like tumor growth.

Usually the description of growth of tumor is carried out at extracellular scale. The mathematical structures are deterministic reaction diffusion equations[55,56,63].

Following Chaplain and Anderson[20], Lavichowicz considered a system of deterministic reaction-diffusion-chemotaxis equations that is able to model the invasive spatial spread of solid tumors. The model is able to capture some aspects of solid tumor growth and invasion at the extracellular scale (tissue level). The model is based on genetic solid tumor growth at the avascular stage, and it describes the interactions between the tumor and surrounding tissue (ECM). The variables in the model are tumor cell density, ρ_1, ECM density, ρ_2, and MDE (certain factors produced by the tumor cells and known as matrix degrading or degrading enzymes) concentration, ρ_3. The model describes one key aspect of tissue invasion, namely the ability of tumors cells to produce and secrete MDEs and their migratory response. Chaplain and Anderson made assumptions that the tumor cells produce MDEs which degrade the ECM locally; the ECM degradation aids in tumor cells motility; movement of tumor cells up to a gradient of ECM is referred as `haptotaxis`; tumor cell motion is driven only by random motility and haptotaxis; the proliferation of tumor cells is not taken into account.

With these assumptions the model (in dimensionless form) of Chaplain and Anderson[20] yields

$$\frac{\partial \rho_1}{\partial t} = d_1 \nabla^2 \rho_1 - \gamma \nabla \cdot (\rho_1 \nabla \rho_1)$$

$$\frac{\partial \rho_2}{\partial t} = -\eta \rho_2 \rho_3 \qquad (6)$$

$$\frac{\partial \rho_3}{\partial t} = d_3 \nabla^2 \rho_3 + \alpha \rho_1 - \beta \rho_3$$

where d_1, γ, η, d_3, α, β are given positive constants (the macroscopic parameters), $d_1 \nabla^2 \rho_1$, $\gamma \nabla \cdot (\rho_1 \nabla \rho_1)$, $\eta \rho_2 \rho_3$, $d_3 \nabla^2 \rho_3$, $\alpha \rho_1$, and $\beta \rho_3$ represent random motility, haptoxis, degradation, diffusion, production and decay respectively. To improve the above model, one should construct cellular model that correspond to the macroscopic model defined by equation (6).

9.2. *Coupling of different scales*

Most existing models focus on one scale. They differ considerably from each other, according to the modeling scale (subcellular, cellular and extracellular) they focus on. While this may provide valuable insight into processes occurring at that scale, it does not address fundamental problems of how phenomena different scales are coupled. This is because one obstacle that must be overcome is the intrinsic multiple scale nature of tumor growth. We present recent research that have been carried with the aim of formulating multiscales model of tumor growth.

In 2004, Alarcon et al.[3] established a modeling framework for developing a realistic multiple scale model of tumor growth. They used the hybrid cellular automaton as a basic theoretical framework to combine models that couple scales ranging from the tissue scale (e.g. vascular structural adaptation) through to the intracellular scale (e.g. cell cycle). This has enabled them to tackle questions such as the effect on tumor growth of blood flow heterogeneity (Alarcon et al.,[2]) and the efficiency of current **chemotherapy** protocols for the treatment of non-Hodgkins lymphomas. In their modeling framework, intercellular processes are represented by ordinary differential equations, extracellular processes by partial differential equations and cell processes by rules in a cellular automaton. Their models are still largely phenomenological and simple, with many processes not included. As more detail is incorporated the computational implementation and analysis become more difficult. The challenge is developing appropriate numerical and analytical techniques in order to efficiently implement, understand, and exploit these models.

In 2005, Jiang et al.[38] presented a mathematical model for avascular tumor growth and development that spans three distinct scales. At the cellular level, a lattice Monte Carlo model describes cellular dynamics (proliferation, adhesion, and viability). At the subcellular level, a Boolean network regulates the expression of proteins that control the cell cycle. At the extracellular level, reaction-diffusion equations describe the chemical dynamics (nutrient, waste, growth promoter, and inhibitor concentrations). Data from experiments with multicellular spheroids were used to determine the parameters of the simulations. Starting with a single tumor cell, this model produces an avascular tumor that quantitatively mimics experimental measurements in multicellular spheroids. Based on the simulations, they predicted:

(1) the microenvironmental conditions required for tumor cell survival, and
(2) growth promoters and inhibitors have diffusion coefficients in the range between 106 and 107 cm^2/h, corresponding to molecules of size 8090 kDa. Using the same parameters, their model also accurately predicted spheroid growth curves under different external nutrient supply conditions.

In 2006, Ayati et al.[6] presented multiscale models of cancer tumor invasion with components at the molecular level (incorporated via diffusion and taxis processes), the cellular level (incorporated via a cell age variable), and the tissue level (incorporated via spatial variables). They provided biological justifications for the model components, present computational results from the models, and discussed the scientific-computing methodology used to solve the model equations. Their models and methodology form the basis for developing and treating increasingly complex, mechanistic models of tumor invasion that will be more predictive and less phenomenological.

10. Conclusions and outlook

The new mathematical models should link all the approaches at different scales in order to gain better insight into dynamics of tumor growth or should be a `multiscale` models. These models will not only replicate experimental observation but also, more importantly, predict behaviors that have not yet been observed.

Acknowledgments

This work was supported by the Department of Mathematical Sciences at Middle Tennessee State University. I would like to thank Dr. Don Hong for introducing me to mathematical modeling in cancer. I also would like to thank the anonymous referee for very constructive comments.

References

1. J.A. Adam, A simplified mathematical model of tumor growth, *Math. Biosci.*, **81** (1986), 229-242.
2. T. Alarcon, H.M. Byrne, and P.K. Maini, A cellular automaton model for tumour growth in inhomogenenous environment, *J. Theor. Biol.*, **225** (2003), 257-274.
3. T. Alarcon, H.M. Byrne, and P.K. Maini, Toward whole-organ modelling of tumour growth, *progress in Biophysics and Molecular Biology*, **85** (2004), 451-472.
4. R.P. Araujo, and D.L.S. McElwain, A history of the study of tumor growth: The contribution of mathematical modeling, *Bull. Math. Biol.*, **66** (2004), 1039-1091.
5. P. Armitage, and R. Doll, The age distribution of cancer and multi-stage theory of carcinogenesis, *Br. J. Cancer*, **8** (1954), 1-12.
6. B.P. Ayati, G.F. Webb, A.R.A. Anderson, Computational methods and results for structured multiscale models of tumor invasion, *Multiscale Model. Simul.*, **5** (2006), 1-20.

7. L.C. Barr, The encapsulation of tumours, *Clin. Exp. Metasis*, **7** (1989), 277-282.

8. L.C. Barr, R.L. Carter, and A.J.S. David, Encapsulation of tumors as a modified wound healing response, *Lancet II*, (1988), 135-137.

9. N. Bellomo, and G. Forni, Dynamics of tumor interaction with the host immune system, *Math. Comput. Model.*, **20** (1994), 107-122.

10. N. Bellomo, and L. Preziosi, Modeling and mathematical problems related to tumor evolution and its interaction with the immune system, *Math. and Comp. Model*, **32** (2000), 413-452.

11. I. Berenblum, The nature of tumour growth, *General Pathology*, (H.E.W Florey, Ed.), Lloyd-Luke, London, 1970.

12. J.M. Brown, Tumor microenvironment and the response to anticancer therapy, *Cancer Biol. Therp.*, **1** (2002),453-458.

13. F. Bussolino, M. Arese, E. Audero, E. Giraudo, S. Marchio, S. Mitola, L. Primo, and G. Serini, Biological aspects of tumour angiogenesis, In: *Cancer Modelling and Simulation*, (L. Preziosi, Ed.), pp. 1-22, Chapman & Hall/CRC Press, London/Boca Raton, FL, 2003.

14. A.C. Burton, Rate of growth of solid tumours as a problem of diffusion, *Growth*, **30** (1966), 157-176.

15. H. Byrne, and M. Chaplin, Modeling the role of cell-cell adhesion in the growth and development of carcinomas, *Math. Comput. Modell.* , **24** (1996), 1-17.

16. H. Byrne, and M. Chaplin, Free boundary value problems associated with the growth and development of multicellular spheroids, *Eur. J. Appl. Math.*, **8** (1997), 639-658.

17. D.P. Cahill, K.W. Kinzler, B. Vogelstein, and C. Lengaurer, Genetic instability and darwinian selection in tumors, *Trends Cell Biol.*, **9** (1999), M57-M60.

18. J.J. Casciari, S.V. Sotirichos, R.M. Sutherland, Variations in Tumor Cell Growth Rates and Metabolism with Oxygen Concentration, Glucose Concentration, and Extracellular pH, *J. cell Physiol.*, **151** (1992), 386.

19. N. Chandasekar, S.R. Jasti, C.R. Arnout, A.L. Lauren, and O. Mandri, Growth characteristics of glioblstoma spheroids, *Int. J. Oncology,* **19** (2001), 1109-1115.

20. M.A.J. Chaplain, and A.R.A. Anderson, Mathematical modelling of tissue invasion, In: *Cancer Modelling and Simulation*, pp.269298, Chapman and Hall, London, 2003.

21. M.A.J. Chaplain and B.D. Sleeman, Modelling the growth of solid tumours and incorporating a method for their classification using nonlinear elasticity theory, *J. Math. Biol.*, **31** (1993), 431-479.

22. P.P. Delsanto, C. Guiot, P.G. Degiorgis, A.C. Condat, Y. Mansury, and T.S. Desiboeck, Growth model for multicellular tumor spheroids, *Appl. Phys. Lett.*, **85** (2004), 4225-4227.

23. S. Dormann, and A. Deutsch, Modeling of self-organized avascular tumor growth with a hybrid cellular automaton, *Silico Biology*, **2** (2002), 35.

24. W.F. Enneking, *Musculoskcletal Tumour Surgery* ,Edniburgh Churchill Livingstone, 1983.

25. J. Ewing, *Neoplastic Diseases*, Saunders, Philadelphia, PA, 1940.
26. J.P. Freyer, P.L. Scholar, and A.G. Saponara, Partial purification of a protein growth inhibitor from multicellular spheroids, *Biochem. Biophys. Res. Comm.*, **152** (1988), 463-368.
27. J. Freyer, and R. Sutherland, Selective dissociation and characterization of cells from different regions of multicell spheroids during growth, *Cancer Research*, **40** (1980), 3956-3965.
28. J. Freyer, and R. Sutherland, Regulation of growth saturation and development of necrosis in EMT6/RO multicellular spheroids induced by the glucose and oxygen supply, *Cancer Research*, **46** (1988), 3504-3512.
29. A. Friedman, A hierarchy of cancer models and their mathematical challenges, *Discr. Contin. Dyn. Systems*, **4** (2004), 147-159.
30. H.P. Greenspan, Models for the growth of a solid tumour by diffusion, *Stud. Appl. Math.*, **52** (1972),317-340.
31. C. Guiot, P.P. Delsanto, A. Carpintari, N. Pugno, Y. Mansury, and T.S. Deisboeck, The dynamic evolution of the power exponent in a universal growth model of tumors, *J. Theor. Biol.*, **240** (2006), 459-463.
32. C. Guiot, P.G. Delsanto, P. Gabriele, and T.S. Deisboeck, Does tumor growth follow a "Universal law"? *J. Theor. Biol.*, **225** (2003), 147-151.
33. D. Hanahan, and R. Weinberg, The hallmarks of cancer, *Cell*, **100** (2000), 57-70.
34. G. Helmlinger, P.A. Netti, H.C. Lichtenbeld, R.J. Melder, and R.K. Jain, Solid stress inhibits the growth of multicellular tumor spheroids, *Nature Biotech.*, **15** (1997), 778-783.
35. L. Hlatky, R.K. Sachs, and E.L. Alpen, Joint oxygen-glucose deprivation as the cause of necrosis in a tumor analog, *J. Cell. Physiol.*, **134** (1988), 167-168.
36. T.L. Jackson, Vascular tumor growth and treatment: consequences of polyclonality, competition and dynamic vascular support, *J. Math. Biol.*, **44** (2002), 201-226.
37. T.L. Jackson, and H.M. Byrne, A mathematical model of tumour encapsulation. *J. Math. Biosc.*, **180** (2002), 307-328.
38. Y. Jiang, J.P. Grbovic, C. Cantrell, and J.P. Freyer, A Multiscale Model for Avascular Tumor Growth, *Biophys. J.*, **89** (2005), 3884-3894.
39. A.R. Kansal, S. Torquato, G.R. Harsh IV, E.A. Chioca, T.S. Deisboeck, Simulated brain tumor growth dynamics using a three-dimensional cellular automaton, *J. theor. Biol.*, **203** (2000), 367-382.
40. A.R. Kansal, S. Torquato, E.A. Chiocca, and T.S. Deisboeck, Simulated Brain Tumor Growth Dynamics Using a Three-Dimensional Cellular Automaton, *J. theor. Biol.*, **207** (2000), 431-382.
41. K. Kiberstis, and et al., Frontiers in cancer research, *Science*, **278**(1977), 1035.
42. J.E. Klaunig, and L.M. Kamendulus, The role of oxidative stress in carcinogenesis, *Ann. Rev. Pharmacol. Toxxixol.*, **44** (2004), 239-267.
43. M. Lachowicz, Describing competitive systems at the level of interacting individuals, *Proc. of the Eight Nat. Confer. Appl. Math. Biol. Medicine*, Lajs, pp. 95-100, 2002.

44. M. Lachowicz, From microscopic to macroscopic descriptions of complex systems, *Comp. Rend. Mecanique(paris)*, **331** (2003), 733-738.
45. M. Lachowicz, On bilinear kinetic equations, Between micro and macro descriptions of biological populations, *Banach Center Publ.*, **63** (2004), 217-230.
46. M. Lachowicz, General population systems, Macroscopic limit of a class of stochastic semigroups, *J. Math. Anal. Appl.*, **307** (2005), 585.
47. M. Lachowicz, Stochastic semigroups and coagulation equations, *Ukrainian Math. J.*, **57** (2005), 913-922.
48. A. Lasota, M.C. Mackey, Chaoes, Fractals, and Noise, Springer, New York, 1994.
49. M. Lachowicz, and D. Wrzosek, Nonlocal bilinear equations, Equilibrium solutions and diffusive limit, *Math. Models Appl. Sci.*, **11** (2001), 1375-1390.
50. D.C. Mallet, Mathematical modeling of the role of haptotaxis in tumour growth and Invasion. Ph.D. Thesis, Queensland University of Technology, Brisbane, Australia, 2004
51. Y. Mansury, and T.S. Deisboeck, Simulating 'structure function' patterns of malignant brain tumors, *Physica A*, **331** (2004), 219-232.
52. M. Marusic, Z. Bajzer, J.P. Freyer, and S. Vuk-Pavlovic, Modeling autostimulation of growth in multicellular tumor spheroids, *Int. J. Biomed. Comput.*, **29** (1991), 149-158.
53. M. Marusic, Z. Bajzer, J.P. Freyer, and S. Vuk-Pavlovic, Analysis of growth of multicellular tumour spheroids by mathematical models, *Cell Prolif.*, **27** (1994), 73-94.
54. W. Mueller-Klieser, Tumor biology and experimental therapeutics, *Oncol. Hematol.*, **36** (2002), 123-139.
55. J.D. Murray, *Mathematical biology*, Springer, New York, 2003.
56. P.A. Netti, Y. Coucher, R.K. Skalak, and R.K. Jain, A poroelastic model for intersttial pressure in tumor, *Biorheology*, **32** (1995), 346.
57. P.C. Nowell, The clonal evolution of tumor cell populations, *Science*, **194** (1976), 23-28.
58. H. Osada, and T. Takahashi, Genetic alterations of multiple tumor supressors and oncogenes in the carcinogenesis and progression of lung cancer, *Oncogene*, **21** (2002), 7421-7434.
59. M.R. Owen, and J.A. Sherratt, Pattern formation and spatiotemperal irregularity in a model for macrophase-tumor interactions, *J. Theor. Biol.*, **189** (1997), 63-80.
60. A.J. Perumpanani, J.A. Sherratt, and J. Norbury, Mathematical modeling of capsule formation and multinodularity in benign tumor growth, *Nonlinearity*, **10** (1997), 1599-1614.
61. G.J. Pettet, C.P. Please, M.J. Tindall, D.L.S. McElwain, The migration of cells in multicell tumor spheroids, *Bull. Math. Biol.*, **63** (2001), 231-257.
62. M.J. Renan, How many mutations are required for tumorigenesis? implications from human cancer data, *Mol. Carinogen*, **7** (1993), 139-146.
63. J.A. Sherratt, Traveling wave solutions of a mathetical model for tumor encapsulation, *SIAM J. Appl. Math*, **60** (1999), 392-407.
64. J. Smoller, *Shock waves and reaction-diffusion equations*, New York (1994).

65. S.L. Spencer, M.J. Berryman, J.A. Garc ia, and D. Abbott, An ordinary differential equation model for the multistep transformation for cancer, *J. Theor. Biology*, **231** (2004), 515-524.

66. A. Stevens, A stochastic cellular automaton modeling gliding aggregation of Myxobacteria, *SIAM J. Appl. Math*, **61** (2000), 172-182.

67. Z. Vager, R. Naaman and E.P. Kanter, Coulomb explosion imaging of small molecules, *Science*, **244** (1989), 426-431.

68. P. Vaupel, and M. Hockel, Blood supply, oxygenation status and metabolic micromilieu of breast cancers: characterization and therapeutic relevance, *Int. J. Oncol.*, **17** (2000), 869-879.

69. J.P. Ward, and J.R. King, Mathematical modeling of avascular tumour growth, *IMA. J. Math. Appl. Med. Biol.*, **14** (1997), 39-69.

70. J.P. Ward, and J.R. King, Mathematical modelling of avascular-tumour growth II: modelling growth saturation, *IMA. J. Math. Appl. Med. Biol.*, **16** (1999), 171-211.

UNIT V

COMPUTING AND VISUALIZATION

CHAPTER 15

ARTIFICIAL NEURAL NETWORKS FOR DATA MINING AND FEATURE EXTRACTION

Jeff Knisley[a], Lloyd Lee Glenn, Karl Joplin, and Patricia Carey

The Institute for Quantitative Biology,
East Tennessee State University,
P. O. Box 70663, Johnson City, TN 37614-0663, USA
E-mail: [a]knisleyj@etsu.edu

Artificial Neural Networks are models of interacting neurons that can be used as classifiers with large data sets. They can also be used for feature extraction and for reducing the dimensionality of large data sets. Dendritic electrotonic models can be used to suggest more robust artificial neural network models that are amenable to data mining and feature extraction.

1. Introduction

The very large data sets now being produced by modern scientific instruments often require data mining techniques which go beyond the usual methods of statistical analysis. Among the most popular data mining algorithms used to classify unknown data are the techniques of clustering analysis, principal components analysis, linear discriminant analysis, decision trees, **support vector machines**, and **artificial neural networks**[1]. The majority of these techniques are applied to unclassified data sets in order to *extract features* from the data that cannot be directly observed. For example, in a *clustering analysis,* subgroups of the data are classified so that members of a subgroup are relatively close to each other while remaining relatively far away from elements in other subgroups[2].

However, if some or all of the data is classified a priori–for example, if a data set can be classified as coming either from an experimental group or from a control–then support vector machines (SVM) and artificial neural networks (ANN) are often the tools of choice. In both cases, data sets for known classifications are used to *train* the SVM or ANN so that it can predict the classification of an unknown data set. In such *classification* problems, it is natural to ask which features of the underlying data set are most responsible for the prediction of the classification of a data set. Artificial neural networks (ANN) can be used to address this question in a natural and straightforward manner[3]. Although there are methods of addressing this question with SVM's, this article will focus on the use of ANN's as *classifiers* which can also reveal features of the underlying data set most responsible for that classification.

There are many different neural network algorithms that are used for classification and feature extraction, including Self Organizing Machines, the Self Organizing Tree Algorithm, perceptron networks, and multilayer perceptron networks (MLP)[4]. These algorithms are being used in an ever increasing number of different applications. For example, artificial neural networks have been used to predict protein structures[5], to diagnose lymphoma[6], to perform clustering analyses[7], and to interpret protein threading scores[8], to name a few. The list is far from exhaustive, but it illustrates the diversity of applications of neural networks for classifying and interpreting data.

This article describes the use of neural networks for classification and feature extraction, with an emphasis on applications to microarray data. The emphasis is on perceptron models, especially as they are used to classify gene expression in microarray data[3]. Section 2 introduces and explores artificial neural networks. Section 3 presents algorithms suitable for classification and feature extraction, and section 4 suggests methods for improving ANN algorithms based on mathematical models of dendritic electrical activity.

2. Artificial Neural Networks

A neuron is known to collect information in the dendrites in the form of variations in membrane resistance and ion channel interactions at synaptic junctions. If the resulting variation in membrane potential is not large, then the potential decays exponentially to a resting potential of about -70 mV. However, if the potential at the soma surpasses a certain threshold, then the neuron "fires", by which we mean that an action potential propagates along the axon to the synapses of the neuron.

The mechanics of this process are described by the Hodgkin-Huxley (HH) equations and by dendritic cable models with a lumped soma boundary condition[10]. Because the HH equations are highly nonlinear and nearly

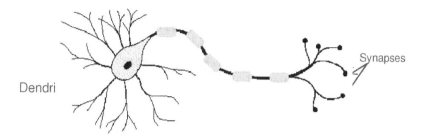

Dendri

Synapses

Fig. 1.   Schematic of a Neuron

intractable, models such as the Fitzhugh-Nagumo model have been created as qualitative models of dendritic-somatic-axonal interactions[11]. An **artificial neuron** is a minimalist qualitative model that suggests that a neuron integrates variations in potential over time and fires if a threshhold is exceeded. An **Artificial Neural Network (ANN)** is a network of interconnected artificial neurons.

Specifically, in an ANN, axonal action potentials are represented by *activations* which are considered to be in $[0,1]$, and synaptic activity is considered to be governed by a parameter known as a *synaptic weight*. If x_j denotes the activation from the jth neuron in a network, and if w_{ij} is the synaptic weight of the connection between the ith and j^{th} artificial neuron, then the activation of the ith neuron is

$$x_i = \sigma \left(\sum_{j \neq i} w_{ij} x_j - \theta_i \right) \tag{1}$$

where the activation function $\sigma\left(\cdot\right)$ is of the form

$$\sigma\left(t\right) = \frac{1}{1 + e^{-\kappa t}}$$

where $\kappa > 0$ is a parameter[12].

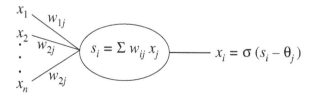

Fig. 2.   An Artificial Neuron

An input neuron is a neuron which takes a single stimulus I as input and returns an activation of the form $x = \sigma(I)$. A multi-layer perceptron (MLP) has a input layer which is connected to one or more *hidden layers*, with the last hidden layer being connected to an output layer. Subsequent layers are completely connected, but there are no connections between two neurons in the same layer or between neurons that are not in subsequent layers. A 3-layer MLP has r input neurons connected to m neurons in a

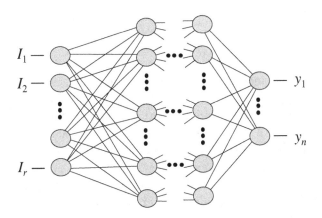

Fig. 3.   A Multi-Layer Perceptron

single hidden layer which are connected to n neurons in an output layer. It has been shown that a 3-layer MLP can approximate any absolutely integrable mapping of the type

$$f(I_1, \ldots, I_r) = (y_1, \ldots, y_n)$$

to within any $\varepsilon > 0$, where I_j is the stimulus presented to the jth input neuron and y_k is the activation from the kth output neuron[13].

If we let $\mathbf{x} = (x_1, \ldots, x_r)$ denote the vector of activations from the input to the hidden layer, then $y_j = \sigma(s_j - \theta_j)$, $j = 1, \ldots n$ and

$$s_j = \sum_{k=1}^{m} \alpha_{jk} \sigma(\mathbf{w}_k \cdot \mathbf{x} - \theta_k)$$

where $\mathbf{w}_k = (w_{k1}, \ldots, w_{kr})$ denotes the vector of weights between the input layer and the kth hidden neuron, $\cdot$ denotes the standard inner product, and α_{jk} denotes the weight between the kth hidden neuron and the jth output neuron.

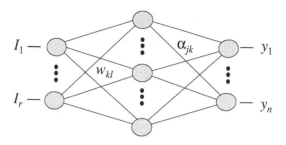

Fig. 4. A 3 Layer MLP

If the output $\mathbf{q} = (q_1, \ldots, q_n)$ for a given input $\mathbf{p} = (p_1, \ldots, p_r)$ is known, then the pair $(\mathbf{p}, \mathbf{q})$ is known as a **training pattern** because the pair can be used to estimate the weights w_{kl} and α_{jk} necessary for the stimulus $\mathbf{p}$ to predict a **classification** of $\mathbf{q}$. The **energy** function for a collection $(\mathbf{p}^1, \mathbf{q}^1), \ldots, (\mathbf{p}^r, \mathbf{q}^r)$ of training patterns is defined

$$E = \frac{1}{2} \sum_{i=1}^{t} \left\| \mathbf{y} - \mathbf{q}^i \right\|^2$$

where $\mathbf{y} = (y_1, \ldots, y_n)$ and where the norm is defined by the corresponding dot product. The network is *trained* to a collection of training patterns if

$$\frac{\partial E}{\partial w_{kl}} = 0 \ \ and \ \ \frac{\partial E}{\partial \alpha_{jk}} = 0$$

at the inputs $\mathbf{p}^i$ for all $l = 1 \ldots r$, $k = 1 \ldots m$, and $j = 1 \ldots n$. Because these equations cannot be solved directly, a gradient-following method called the **backpropagation** algorithm is used instead. The algorithm is based on the observation

$$\sigma' = \kappa \sigma (1 - \sigma),$$

which can be used to simplify $\partial E / \partial \alpha_{jk}$ and $\partial E / \partial w_{kl}$. In particular, for each **training pattern** $(\mathbf{p}_i, \mathbf{q}_i)$, a 3-layer MLP first calculates $\mathbf{y}$ as the output to $\mathbf{p}_i$, which is the *feedforward* step. The weights α_{jk} are subsequently adjusted using

$$\alpha_{jk} \rightarrow \alpha_{jk} + \lambda \delta_j \xi_k$$

where $\xi_k = \sigma (\mathbf{w}_k \cdot \mathbf{x} - \theta_k)$, where $\lambda > 0$ is a fixed parameter called the *learning rate*, and where

$$\delta_j = \kappa y_j (1 - y_j) (q_j^i - y_j).$$

The weights w_{kr} are adjusted using

$$w_{kl} \to w_{kl} + \lambda \varepsilon_k \; x_l,$$

where $x_l = \sigma \left(p_l^i - \theta_l \right)$ and where

$$\varepsilon_k = \kappa \xi_k \left(1 - \xi_k \right) \sum_{j=1}^{n} \alpha_{jk} \delta_j.$$

Before any training sessions begin, the weights α_{jk} and w_{kr} should be initialized to small random values and λ should be chosen close enough to 0 to allow the backpropagation algorithm to converge. In each training session, the patterns should be randomly permuted to avoid bias, and training should continue until E is sufficiently close to 0. The backpropagation algorithm is well-established and can be found in many textbooks and monographs. See, for example, Bose and Liang[12] for additional information about the backpropagation algorithm.

3. Data Mining and Microarrays

Microarrays capture gene expression data for a given state by comparing mRNA from a population in that state (sample) with mRNA from a population not in that state[1]. If M_l is the base 2 logarithm of the ratio of the intensity of the sample to the intensity of the reference for the lth gene, then on average $M_l \approx 0$ for unregulated genes and $|M_l| >> 0$ for regulated genes.

More generally, if there are N different classifications for a collection of training patterns, then for each $i = 1, \ldots, N$ there is a pattern vector $\pi^i = \left(\pi_1^i, \ldots, \pi_r^i \right)$, where

$$\pi_l^i = \begin{cases} 1 & \text{if gene } l \text{ is regulated} \\ 0 & \text{otherwise} \end{cases}$$

Data sets for the classifications are of the form $\left(\mathbf{p}^i, \mathbf{q}^i \right)$, $i = 1, \ldots, t$, where each $\mathbf{q}^i$ is one of a fixed set of output vectors $\mathbf{o}_1, \ldots, \mathbf{o}_N$ and the corresponding $\mathbf{p}^i = \left(p_1^i, \ldots, p_r^i \right)$ are given by

$$p_l^i = R_l + M_l \; \pi_l^j$$

where R_l and M_l are random variables with $\bar{R}_l = 0$ and $\left| \bar{M}_l \right| >> 0$ for each $l \in \{1, \ldots, r\}$. Similar to a microarray analysis, the problem is that of using the training set to predict the pattern π^j for each $j = 1, \ldots, N$.

For microarray data, there is only one classification (i.e., the "sample"), which means that classification and feature extraction of microarray

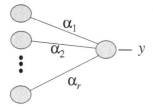

Fig. 5.   The Perceptron

data can be accomplished with a perceptron, which is an MLP with no hidden layers and only one output neuron[3]. In analyzing microarray data, the pattern vector $\pi = (\pi_1, \ldots, \pi_r)$ represents the genetic expression of the condition observed in the sample.

The `backpropagation` algorithm implies that after a large number of training sessions, the weights are of the form

$$\alpha_l = \mu_l + \lambda\kappa \sum_{\{i \mid q^i=1\}} y\left(\mathbf{p}^i\right)\left(1 - y\left(\mathbf{p}^i\right)\right)^2 p_l^i - \lambda\kappa$$

$$\times \sum_{\{i \mid q^i=0\}} y\left(\mathbf{p}^i\right)^2 \left(1 - y\left(\mathbf{p}^i\right)\right) p_l^i$$

where μ_l is a random initial offset that is very close to 0. It follows that

$$\mu_l - \sum_{\{i \mid q^i=1\}} p_l^i \le \alpha_l \le \mu_l + \sum_{\{i \mid q^i=1\}} p_l^i$$

so that if $\pi_l = 0$, then we have

$$\mu_l - \bar{R} \le \alpha_l \le \mu_l + \bar{R}$$

or equivalently, $\alpha_l \approx \mu_l$. That is, input neurons (genes) not in the pattern π will on average correspond to weights α_l which are close to 0 (given that μ_l is chosen to be close to 0 as well).

When combined with a simple genetic algorithm that eliminates the input neurons corresponding to the α_l with the smallest magnitudes, the result is a process for *reducing the dimensionality* of the classification data $\left(\mathbf{p}^i, \mathbf{q}^i\right)$. A naive implementation of this process can be described as follows:

(1) Let $\left(\mathbf{p}_0^i, \mathbf{q}_0^i\right), i = 1, \ldots, N$ denote the original training set.
(2) For $k = 0, 1, 2, \ldots$

(a) Train the network with the data $\left(\mathbf{p}_k^i, \mathbf{q}_k^i\right)$ until the error E is sufficiently close to 0.

(b) Remove a small number of input neurons (genes) with weights closest to 0 to create a reduced data set $\left(\mathbf{p}_{k+1}^i, \mathbf{q}_{k+1}^i\right)$, $i = 1, \ldots, N$

The support of $\mathbf{p}_k^i$ is a prediction of the input pattern π (i.e., the expressed genes). As a variation on this procedure, it may be more appropriate to remove a fixed percentages of genes which correspond to weights that are large in magnitude and then continue until convergence becomes very poor or no weights remain with magnitudes sufficiently distant from 0.

Perceptrons can be used as classifiers only on data which can be divided into separate classes by a hyperplane[12], thus making it desirable to use an MLP instead. Although there is no obvious correspondence between input neurons and weights in an MLP, there are strategies for using MLP's to reduce the dimensionality of the classification data.

Let's begin by deriving a simple algorithm for feature extraction in multilayer perceptrons. To do so, let us notice that in the back propagation algorithm, the change in the weights w_{kl} is

$$\Delta w_{kl} = \lambda \varepsilon_k \, x_l$$

so that if $x_l = p_l^i$ and if $\pi_l = 0$, then after some large number of training sessions we have

$$\Delta w_{kl} = \sum \lambda \varepsilon_k R_l$$

where the sum is over the training sessions. If λ is chosen so that $|\lambda \varepsilon_k| < 1$, then Δw_{kl} is close to 0 when the lth neuron is not in the pattern. Such a criteria in combination with the algorithm above allows the use of a MLP in reducing the dimensionality of a set of classified data.

This method is similar to methods that use sensitivity analysis to predict the relative importance of a given input neuron. Specifically, for each $i = 1, \ldots, n$ and $l = 1, \ldots, r$, the partial derivative

$$\frac{\partial y_j}{\partial x_l} = \kappa^2 y_j \left(1 - y_j\right) \sum_{k=1}^m \alpha_{jk} w_{kl} \xi_k \left(1 - \xi_k\right)$$

measures the sensitivity of the output neuron y_j to variations in the input neuron x_l (see [15]). Given a training set $\left(\mathbf{p}^i, \mathbf{q}^i\right)$, $i = 1, \ldots, N$, the significance of the lth input neuron is defined to be

$$\Phi_l = \max_{i \in \{1, \ldots, N\}} \left(\frac{1}{n} \sum_{j=1}^n \left| \frac{\partial y_j}{\partial x_l} \right|_{\mathbf{y}=\mathbf{q}^i, x_l = \sigma\left(p_l^i - \theta_l\right)}^2 \right)^{1/2}.$$

Large Φ_l predict input neurons (genes) most significant to the training of the network, while small Φ_l predicts neurons with lesser significance[16].

Both cases imply a natural criteria for pruning input neurons with lesser significances. Thus, a general algorithm for dimensionality reduction and feature extraction is to alternately train the network to predict classifications and prune weights which are relatively unchanged over large periods of time.

4. Neuron Inspired Neural Networks

Neural networks are powerful tools for exploring mining data, but there are also many problems that can arise. It is necessary in Cybenko's theorem for the hidden layer to become arbitrarily large, which may also lead to networks that converge poorly and slowly at best. Overfitting is problematic, as it so often is with nonlinear techniques. A training set in which some $(\mathbf{p}, \mathbf{q})$ pairs are errantly associated with each other (mislabeled data) may also lead to slow convergence of the back propagation algorithm. Mislabeled data can also produce errant classifications in general.

Many of these issues are addressed in the literature by using known mathematical techniques to modify ANN algorithms to address such difficulties. However, we conclude by suggesting how models of real-world neurons can be used to suggest modifications to artificial neurons.

In particular, models have been developed which incorporate ion channels (i.e., active properties) into dendritic electrotonic cable models[17]. In these models, the dendritic membrane voltage $V(X,t)$ at a dimensionless distance X from the soma and at time t satisfies

$$V(X,t) = V_{initial} + \sum_{j=1}^{n} \int_0^t G(X, X_j, t - \tau) I_j(\tau) d\tau$$

where X_j corresponds to the location of an ionic channel, $I_j(\imath)$ is the activation at that channel, and $G(X, X_j, t)$ is a multi-exponential decay[18]. Since $V(0,t)$ is the voltage at the soma and since $G(X, X_j, t)$ is a multi-exponential decay, the somatic voltage is of the form

$$V_{soma} = V_{initial} + \sum_{j=1}^{n} \sum_{s=1}^{\infty} w_{js} C_{js} e^{-\beta_{js} t} \int_0^t e^{\beta_{js}\tau} I_j(\tau) d\tau \tag{2}$$

where β_{js} is the sth rate of decay at the jth synaptic channel.

Broadly interpreted, this means that an artificial neuron can be considered to be of the form

$$x_i = \sigma \left(\sum_{j=1}^{n} w_{ij} \sum_{s=1}^{v} X_{js} - \theta_i + \mu_i \right)$$

where X_{sik} is some transformation of x_i and where μ_i is a small random number modeling fluctuations in $V_{initial}$. For example, if $I_j(\tau)$ is constant in (2), then

$$e^{-\beta_{js}t} \int_0^t e^{\beta_{js}\tau} I_j(\tau)\, d\tau = \beta_{js}^{-1} \left(1 - e^{-\beta_{js}t}\right) I_j$$

and the corresponding artificial model is

$$x_i = \sigma \left(\sum_{j=1}^{n} \sum_{s=1}^{v} w_{ij}\gamma_{sj}x_j - \theta_i + \mu_i \right)$$

where $\gamma_{sj} = C_{js}\beta_{js}^{-1}\left(1 - e^{-\beta_{js}T}\right)$ for some fixed $T > 0$. Although this model is mathematically equivalent to (1)—thus allowing back propagation training—comparison to (2) suggests that the γ_{sj} should be trained at different "time scales" and that small amounts of "noise" may be added at each iteration.

This confirms recent models obtained without biological inspiration in which Monte Carlo techniques and extensions of the back propagation training method have been used to improve neural network performance[14,19]. Conversely, it suggests that more recent models of the neuron can produce improved artificial neural network models. If vision is interpreted to be feature extraction on a grand scale, then real world neural networks can be considered to be the ultimate data mining tools, behooving us to continually revisit our understanding of real neurons in our quest to develop suitable artificial models designed to perform similar tasks.

Acknowledgements

The authors wish to thank the referees for their several excellent suggestions. This research was supported in part by the National Science Foundation under Grant No. 0126682.

References

1. W. Dubitzky, M. Granzow, and D. Berrar, Data Mining and Machine Learning Methods for Microarray Analysis, In: *Methods of Microarray Data Analysis - Papers from CAMDA 2000*, (S.M. Lin, K.F. Johnson, Eds.), pp. 5-22, Kluwer Academic Publishers, 2001.

2. M.P.S. Brown, W.N. Grundy, D. Lin, N. Cristianini, C. Sugnet, T.S. Furey, M. Ares, Jr., and D. Haussler, "Knowledge-based analysis of microarray gene expression data using support vector machines." *Proceedings of the National Academy of Science*, **97** (2000), 262-267.

3. A. Narayanan, A. Cheung, J. Gamalielsson, E. Keedwell, and C. Vercellone, Artificial Neural Networks for Reducing the Dimensionality of Gene Expression Data in Bioinformatics using Computational Intelligence, Seiffert. U., 2004.

4. J. Herrero, A. Valencia, and J. Dopazo, A hierarchical unsupervised growing neural network for clustering gene expression patterns, *Bioinformatics*, **17** (2001), 126-136.

5. S.R. Holbrook and S.M. Muskal, Predicting Protein Structural Features With Artificial Neural Networks, *Artificial Intelligence and Molecular Biology*, (L. Hunter, ed.), AAAI Press, 1993.

6. M.C. O'Neill and L. Song, Neural network analysis of lymphoma microarray data: prognosis and diagnosis near perfect, *BMC Bioinformatics*, **4** (2003), 4:13.

7. P. Tomsich, A. Rauber, and D. Merkl, Optimizing the parSOM Neural Network Implementation for Data Mining with Distributed Memory Systems and Cluster Computing, DEXA Workshop (2000), 661-668.

8. Y. Xu, D. Xu, and V. Olman, A Practical Method for Interpretation of Threading Scores: An Application of Neural Network, *Statistica Sinica* **12** (2002), 159-177.

9. F. Rossia, N. Delannay, B. Conan-Gueza, and M. Verleysen, Representation of functional data in neural networks, *Neurocomputing*, **64** (2005), 183-210.

10. J.J.B. Jack, D. Noble, and R.W. Tsien, Electric current flow in excitable cells, Clarendon Press, Oxford, 1975.

11. H.C. Tuckwell, Introduction to theoretical neurobiology: volume 1 linear cable theory and dendritic structure, Cambridge University Press, New York, 1988.

12. N.K. Bose and P, Liang, Neural Network Fundamentals with Graphs, Algorithms, and Applications, McGraw-Hill, New York, 1996.

13. G. Cybenko, Approximation by Superpositions of a sigmoidal function, *Mathematics of Control, Signals, and Systems*, **2**(4) (1989), 303-314.

14. A. Engelbrecht, L. Fletcher and I. Cloete, Variance Analysis of Sensitivity Information for Pruning Feedforward Neural Networks, IEEE International Joint Conference on Neural Networks, Washington DC, USA, paper 379, 1999. 13.

15. A. Engelbrecht and I. Cloete, Feature Extraction from Feedforward Neural Networks using Sensitivity Analysis, International Conference on Systems, Signals, Control, Computers, Durban, South Africa, 2, 1998, 221-225.

16. A. Engelbrecht, Sensitivity Analysis for Selective Learning by Feedforward Neural Networks, *Fundamenta Informaticae*, **45** (2001), 295-328.

17. R.R. Poznanski and J. Bell, A dendritic cable model for the amplification of synaptic potentials by an ensemble average of persistent sodium channels, *Mathematical Biosciences*, **166** (2000), 101-121.

18. L. Glenn and J. Knisley, Voltage Transients in Branching Multipolar Neurons With Tapering Dendrites and Sodium Channels, In: *Modeling in the Neurosciences: From Proteomics to Robotics*, (K.A. Lindsay, R.R. Poznanski, and J.R. Rosenberg, Eds.), Taylor and Francis, London, 2003.

19. J.F.G. de Frietas, M. Niranjan, A.H. Gee, and A. Doucet, Sequential Monte Carlo Methods to Train Neural Network Models, *Neural Computation*, **12** (2000), 955-993.

CHAPTER 16

MULTIFRACTAL DISCRIMINATION MODEL (MDM) OF HIGH-FREQUENCY PUPIL DIAMETER MEASUREMENTS FOR HUMAN-COMPUTER INTERACTION

Bin Shi

The MathWorks, Inc.,
3 Apple Hill Dr., Natick, MA 01760, USA
E-mail: bin.shi@mathworks.com

Kevin P. Moloney, V. Kathlene Leonard, Julie Jacko,
François Sainfort and Brani Vidakovic

Health Systems Institute,
Wallace H. Coulter Department of Biomedical Engineering,
Georgia Institute of Technology,
313 Ferst Dr. NW, Atlanta, GA 30332-0535, USA
E-mails: {moloney, leonard, jacko, sainfort, brani}@hsi.gatech.edu

Multifractality present in high-frequency pupil diameter measurements, usually connected with the irregular scaling behavior and self-similarity, is modeled with statistical accuracy and discriminatory power. The Multifractal Discrimination Model (MDM) is proposed to determine ocular pathology based on the pupillary response behavior (PRB) exhibited by older adults with and without ocular disease during the performance of a computer-based task. The MDM consists of two parts: (1) a discriminatory summary of the multifractal spectrum and (2) a combined k-nearest-neighbor classifier. The multifractal spectrum is used to discriminate the PRB from four groups of older adult users, differing in ocular pathology. Spectral Mode, Broadness, and left Slope (the **M.B.S.** summary), three measures characterizing the multifractal spectrum of observations, are proposed as distinguishing features of PRB across the groups. The combined k-nearest neighbor classifier is shown to be a valid classifier for the accurate prediction of ocular pathology from the PRB measurements.

1. Introduction

The discipline of human-computer interaction (HCI) strives to evaluate and improve user performance and interaction with information technologies for users with varying abilities and needs across many different contexts. Mental workload has long been recognized as an important component of human performance during interaction with complex systems [1], such as computers. Notably, extreme levels of workload (high and low) have been shown to be predictive of performance decrements for different users under different conditions. To this end, this study examines the workload experienced by users with visual impairments during the performance of a computer-based task.

Previous investigations have examined the interactions of users with visual impairment related to Age-related Macular Degeneration (AMD) [2,3,4]. AMD is one of the leading causes of visual impairment and blindness for individuals 55 years of age and older [5]. Since the majority of information offered by computers is presented visually on a screen, these users are at a clear disadvantage. Research efforts directed towards the characterization of computer interaction for users with visual impairments can provide designers with the knowledge to better anticipate user needs in the development of information technologies.

AMD affects central, high-resolution vision, which has a large impact on an individual's ability to perform focus-intensive tasks, such as using a computer [6]. Researchers have found that users with AMD tend to perform worse than normally-sighted users, as measured by performance metrics such as task times and errors, on simple computer-based tasks [2,3,4]. However, little work has been done to examine how these performance decrements are affected by increases in mental workload due to sensory impairments.

Measures of workload can be performance-based, survey-based, or physiologically assessed. Pupil diameter is a well-documented, physiological measure of mental workload [7,8]. While research has shown pupillary response behavior (PRB) to be related to changes in mental workload and task difficulty in a number of domains [9,10,11,12], the complex control mechanism of the pupil has made it difficult to extract the small, meaningful signals, related to changes in mental workload from the larger, overall noisy signal of PRB [13].

Additionally, research in ophthalmology has shown that ocular disease affecting the central visual field – such as AMD – also has an effect on the physiological mechanism controlling PRB [14,15]. This makes the PRB of individuals with ocular disease particularly noisy and difficult to use in data analyses. This being said, it is necessary to develop analytical techniques that can isolate these small changes in PRB. A more comprehensive analysis of PRB may provide a solution to this problem and provide a unique characterization of interaction for individuals with AMD.

The development of analytical tools for high-frequency data lends strong support to the analysis of PRB data. The high-frequency PRB measurements share many important features with other extensively studied measurements, such as the turbulence [16], internet traffic [17] and high-frequency financial time series [18]. These types of measurements are considered as fractal processes. Fractal processes are usually divided into two classes – monofractal processes and multifractal processes. Recent work of Moloney and colleagues [19] shows the advantages of multifractal process models in overcoming the data complexity of PRB.

This chapter proposes a Multifractal Discrimination Model (MDM) to predict ocular pathology from PRB measurements. We describe a multifractal spectral model to fit the PRB measurements and then extract features from this model in order to discriminate the measurements coming from different visual acuity groups. The challenge of this problem is due to the complexity of PRB, the non-Gaussian distribution of the multifractal spectral characteristics and the difficulty of building a stable classifier for multi-class data. The choice of taking the multifractal spectral characteristics as the classifier input is supported by the descriptive statistics. To build a predictive multi-class classifier for non-Gaussian data, the combination of k-nearest-neighbor classifier is employed to improve the predictive accuracy.

The chapter is organized as follows. The dataset is described in Section 2. Section 3 includes the description of The multifractal spectrum model and the features based on the multifractal spectrum. Discriminate analysis of PRB data using the multifractal model is presented in Section 4. Section 5 provides conclusions.

2. PRB Measurement

In this section, we briefly describe the datasets and how the data is preprocessed to fit the further analysis.

2.1. *Datasets description*

The equipment used to collect PRB data during this study was the Applied Science Laboratories (ASL) Model 501 head-mounted optics system. Pupil size was recorded at a rate of 60 Hz for each participant over 105 trials of a computer-based task using a graphical user interface (GUI). A camera records the pupil image, which has been distinguished by a near-infrared beam that illuminates the interior of the eye. Pupil size is assessed as the number of pixels attributed to the pupil's image, which has been determined by real-time edge detection processing of the image. Actual pupil diameter measurements (in millimeters) are then calculated by multiplying each pixel value by a scaling factor that is based on the physical distance of the camera from each participant's eye.

The dataset is comprised of PRB data streams for 36 individuals, as described in Table 1. In this table, N refers to the number of individuals comprising this user group. Visual acuity refers to the range of Snellen visual acuity scores (assessed by ETDRS) of the better eye for participants of each group. AMD? refers to the presence (Yes) or absence (No) of this ocular disease in individuals within each group. Number of data sets refers to the number of 2048-length data sets that were obtained from the data streams for each group. For this study, data was collected from four groups of individuals, classified by visual acuity and the presence or absence of age-related macular degeneration (AMD). Visual acuity, an individual's ability to resolve fine visual detail, was assessed via the protocol outlined in the Early Treatment of Diabetic Retinopathy Study (ETDRS) [20]. The experimental protocol from this study is fully described in studies by Jacko and colleagues [3,19].

Table 1.   Group characteristics summary

Group	N	Visual Acuity	AMD?	Number of Data Sets
Control	19	20/20 - 20/40	No	111
#1	6	20/20 - 20/50	Yes	59
#2	5	20/60 - 20/100	Yes	57
#3	6	20/100	Yes	124

2.2. *Preprocessing*

Studies of PRB are faced with the problem of how to remove blink artifacts. A blink generally lasts about 70-100 msec. (producing an artifact spanning

4-6 observations under 60 Hz sampling) during which time the camera registers loss and a pupil diameter of zero is recorded. Thus, the detection and elimination of these contiguous zero observation artifacts from the PRB records is relatively straightforward. However, on either side of a blink, one may also observe highly unusual recordings because the pupil may be measured inaccurately as the eyelid partially obscures the pupil. The result may be an impossibly small value for the pupil's size.

To ensure that the analysis is conducted on pupil constriction or dilation and not on misleading discontinuities caused by blinks or partial blinks, one must either remove the blink observations from the data entirely or replace them with linearly interpolated values. Blinks (i.e., zero recordings) have been found to account for approximately 3-4% of all observations. Partial blinks account for another 1% of the total number of observations. The blink-removal procedure removes all observations having zero values (i.e., the blink) as well as any extreme values that occur within six additional observations on either side of the zero value (i.e., partial blinks). Figure 1 presents a preprocessed result of the typical measurements of subjects from four different vision ability categories.

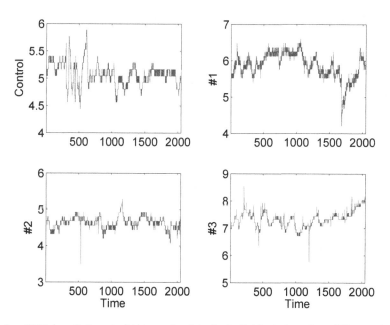

Fig. 1. PRB (pupil diameter) time series data for individuals from four different vision ability categories.

Because of difficulty of collecting the measurements, especially from individuals with AMD, the original datasets were cut into equal length pieces to exploit their usage. Another reason of the segmentation is that the original measurements are not equally long. The segmentation is conducted after the 'Six Law' filtering, as mentioned above. The dataset contains the sum of 351 segments of measurements after segmentation and necessary outlier detection and each have the length of 2048. The distribution of the number of the segments among the four groups (Control, #1, #2 and #3) is reported in Table 1.

3. Multifractality Features

In this section, we discuss the concept of multifractality and the definition of the multifractal spectrum and analyze the features of the multifractal spectrum from the perspective of discrimination.

3.1. *Scaling and multifractal spectrum*

Many measurements encountered in nature, industry, and science are characterized by complex scaling behavior, namely multifractality. Multifractals are processes that possess a continuous range of irregularity indices, rather than a single irregularity index H (usually the worst overall index of irregularity) typical of monofractality. Prime examples of multifractals are turbulence measurements where the deviation from the constant scaling, characterized by a Hurst exponent of $1/3$ and called the Kolmogorov K41 law, is explained by multifractality of such measurements [21].

The wavelet-based energy spectrum is a commonly used tool to check the scaling behavior of the process. This spectrum describes the second order statistics (i.e., variance) of the process at different scales (frequency points). The linearity (or curvature) of this spectrum reflects the fractality of the process and this connection could be utilized to the estimation of the Hurst exponent of the process. The exact definition of the wavelet-based energy spectrum and its estimation could be found in the monograph of Vidakovic [22]. Figure 2 shows the wavelet-based energy spectrum of typical PRB measurement. This spectrum suggests that fractal behavior exists in PRB and that the multifractal model can be used to identify the inherent features within the PRB signals of different individuals.

The measure of multifractality is given by the multifractal spectrum, which describes the "richness" of the process in terms of various regular-

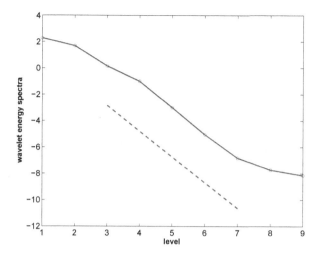

Fig. 2. Wavelet-based energy spectrum for PRB from a Control subject. The slope in the intermediate scales is found to be -1.9484 corresponding to the Hurst exponent of 0.4742. The "hockey-stick" effect in the finest two scales is caused by quantization and possible smoothing of high frequencies of the measuring instrument.

ity indices. The term spectrum connotes the spectral decomposition of the process into components characterized by their irregularity. Thus, multifractal analysis is not focused on the irregularity/self-similarity of the data set as measured by a single parameter, but rather on a measure of inhomogeneity of such a parameter. In recent years, the multifractal formalism is implemented with wavelet tools [23,24] and hence could be efficiently used in practice. The wavelet-based multifractal spectrum is based on the local singularity strength measure:

$$\alpha(t) = \lim_{k2^j \to t} \frac{1}{j} \log_2 |d_{j,k}| \tag{1}$$

where $d_{j,k}$ is the wavelet coefficient at scale j and location k. It has been shown that the wavelet coefficients can carry the scaling behavior of the process if the wavelet is more regular than the process [25] and the local singularity strength measure (1) converges to the local irregularity index the process at time t. As the name tells, $\alpha(t)$ indicates the oscillation of the process at time t, with small values of $\alpha(t)$ reflecting the more irregular behavior at time t. It can be imagined that any inhomogeneous process has a collection of local singularity strength measures and their distribution $f(\alpha)$ formulates the multifractal spectrum. The detailed estimation procedure of the wavelet-based multifractal spectrum is outlined in the seminal work by

Gonçalvès and colleagues [26].

3.2. *Features based on multifractal spectrum*

Theoretically, the multifractal spectrum of fBm (a representative of mono-fractal) consists of three geometric parts: the vertical line, the maximum point and the right slope. The spectral **Mode** corresponds to the Hurst exponent and the vertical line is thought to be an inherent feature, which distinguishes fBm from the multifractal process. However, it is rare to obtain such a perfect spectrum in practice. Due to the error of estimation, the spectrum generated from an accurately simulated may even deviate from the theoretical form, as shown in Figure 3. Even with the lack of precise estimation of the spectrum, the deviation from the vertical line can still be utilized in the discrimination between the monofractal and multifractal processes. In Figure 3, two type processes are presented in the multifractal spectra. One is the fBm and the other is the turbulence measurement, which is widely believed to be a multifractal process. Comparing with the turbulence measurement, the fBm is much closer to the vertical line and this closeness may be quantified by the left **S**lope of the spectra. Another important difference between these two spectra is the width spread of the spectra. It is obvious that the width spread of the fBm is much smaller than that of the turbulence measurement.

Despite the existence of the estimation error, the spectrum can be approximately described by two slopes and one point without loss of the discriminant information. Alternatively, we can also approximate the spectrum by the left **S**lope, the maximum point and the width spread. A typical multifractal spectrum, described in this way, is shown in Figure 4.

The left and right slopes can be obtained easily using the linear regression technique. However, it is not as straightforward to define the width spread automatically. The difficulties are related to two aspects – one being how to locate the start and end points of the width spread, while the other is what to do with the discreteness of the spectrum. It is easy to see that the former is difficult conceptually, while the latter is difficult computationally. There are many ways to define the width spread. In this chapter, we give one definition of width spread, which we name the **broadness** of the spectrum.

Definition 1: Suppose that α_1 and α_2 are two roots which satisfy the equation $f(\alpha) + 0.2 = 0$ and $\alpha_1 < \alpha_2$, the **B**roadness of multifractal spectrum is defined as $B = \alpha_2 - \alpha_1$, where $f(\alpha)$ is the spectrum function

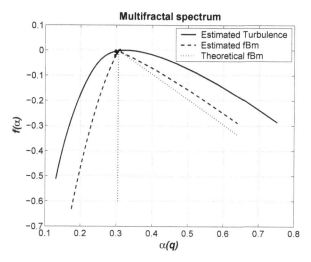

Fig. 3. Multifractal Spectra for mono- (dashed line) and multi-fractal (solid line) processes. The dotted line indicates the theoretical slope of the spectrum for an fBm process (mono-fractal) with a Hurst exponent of 1/3

in terms of Holder regularity indices α's.

This definition is also graphically presented in Figure 4. The deviation from the monofractal could be fairly quantified using this **B**roadness measure since it posts a universal standard on the width spread. It is worth to point out the threshold value 0.2 used in this definition could be adjusted empirically in the practice analysis to ensure that this measure is well defined for all analyzed processes.

As mentioned earlier, the discreteness may produce difficulties in the computation. The problem is that it may be hard to find the exact roots of the equation $f(\alpha) + 0.2 = 0$ among the discrete values of α's. To get around this, we try to find the minimum value of $|f(\alpha) + 0.2|$ with respect of α instead of solving the equation directly.

Applying our idea about extracting the spectral features to the PRB measurements, we obtain the **B**roadness, spectral **M**ode (Hurst exponent), and left **S**lope for each measurement. Table 2 summarizes the spectral characteristics of the PRB datsets that we are using in our study. We will use this result in Section 4.

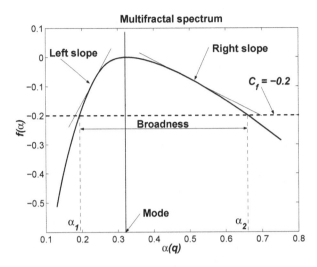

Fig. 4. Canonical features of the multifractal spectrum , including the left Slope, Broadness, and spectral Mode measures.

Table 2. Summary statistics of the multifractal spectral characteristics for our PRB datasets

Group		Left Slope	Spectral Mode	Broadness
Control	Mean	0.5053	0.4177	0.8591
	Median	0.4725	0.4153	0.7668
	Std.	0.1658	0.1517	0.4956
#1	Mean	0.3787	0.3561	0.8404
	Median	0.3701	0.3214	0.7266
	Std.	0.0738	0.1511	0.6796
#2	Mean	0.4049	0.4233	0.6989
	Median	0.3908	0.4104	0.6804
	Std.	0.1105	0.0985	0.1655
#3	Mean	0.484	0.3965	1.348
	Median	0.4608	0.3926	0.8562
	Std.	0.139	0.1723	1.1761

4. PRB Data Analysis

As mentioned previously, we attempt to find the inherent features which can separate the measurements with different ocular pathologies from each other. The empirical evidence (e.g., wavelet-based energy spectrum) has shown that PRB measurements possess self-similarities and fractalities. Hence, it is natural to apply multifractal spectra to discriminate these measurements.

We have discussed the features of multifractal spectra in section 3. The most important feature of the spectrum is the spectral Mode, which corresponds to the Hurst exponent if the process is monofractal. The Hurst exponent is a measure of "roughness" of the self-similar process. The Hurst exponent coincides with the Holder regularity index, and processes with H close to 0 look quite irregular and intermittent, while for H close to 1 the processes look smooth. Such an important property of the spectral Mode enables us to explain the dynamics of PRB.

Informally speaking, large values of spectral Mode correspond to less dynamic changes in pupil size ("frozen eye") while low values of the exponent indicate bursty and frequent changes. Therefore, the spectral Mode could discriminate the measurements. The boxplots of spectral modes for the four groups are shown in Figure 5. According to this figure, the group #1 have spectral Modes much lower than the Control group, which reflects that the individuals from this group have more irregular PRB than those from the Control group.

As can be seen in Figure 5, the spectral Mode could not completely discriminate the groups. This motivates us to introduce other discriminatory quantities. Another measure we just defined is the Broadness, which is able to quantify the level of deviations from mono-fractality. The Broadness measure describes the richness in the distribution of local singularity indices.

PRB measurements with narrow multifractal spectra are close to monofractals (i.e., the scaling is quite uniform over all scales). The boxplot of Broadness measures are given in Figure 6. It is very hard to tell the difference among the four groups. However, the last group #3 significantly differs in terms of the Broadness from other experimental groups (#1, #2). Group #3 has relatively high large Broadness measures, which indicates that the PRB of the individuals from this group deviates from mono-fractal much more than groups #1 and #2. Physiologically speaking, more change patterns of the PRB dynamics exist in group #3.

Neither the spectral Mode nor the Broadness measure is able to achieve the complete discrimination by itself, but each of them distinguish the PRB from different perspectives.

Thus, we need to combined these two measures, characterizing the data with both measures. Figure 7 presents the centroid points for the four groups. These four points look nearly evenly distributed on the plane. From this figure, we can see that the spectral Mode from the Control group is relatively large although it is not the largest. Only group #2 has a larger

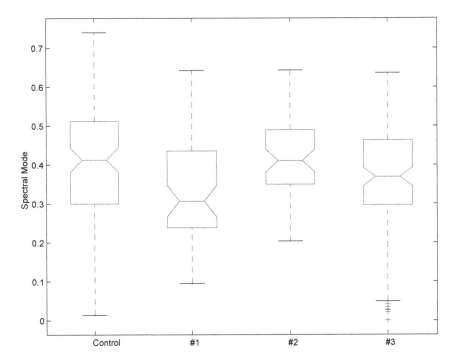

Fig. 5.   Boxplot for spectral modes of multifractality.

spectral Mode than the Control group. Comparing these two groups, we can tell that the PRB from the Control group is further from monofractal than group #2 since the Broadness measure of group #2 is the smallest. Therefore, we can claim that the PRB of individuals from the Control group is very smooth although the fractal properties are relatively inhomogeneous, which implies the causes of the regularity are quite rich. Group #1 is located on the very left-bottom side of the plane and hence it represents measurements with much more irregular dynamics and homogeneous fractal properties, which indicates the cause of the irregularity is relatively simple. Group #3 located near the top left side signifies that the measurements are quite irregular and have inhomogeneous fractal properties, which indicates the cause of the irregularity is not single.

Another important task in the analysis of these measurements is the classifier building. Among the many candidates, the k-nearest-neighbor classifier is chosen because of its inherent nonparametric characteristic.

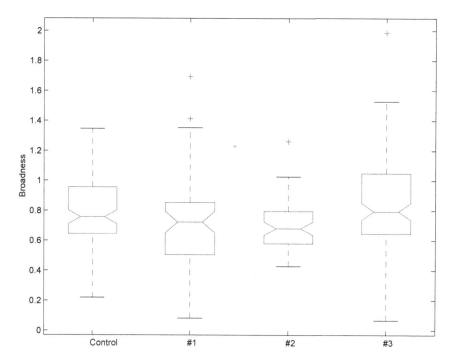

Fig. 6.   Boxplot for **B**roadness measures of multifractality.

Neither theoretical guidance or empirical evidence is absent to convince
the choice of linear classifier and other parametric classifiers for our PRB
measurements. Therefore, the nonparametric model, like k-nearest-neighbor
classifier, is preferred in this problem for the sake of better modeling accuracy. As usual, it is very easy to build a nonparametric mode with poor
predictive properties if the model is not tuned very well. To get around
this, cross validation (CV) strategy is often used to ensure the relative good
model is selected. The idea of CV is to divide the dataset into the training
set and test set. The former is used to estimate the model parameters and
the latter is used to validate the predictive accuracy of the model. In our
problems, the original PRB measurements are divided into two parts for
each group, one of them is assigned to training set and the other is used
to test the trained classifier. The training set includes a 90% randomly selected sample of each group from the whole datasets and the rest is taken
to be the test set.

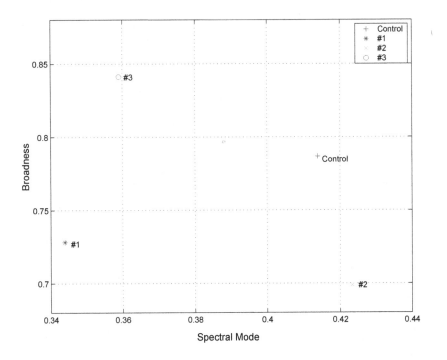

Fig. 7.   Centroid points for bivariate measures: Spectral Mode and Broadness Measures.

To choose the nearest neighbor parameter k, the classifier is built as a learning process. The learning curve, which includes the test error and training error corresponding to different parameters k, is given in Figure 4. Although, relatively low training error could be achieved by choosing small k, the test error is too big for a practically useful classifier. To overcome these drawbacks, we adapt the model by combining techniques. Model combining is a technique of combining the predictions from different classifiers. The results have shown to be promising. For the details of this combining technique, the reader is directed to Xu and colleagues [27]. The advantage of using model combining is due to its ability of overcoming the instability of the single classifier. In fact, Shi and colleagues [28] provides a Bayesian justification of the correctness of model combining. In our study, the single k-nearest-neighbor classifier is not very accurate and robust according to Figure 8. By applying the model combining technique to these k-nearest-neighbor classifiers ($3 \leq k \leq 10$), the test errors get much smaller as we

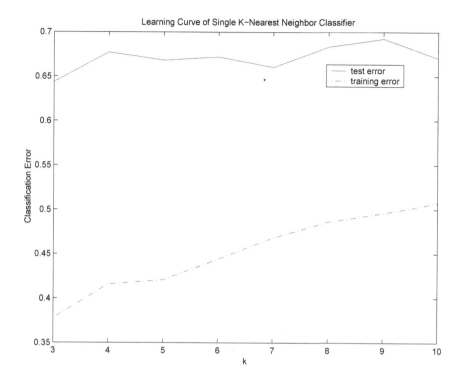

Fig. 8.   Learning curve of k-nearest neighbor (KNN) classifier.

can see from Table 3. Although the combining rules do not make much differences from each other, the result from mean-combining rule is shown to be optimal among the alternatives. Up to now, our classifier is based on only two features: the spectral **Mode** and **Broadness** measures. To demonstrate how an additional measure may affect the classification accuracy, we add the left **S**lope into the feature vector and the classification results are reported in Table 4. It is apparent that both the test and training errors decrease a lot as the new feature is added (e.g. the test errors drops down about 6%).

5. Conclusions

The overreaching goal of this detailed analysis was to determine if individuals with different ocular pathologies exhibit quantifiable differences in their interaction with graphical user interfaces. These distinctions between

Table 3. Error rate after combining the nearest neighbor classifiers

	rule	mean	median	max	min	majority voting
Training	mean	0.42	0.43	0.44	0.42	0.46
Errors	std. dev.	0.01	0.01	0.02	0.02	0.01
Test	mean	0.51	0.53	0.52	0.52	0.55
Errors	std. dev.	0.09	0.07	0.08	0.09	0.07

Table 4. Error rate after combining the nearest neighbor classifiers(with the Left Slope feature added)

	rule	mean	median	max	min	majority voting
Training	mean	0.407	0.414	0.417	0.401	0.432
Errors	std. dev.	0.013	0.012	0.015	0.015	0.013
Test	mean	0.446	0.450	0.439	0.459	0.475
Errors	std. dev.	0.051	0.045	0.048	0.057	0.050

classes of users can enable developers to design improved interfaces for more efficient and effective human-computer interactions. PRB is an informative, yet complex, means of quantifiably assessing differences in the interaction behaviors of users.

Using measurement of PRB during task performance is one way to study the effects of mental workload on users. However, the inherent complexity of PRB requires that robust and valid measures should be developed to extract the meaningful components of the data stream in order to characterize those changes in PRB that distinguish changes in mental workload. In this way, the relative mental workload of users with different visual capabilities can be examined. These distinctions between user needs can be used to modify visual interfaces and interaction paradigms in order to best adapt information technologies for users with visual impairments.

In this chapter, we study how to incorporate characteristics of the multifractal spectrum into the modeling and discrimination of the PRB highfrequency measurement. The multifractal process was validated to be appropriate in the analysis of the PRB data. The feature extraction is discussed in the context of decomposing the spectrum into describable parts. The concepts of the spectral Mode, Broadness, and left Slope measure (the M.B.S. summary) of a multifractal spectrum were defined. The analysis based on the spectal Mode and Broadness measures gave distinguishable characteristics of the PRB from the individuals with different visual acuity ranges. The model-free classification method, k-nearest-neighbor classifier, is applied with the model combining technique to build a robust and accurate classifier.

References

1. D. Gopher and E. Donchin, in *Handbook of Perception and Human Performance*, (K.R. Boff, L. Kaufman, and J.P. Thomas, Eds.), pp. 41-49, John Wiley and Sons, New York, NY, 1986.

2. J.A. Jacko, I.U. Scott, A.B. Barreto, H.S. Bautsch, J.Y. Chu, and W.B. Fain, in *Proceedings of the 9th International Conference on Human-Computer Interaction*, pp. 423-427, New Orleans , LA 2001.

3. J.A. Jacko, I.U. Scott, F. Sainfort, L. Barnard, P.J. Edwards, V.K. Emery, T. Kongnakorn, K.P. Moloney, and B.S. Zorich *CHI Letters*, **5(1)** (2003), 33-40.

4. J.A. Jacko, I.U. Scott, F. Sainfort, L. Barnard, K.P. Moloney, T. Kongnakorn, B.S. Zorich and V.K. Emery, *Lecture Notes in Computer Science (LNCS)*, **2615** (2003), 3-22.

5. The Schepens Eye Research Institute, Harvard Medical School, Harvard University. Macular degeneration: Your questions answered. Retrieved November 12, 2002, from http://www.eri.harvard.edu/htmlfiles/md.html

6. The Center for the Study of Macular Degeneration, University of California, Santa Barbara. (2002, January 25). Biology of AMD. Retrieved October 15, 2002, from http://www.csmd.ucsb.edu/faq/faq.html

7. I.E. Loewenfeld, *The pupil: Anatomy, physiology, and clinical applications* (2nd ed.), Oxford, UK: Butterworth-Heinemann (1999).

8. J.L. Andreassi, *Psychophysiology: Human behavior & physiological response*, (4th ed.), Lawrence Erlbaum Associates, Mahwah, NJ, 2000.

9. R.W. Backs and L.C. Walrath, *Applied Ergonomics*, **23** (1992), 243-254.

10. D. Kahneman, *Attention and Effort*, Prentice-Hall, Englewood Cliffs, NJ, 1973.

11. J. Beatty, *Psychological Bulletin,* **91** (1982), 377.

12. S.P. Marshall, C.W. Pleydell-Pearce, and B.T. Dickson, In *Proceedings of the 36th Hawaii International Conference on System Sciences* (HICSS '03), 2002.

13. J.L. Barbur, in *Learning from the pupil - studies of basic measurement mechanisms and clinical applications*, (L.M. Chalupa and J.S. Werner, Ed.), MIT Press, Cambridge, MA, 2003.

14. I.E. Loewenfeld, *The Pupil: Anatomy, Physiology, and Clinical Applications*, (2nd ed., Vol. 1), Butterworth-Heinemann, Oxford, UK, 1999.

15. O. Bergamin and R.H. Kardon, *Ophthalmology*, **109(4)** (2002), 771-780.

16. B. Shi, B. Vidakovic, G. Katul, and J. Albertson, *Physics of Fluids*, **17**(2005), 055104 (12 pages).

17. P. Abry and D. Veitch, *IEEE Transactions on Information Theory*, **44** (1998), 2-15.

18. B.B. Mandelbrot, L. Calvet, and A. Fisher, *A Multifractal Model of Asset Returns*, Working Paper, Yale University, Cowles Foundation Discussion Paper #1164 (1997).

19. K.P. Moloney, B. Shi, V.K. Leonard, J. Jacko, B. Vidakovic, and F. Sainfort, *ACM transactions on Computer Human Interaction (TOCHI)*, forthcoming (2006).

20. University of Maryland School of Medicine, Department of Epidemiology and Preventative Medicine, *Early treatment diabetic retinopathy study, Manual of Operations*, pp. 1-15, ETDRS Coordinating Center, Baltimore, MD, 2002.

21. B.B. Mandelbrot, *SIAM review*, **10** (1968), 422.

22. B. Vidakovic, *Statistical Modeling by Wavelets*, John Wiley & Sons, Inc., New York, 1999.

23. A. Arneodo, E. Bacry, S. Jaffard, and J.F. Muzy, *Journal of Fourier Analysis and Applications*, **4(2)** (1998), 159-174.

24. R. Riedi, *Multifractal Processes, Long range dependence: Theory and Applications*, preprint, (2002).

25. S. Jaffard, *Contemporary Mathematics*, **189** (1995), 287.

26. P. Gonçalvès, R.H. Riedi and R.G. Baraniuk, *Proceedings of the 32nd Conference on Signals, Systems and Computers*, Asilomar, November 1998.

27. L. Xu, A. Krzyzak, and C.Y. Suen, *IEEE Trans. SMC*, **22**, 418 (1992).

28. B. Shi, Y. Pan, P.K.P. Moloney, V.K. Emery, J. Jacko, F. Sainfort, and B. Vidakovic, *Journal of Statistical Computation and Simulation*, **76** (2006), 431.

INDEX